C000110031

HERBAL MEDICINE AND
REPRODUCTIVE HEALTH

HERBAL MEDICINE AND REPRODUCTIVE HEALTH

Natural approaches to male and female reproductive health problems and improving fertility

Marie Reilly MSc, MNIMH, DipCoun

AEON

First published in 2021 by
Aeon Books
PO Box 76401
London W5 9RG

Copyright © 2021 by Marie Reilly

The right of Marie Reilly to be identified as the author of this work has been asserted in accordance with §§ 77 and 78 of the Copyright Design and Patents Act 1988.

All rights reserved. No part of this publication may be reproduced, stored in a retrieval system, or transmitted, in any form or by any means, electronic, mechanical, photocopying, recording, or otherwise, without the prior written permission of the publisher.

British Library Cataloguing in Publication Data

A C.I.P. for this book is available from the British Library

ISBN-13: 978-1-91280-722-2

Typeset by Medlar Publishing Solutions Pvt Ltd, India
Printed in Great Britain

www.aeonbooks.co.uk

For my mother

TABLE OF CONTENTS

PART II: REPRODUCTIVE HEALTH PROBLEMS IN MEN

ACKNOWLEDGEMENTS

I would like to thank all my teachers, past and present, for generously sharing their wisdom and expertise, and for being such a source of inspiration; and all my patients and students, who have also been such wonderful teachers over the years, and given me the motivation to research and to learn.

I am also eternally grateful to my colleagues at the clinic where I work, who support me in so many ways, both personally and professionally; and to all my colleagues in herbal medicine, whose different knowledge and varied approaches bring such variety and richness to the tapestry of our profession.

And finally I must express my sincere gratitude to my family, to my mother, Josephine Reilly, and my partner, Bren Ó Ruaidh, for their incredible support, and to my beautiful children, Daisy, Lily, and Holly for their incredible patience and encouragement.

ABOUT THE AUTHOR

Marie Reilly is an experienced medical herbalist and teacher. She qualified from the College of Phytotherapy in 2004 and subsequently completed the Scottish School of Herbal Medicine Master's Degree Programme, having conducted her research dissertation on the treatment of female functional infertility with herbal medicine. She has also studied endobiogenic medicine with Dr Jean Claude Lapraz, and Ayurveda with Dr Vasant Lad. She currently runs a busy multidisciplinary clinic in Lismore, Ireland.

Marie has taught on the BSc Herbal Sciences course at Cork Institute of Technology, the Clinical Practitioner Training Programme at the Irish Plant Medicine School, the Excelsior School of Herbal Medicine, the Betonica Medical Herbalist Training Programme, and the Heartwood Professional Herbal Medicine Course. She has lectured at the Cork Institute of Technology Herbal Science Symposium, at Botanica 2014 (Trinity College Dublin), and at the National Institute of Medical Herbalists Annual Conference. She also regularly provides numerous CPD seminars on various subjects for practitioners of herbal medicine, nutrition, and other forms of health care.

Marie is also a qualified emergency first responder, and works in conjunction with a medical doctor and paramedic to provide emergency first aid in the local community as part of the Lismore Community First Response Team, a voluntary service.

INTRODUCTION

Not everyone wants to become a parent, but for those who do, the idea of having children feels like a fundamental part of life. Most of us spend the earlier part our lives trying to avoid an unplanned pregnancy, and assume that if and when we are ready to start a family, it will happen without any problem.

In recent times, people are increasingly deciding to delay having children until they feel the time is right and they are in a position to provide a secure environment and future for their children. There also seems to be a societal expectation that women can, or should, have children later in life.[1] In the decade between 2004 and 2014, the number of births to mothers over forty climbed by almost 75%, and the average age of first-time mothers increased from twenty-eight to thirty.[2]

A woman's fertility peaks in her mid-twenties, at a time when she may be still trying to establish a career, or a secure home and a stable relationship (or other support network), within which to raise a family. Young people are also increasingly burdened by debt, and there is little support for women to become mothers earlier in life.[3] Unfortunately, from the age of thirty, the point at which the average woman starts having children, female fertility begins to decline (at a rate of around 3% a year), and after thirty-five, the rate of decline accelerates even more.[4]

Therefore, more and more women are facing difficulties in conceiving when they feel the time is right for them to have children.

There is a myth that age does not affect fertility in men. However, while some men are able to conceive into their seventies, age can in fact have a significant impact on male fertility, and most men will have reduced sperm motility and less genetic integrity from their late forties.[5]

Even where individuals and couples don't attempt to delay having children, and start trying to conceive early, many still experience difficulty. An array of hormonal, structural, and functional problems affecting the reproductive system, together with environmental, nutrition, and lifestyle factors, may contribute to infertility in both men and women of all ages.

For those who want children, being unable to conceive is a very painful and difficult issue, and watching friends and family members announce pregnancies, give birth, and raise children only increases the sense of failure and loss. Infertility can cause tremendous stress for individuals and couples, and may be heightened by pressure from family friends, and society as a whole, to have children.

Infertility is clinically defined as the inability to conceive a child within one year of unprotected intercourse.[6,7] Individuals who have never conceived are described as having *primary infertility*, while those who have previously conceived, but have difficulty conceiving again, are said to be suffering from *secondary infertility*.[8] This is often a source of confusion, since in the case of other health conditions, a "primary" problem is a term that is generally used to describe a health problem that has no other underlying cause, while "secondary" problems usually refer to those that are the result of another health condition. However, in the case of infertility, the classification is somewhat different.

Overall, 15%–20% of couples experience difficulty conceiving, and in up to 30% of these cases the cause of infertility remains unexplained.[9,10,11] In the vast majority of these cases, the woman alone is offered conventional treatment,[12] and it is not unheard of for women to be prescribed fertility drugs by GPs without their partners ever having been tested for male factor infertility.

For individuals who experience conditions which lead to infertility, such as primary ovarian insufficiency, PCOS, and endometriosis, orthodox medicine has very little to offer in terms of safe, effective treatments, particularly for those who wish to become pregnant. Hormone-containing medications and endogenous hormone antagonists used to treat problems affecting the female reproductive system may have unpleasant side effects, are frequently associated with significant risk factors, and in many cases preclude pregnancy. Likewise, orthodox medicine has little to offer for improving sperm count, motility, and morphology in men.

The success rate of assisted reproduction techniques (for each cycle) ranges from less than 10% with the drug clomiphene citrate, to 20%–25% for in-vitro fertilisation (IVF).[13] The cost of IVF treatment in Ireland ranges from €4000 to €7000 per cycle.[14] In most cases, these interventions pay little or no attention to issues that may affect the outcome of the treatment, such as the overall health of the couple, their stress levels, the quality of oocyte and sperm, or various factors influencing implantation and maintenance of pregnancy. In some cases, infertility treatments may be associated with side effects, such as increased risk of multiple pregnancy, ovarian hyper stimulation syndrome, and ovarian cancer,[15] and the psychological effects of infertility treatment, and mood disturbances associated with hormonal manipulation can be as significant as the medical complications.[16]

While some people may need to undergo orthodox fertility treatment in order to conceive, for many, subfertility is simply due to an issue such as minor hormone imbalance, poor blood flow, suboptimal health of the pelvic organs, or various environmental, dietary, and lifestyle factors which may be improved with natural approaches such as nutrition and lifestyle modification, herbal medicine, and other complementary and alternative approaches, without the need for orthodox assisted reproduction techniques.

This book focuses on improving reproductive health and fertility with Western herbal medicine, nutrition, and lifestyle modification. However, there are other complementary and alternative approaches, including acupuncture and various bodywork treatments (such as chiropractic), which can be used in combination with herbal medicine and orthodox fertility treatments where necessary. These approaches can help to improve fertility, reduce levels of stress that are often associated with trying to conceive, alleviate some of the side effects of orthodox fertility treatments, and increase feelings of hopefulness and control over the process.[17]

Of course individuals who do not wish to conceive a child are just as likely to suffer from reproductive health problems as those who do. Conditions such as amenorrhoea, PCOS, fibroids, endometriosis, dyspareunia, and premenstrual syndrome (PMS), apart from causing infertility, are associated with an array of distressing symptoms; and women who do not wish to have children may still prefer to manage these conditions with natural medicine. To be able to help people to overcome reproductive health problems, from which they may have been suffering for many years, is incredibly rewarding in its own right.

Equally, men who are not interested in having children also suffer from conditions such as erectile dysfunction or premature ejaculation, and may choose natural approaches to help address these problems. Fertility is basically the result of achieving and maintaining a balanced and healthy reproductive system. Therefore this book is not just about improving fertility, but also about understanding and treating a wide range of reproductive health problems, whether or not the individual wishes to conceive a child.

Throughout this book, reference is made to "men" and "women" when discussing health problems that affect the male and female reproductive systems respectively. However, it is also acknowledged that there are people of other genders (such as trans men or non-binary individuals, for example), who menstruate, and may therefore be equally affected by symptoms of oestrogen or progesterone imbalance, or suffer from conditions such as endometriosis or fibroids. Similarly, trans women, and those with other gender identities, may experience testicular problems (such as varicocele, for example), so it is important to recognise this, and to respect the gender identity of the individual patients that we treat.

Integrated or integrative medicine involves incorporating complementary and alternative medicine (CAM) with orthodox medicine into a comprehensive and holistic treatment plan.[18,19,20] It focuses on health and healing rather than disease and treatment, and encourages the patient to take individual responsibility for his or her own health.[21,22] Integrated medicine is becoming increasingly popular among both patients and clinicians, many of whom consider the narrowly focused biological approach of orthodox medicine to be inadequate.[23,24]

The strictly biomedical approach of many orthodox clinicians allows minimal scope for the discussion of emotional issues or lifestyle strategies, which is in contrast with the more holistic therapeutic relationship found in many CAM therapies. Herbal medicine and other CAM approaches also have an important role to play in management of the side effects of orthodox interventions,[25] including assisted reproduction techniques.

At least 40% of the population of industrialised countries now regularly use one or more forms of complementary and alternative medicine, including herbal medicine. Patients frequently combine conventional treatment and CAM approaches rather than using one or the other exclusively, and the majority of people who use CAM do so because they consider it to be more congruent with their values and beliefs, rather than because of dissatisfaction or negative attitudes towards conventional medicine.[26] Many people who decide to use orthodox assisted reproduction techniques (ART) choose to combine these orthodox interventions with natural approaches. The high cost and relatively poor success rate of assisted reproduction techniques mean that many people will turn to CAM therapies, in order to try to increase their chance of success.

Therefore, herbalists and other complementary and alternative healthcare practitioners are very well placed to be able to help individuals and couples to improve not only their reproductive health and fertility, but also their general health and well-being, thereby increasing their chances of conceiving naturally, and maximising the success of assisted reproduction techniques where necessary. Indeed, for many practitioners, helping people to overcome health problems, which they may have been suffering with for many years, and helping individuals and couples to fulfil their dreams of becoming parents, can be among the most rewarding aspects of practising natural medicine.

Notes

1. Fertility, S. A. (2019). The top 3 reasons infertility is on the rise [online]. Available from fertilitysa.com.au (accessed 10 November 2019).
2. Central Statistics Office (2016). *Central Statistics Annual Report 2014* [online]. Available from https://cso.ie/en/releasesandpublications/ep/p-vsar/vsar2014/ (accessed 10 November 2018).
3. Fertility, S. A. (2019). The top 3 reasons infertility is on the rise [online]. Available from fertilitysa.com.au (accessed 10 November 2019).
4. Keane, D. (2016). Age & Fertility [online]. Available from https://vhiblog.ie/2016/12/02/age-fertility/ (accessed 10 November 2018).
5. Keane, D. (2016). Age & Fertility [online]. Available from https://vhiblog.ie/2016/12/02/age-fertility/ (accessed 10 November 2018).
6. Abma, J. C., Chandra, A., Mosher, W. D., Peterson, L., & Piccinino, L. (1997). Fertility, family planning and women's health: estimates from the National Survey of Family Growth. *Vital and Health Statistics*, 23: 1–14.
7. Hummel, W. P. (2005). *Miscarriage and the Successful Pregnancy: A Woman's Guide to Infertility and Reproductive Loss.* iUniverse.
8. Storck, S. (2010). *Infertility*. Medline Plus [online]. Available from http://nlm.nih.gov/medlineplus/ency/article/001191.htm (accessed 15 June 2010).

9. Cahill, D. J., & Wardle, P. G. (2002). Management of infertility. *British Medical Journal*, 325: 28–32.
10. Forti, G., & Krausz, C. (1998). Evaluation and treatment of the infertile couple. *Journal of Clinical Endocrinology & Metabolism*, 83(12): 4177–4188.
11. Hart, R. (2003). ABC of subfertility: Unexplained infertility, endometriosis and fibroids. *British Medical Journal*, 327: 721–724.
12. Gascoigne, S. (2001). *The Clinical Medicine Guide: A Holistic Perspective*. Clonakilty, Ireland: Jigme.
13. Beers, M. H., & Berkow, R. (1999). *The Merck Manual of Diagnosis and Therapy*. Kenilworth, NJ: Merck.
14. Clane General Hospital (2008). *IVF Fee Schedule* [online]. Available from http://www.clanehospital.ie/ivfprices (accessed 13 February 2009).
15. Templeton, A. (2000). Infertility and the establishment of pregnancy—overview. *British Medical Bulletin*, 56(3): 577–587.
16. Rosene-Montella, K., Keely, E., Laifer, S. A., & Lee, R. V. (2000). Evaluation and management of infertility in women: the internists' role. *Annals of Internal Medicine*, 132(12): 973–981.
17. Miner, S. A., Robins, S., Zhu, Y. J., Keeren, K., Gu, V., Read, S. C., & Zelkowitz, P. (2018). Evidence for the use of complementary and alternative medicines during fertility treatment: a scoping review. *BMC Complementary & Alternative Medicine*, 18(1): 158.
18. Leach, M. J. (2006). Integrative health care: a need for change? *Journal of Complementary and Integrative Medicine*, 3(1) [online]. Available from http://bepress.com/jcim/vol3/iss1/1 (accessed 24 July 2009).
19. Rakel, D. (2007). *Integrative Medicine* (2nd edn). Philadelphia, PA: Saunders.
20. Rees, L., & Weill, A. (2001). Integrated medicine imbues orthodox medicine with the value of complementary medicine. *British Medical Journal*, 322: 191–120.
21. Bendle, C., Fitter, M., & Nohr, K. (2000). *Foxhill Medical Herbalist Project Report* [online]. Available from http://theherbalist.co.uk/foxhill.doc (accessed 7 May 2009).
22. Smith, R. (2001). Editor's choice: Restoring the soul of medicine. *British Medical Journal*, 322 [online]. Available from http://bmj.com (accessed 27 April 2009).
23. Boon, H. S., & Kachan, N. (2008). Integrative medicine: a tale of two clinics. *BMC Complementary and Alternative Medicine*, 8: 32 [online]. Available from http://biomed-central.com/1472-6882/8/32 (accessed 27 April 2009).
24. Sharpe, M. (2001). Letters: Science of the art of medicine does exist. *British Medical Journal*, 322: 1485.
25. Killgrew, S. (1999). Chapter 14: Emotions, boundaries and medical care. In: N. Malin (Ed.), *Professionalism, Boundaries and the Workplace*. Oxford: Routledge.
26. Astin, J. A. (1998). Why patients use alternative medicine: Results of a national study. *Journal of the American Medical Association*, 279: 1548–1553.

PART I

FEMALE REPRODUCTIVE HEALTH

Reproductive health problems leading to infertility in women can be divided into two broad categories: *organic infertility* and *functional infertility.*

Organic infertility is that which is clearly related to an identifiable, underlying medical condition.[27] It is further subdivided into *anovulatory infertility*, in which ovulation does not occur due to an identifiable cause; and *structural infertility*, which is due to a structural abnormality of the reproductive organs, which prevents conception from occurring.[28]

Some cases of organic infertility may require orthodox medical or surgical intervention in order for the woman to conceive, although sometimes the condition may be irreversible. However, in many cases, herbal medicine may be of benefit, either alone, or in combination with other forms of treatment.

Functional infertility on the other hand is due to incorrect *functioning* of the reproductive system, which is not due to any underlying medical condition. It includes improper functioning of the reproductive hormones for which no cause has been identified, as well as unexplained causes of infertility.[29] Herbal medicine and other complementary and alternative approaches have a great deal to offer for women with functional and unexplained infertility, and this is discussed further in Chapter 4 of this book.

For individuals with functional reproductive health problems or unexplained infertility, traditional medicine systems, such as traditional Chinese medicine (TCM) and Ayurveda (the traditional medicine system of India), can often help to provide an explanation for the difficulty in conceiving where orthodox medicine has failed to do so. Traditional diagnostic techniques may be used alongside orthodox investigations to help identify "energetic" patterns of disharmony that contribute to reproductive health problems and infertility, and help practitioners to formulate an approach to treatment, which will improve the chances of conceiving naturally, or increase the success rates of assisted reproduction. These traditional medicine systems and "energetic" patterns of disharmony are discussed in Chapter 6.

Finally, lifestyle factors, such as poor nutrition, lack of exercise, smoking, caffeine and alcohol consumption are significant contributing factors in cases of infertility. These will be covered in Chapter 5.

Organic infertility		*Functional infertility*
Related to an identifiable underlying medical condition		*Not due to any underlying medical condition*
Anovulatory infertility	**Structural infertility**	**Incorrect functioning of the reproductive system**
• Primary amenorrhoea	**Fallopian tube damage or blockage**	**Abnormal blood flow**
• Hypothalamic amenorrhoea	• Pelvic inflammatory disease	**Functional hormone imbalance**
• Hypopituitarism	• Endometriosis	• Oestrogen
• Hyperprolactinaemia	**Uterine, cervical, or vaginal abnormalities**	• Progesterone
• Primary ovarian insufficiency		• Cortisol
		• Prolactin
• PCOS	• Dyspareunia & vaginismus	**Prostaglandin imbalance**
• Being overweight or underweight	• Congenital vaginal obstruction	**Stress**
• Thyroid hormone imbalance	• Cervical factor infertility	**Lifestyle factors**
	• Uterine abnormalities	**Unexplained infertility**
	• Fibroids	

Notes

27. Williams, K. E., Marsh, W. K., & Rasgon, N. L. (2007). Mood disorders and fertility in women: a critical review of the literature and implications for future research. *Human Reproduction Update* [online]. Available from http://humupd.oxfordjournals.org/cgi/content/full/dmm019v1 (accessed 12 June 2010).

28. Liu, W., & Gong, C. (2009). Opening the blockage to reproduction: Infertility. *Traditional Chinese Medicine Information Page* [online]. Available from http://tcmpage.com/hpinfertility.html (accessed 4 July 2011).

29. Indhorn, M., & van Balen, F. (2002). *Infertility around the Globe: New Thinking on Childlessness, Gender, and Reproductive Technologies*. Berkeley, CA: University of California Press.

CHAPTER ONE

Organic infertility: conditions leading to anovulation

In women with anovulatory infertility, ovulation does not occur due to an underlying identifiable medical condition. This chapter discusses the various medical conditions which may result in failure to ovulate, and approaches to treatment with herbal medicine, nutrition, and lifestyle changes.

Amenorrhoea

Amenorrhoea is the absence of menses. It is divided into two categories, *primary amenorrhoea* and *secondary amenorrhoea*.

Primary amenorrhoea

Primary amenorrhoea refers to the absence of menstruation by the age of sixteen years (or fourteen years in cases where there is no development of secondary sexual characteristics).[30] It affects less than 1% of women.[31] Women with primary amenorrhoea have never had a period, usually due to chromosomal abnormalities (such as Turner's syndrome) and/or congenital abnormalities of the reproductive organs (such as imperforate hymen or transvaginal septum).[32] Primary amenorrhoea can usually only be treated with surgery and/or permanent hormone replacement therapy.[33] It generally does not respond to herbal medicine alone;[34] however, herbal medicines and other complementary and alternative approaches may be used in conjunction with orthodox interventions, depending on the needs of the individual patient.

Secondary amenorrhoea

Secondary amenorrhoea is the absence of menstruation for at least three months in a woman with previously normal menstrual cycles; or six months in women with a history of oligomenorrhoea.[35] It is a symptom of an underlying imbalance or disorder, rather than a disease in itself. Therefore it is essential to take a comprehensive medical history to establish the cause of the amenorrhoea, and also to rule out pregnancy.[36] Secondary amenorrhoea may be due to conditions such as hypothalamic amenorrhoea, hypopituitarism, hyperprolactinaemia, primary ovarian insufficiency, or polycystic ovary syndrome.[37]

Hypothalamic amenorrhoea

Hypothalamic amenorrhoea is the most common form of amenorrhoea in pre-menopausal women.[38] It may be caused by marked weight loss, excessive exercise, physical illness, or emotional stress,[39] or it may occasionally occur following the use of oral contraceptives.[40]

Normal reproductive hormone function

During normal functioning of the reproductive system, secretion of gonadotropin-releasing hormone (GnRH) by the hypothalamus, triggers release of follicle stimulating hormone (FSH) by the pituitary. FSH stimulates growth and maturation of the ovarian follicles, and production of oestrogen, which in turn stimulates endometrial growth. Insufficient production of oestrogen by the ovary increases FSH release in order to increase the stimulation of the ovarian follicles, whereas higher levels of oestrogen reduce FSH release as a result of negative feedback. When the ovarian follicle is mature, GnRH causes a surge of luteinising hormone (LH) from the pituitary gland, which triggers egg release. The empty follicle then forms the corpus luteum, which produces progesterone.

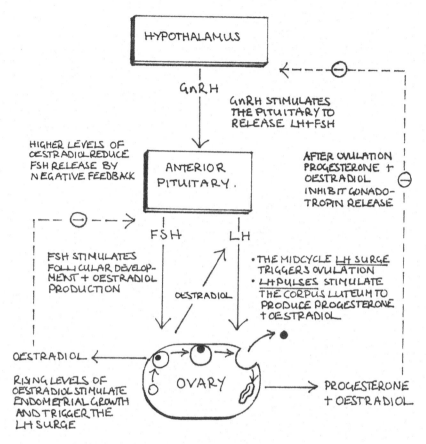

Figure 1: Normal reproductive hormone function.

Reproductive hormone function in hypothalamic amenorrhoea

The absence of menstruation in hypothalamic amenorrhoea is caused by deficient secretion of gonadotropin-releasing hormone (GnRH) by the hypothalamus, resulting in low pituitary secretion of ollicle stimulating hormone (FSH).[41] The lack of stimulation of ovarian follicles by FSH in turn prevents normal follicular growth and maturation, and leads to low levels of oestrogen, and reduced endometrial growth. Deficient GnRH secretion also leads to absence of the pituitary LH surge that normally triggers egg release, leading to anovulation and low progesterone levels.[42] Because the problem lies with the central control of the endocrine system in the hypothalamus, low levels of oestrogen in hypothalamic amenorrhoea do not lead to a compensatory rise in FSH.

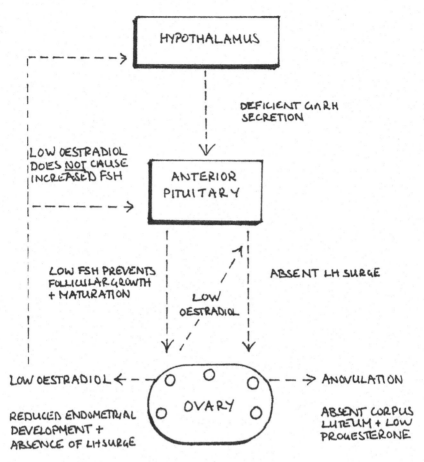

Figure 2: Hypothalamic amenorrhoea.

Hypothalamic amenorrhoea should be differentiated from other forms of amenorrhoea.[43] It differs significantly from amenorrhoea due to primary ovarian insufficiency, or "early menopause" (discussed in more detail later), which occurs when the ovaries cease to function. In the latter case, the failure of the ovarian follicles to secrete oestrogen causes pituitary FSH levels to rise, as a result of a lack of negative feedback inhibition by oestrogen.[44] In other words, premature ovarian insufficiency is associated with low levels of oestrogen and *high levels of FSH*, whereas hypothalamic amenorrhoea is associated with low levels of oestrogen and *low levels of FSH*.

In women experiencing amenorrhoea it is therefore vitally important to request appropriate blood tests, and to obtain copies of the results, in order to establish the correct diagnosis, and devise the most appropriate approach to treatment. (For further information about laboratory testing to assess reproductive health, see Chapter 12.)

In addition to causing infertility, amenorrhoea associated with oestrogen deficiency also poses other risks to women's health, including decreased bone density (which leads to increased fracture risk), increased risk of cardiovascular disease, higher incidence of depression and anxiety, and sexual problems such as reduced libido and vaginal dryness,[45] which may be improved with herbal medicine, nutrition, appropriate exercise, and lifestyle changes (discussed in more detail later in this chapter, in the section on primary ovarian insufficiency).

Treatment of hypothalamic amenorrhoea

Hypothalamic amenorrhoea may be reversed by reducing exercise (particularly if this is excessive in intensity or duration), and by improving nutrition.[46,47] Orthodox treatment of hypothalamic amenorrhoea is also aimed at reversing the underlying causes of amenorrhoea, such as inadequate nutrition, excessive exercise, or physical or emotional stress. Use of oral contraceptives, or bisphosphonate drugs, which are often prescribed in order to prevent bone loss due to lack of oestrogen, are not recommended in hypothalamic amenorrhoea. However, some women may be offered short-term transdermal oestrogen to improve bone density, if there is very long-standing amenorrhoea.[48]

Hypothalamic amenorrhoea is associated with low LH and elevated cortisol levels.[49] Therefore herbs which improve LH secretion (such as *Vitex-agnus castus*),[50] and measures to relieve stress (including stress management techniques, nervines such as *Verbena officinalis*, and herbal adaptogens such as *Withania somnifera*) may help to reverse hypothalamic amenorrhoea.

Lepidium meyenii (maca) is a nutritive, adaptogenic herb that increases secretion of both FSH and LH by the pituitary.[51] This may improve ovarian function in women, and thereby increase ovarian hormone production.

Steroidal saponin-containing herbs may be taken for 10 days of each month to mimic a menstrual cycle.[52] *Dioscorea villosa* (wild yam),

Tribulus terrestris (puncture vine), and *Trigonella foenum graecum* (fenugreek) contain steroidal saponins such as diosgenin, which compete with endogenous oestrogens for hypothalamic oestrogen receptors. They have a weaker effect on hypothalamic oestrogen receptors than endogenous oestrogen, causing the body to respond as if oestrogen levels are lower than they really are, stimulating the pituitary to increase FSH secretion, which in turn increases oestrogen production.[53] Improved levels of FSH also lead to improved ovulation, especially when given on days 5–14.[54]

Energetics

In Ayurveda, amenorrhoea is often associated with *Vata* disturbance, and therefore benefits from consumption of moist, sweet, heavy, and nourishing foods such as root vegetables, soaked nuts, and oils (such as flaxseed oil); and herbs such as *Asparagus racemosus* (shatavari) and *Trigonella foenum graecum* (fenugreek).[55] It is also important to reduce stress levels and to avoid strenuous exercise in order to reduce Vata.[56]

In traditional Chinese medicine (TCM), hypothalamic amenorrhoea is often associated with severe Blood Deficiency,[57] which similarly requires moist, warming, and nourishing foods and herbs, such as *Angelica sinensis* (Dang Gui) and *Rehmannia glutinosa* (Shu Di Huang).[58] For more information about "energetic" approaches to understanding and treating infertility, please see Chapter 6.

Case study

Twenty-seven-year-old female

Presenting complaint
- Amenorrhoea for 4 years after discontinuing oral contraceptives
- Blood tests showed slight leukopenia, neutropenia, and lymphopenia
- LH 2.1 u/L, FSH 5.3 u/L, Oestradiol <50 pmol/L
- Pituitary MRI normal

Medical history
- Low mood since break-up of long-term relationship 3 years ago
- Non-smoker, social alcohol, no current medication
- Exercises for one hour per day at the gym
- Tendency to overwork and perfectionism

BP: 110/75

Pulse: 60 bpm (regular)

Tongue: Pale, red tip

Rx
- *Vitex agnus castus*   (1:3)   15
- *Withania somnifera*   (1:1)   15
- *Glycyrrhiza glabra*   (1:1)   15
- *Verbena officinalis*   (1:3)   30
- *Hypericum perforatum*   (1:3)   30

                                        105 ml   (Sig. 7.5 ml bid)

Rx *Dioscorea villosa*   (1:3)   35 ml   (Sig. 5 ml od for first
                                               10 days of the month)

Rx *Lepidium Meyenii powder*   (Sig. 3 g per day)

Recommendations
- Reduce intensity and duration of exercise
  (yoga, walking 30–50 minutes a day)
- Increase moist, warming and nourishing foods

Follow-up
- After 3 months blood tests showed LH 5.8, FSH 8.1, oestradiol 137
- Menstruation returned to 35 day cycle one month later

Hypopituitarism

Hypopituitarism refers to failure of pituitary gland to secrete one or more of the pituitary hormones. It is a rare disorder, with a prevalence of around 45 cases per 100,000 people.[59] It may be congenital, or may be caused by a tumour, brain injury, subarachnoid haemorrhage, meningitis, haemochromatosis, or cranial radiation or surgery.[60]

Under normal circumstances, low target hormone levels (such as low oestrogen, androgens, thyroxine, or cortisol) stimulate the pituitary gland to increase production of stimulating hormones (such as FSH, LH, TSH, or ACTH [adrenocorticotropic hormone] respectively). However, in hypopituitarism, the pituitary gland response to falling target hormone levels is absent or suboptimal, which results in secondary failure of the target glands (such as the ovaries, thyroid, testes, and adrenal glands).

Therefore, hypopituitarism is associated with *low* levels of oestrogen, thyroxine, and/or cortisol, and *low or normal levels* of pituitary hormones FSH, LH, TSH, ACTH, GH, and/or prolactin. Symptoms of hypopituitarism in women include oligo- or amenorrhoea, infertility, and various other symptoms, depending on the cause of the hypopituitarism and which hormones are affected.[61]

Again, it is very important to ensure that both pituitary hormones (such as FSH, LH, TSH) *and* target hormones (such as oestrogen and thyroxine) are tested, since a low target gland hormone level, yet normal or low pituitary hormone level, suggests pituitary disease, rather than target gland failure. Pituitary causes of infertility and other conditions (such as central hypothyroidism) may be missed by only measuring levels of stimulating hormone.[62]

Treatment of hypopituitarism

Treatment options for hypopituitarism vary depending on the cause. Some individuals with hypopituitarism may need hormone replacement therapy.[63] However, herbal medicines and other complementary and alternative approaches may be used in conjunction with orthodox interventions, to improve health and well-being, depending on the needs of the individual patient.

Hyperprolactinaemia

Hyperprolactinaemia refers to elevated levels of prolactin, the pituitary hormone that is responsible for breast development and lactation.[64] Hyperprolactinaemia may be caused by pituitary trauma, chest wall trauma, stress, various medications (especially those affecting dopamine levels),[65] and hypoglycaemia.[66]

Approximately 30% of cases of hyperprolactinaemia are caused by prolactin-secreting tumours (prolactinomas), which are usually benign. Prolactin production can also be stimulated by thyrotropin-releasing hormone (TRH), therefore primary hypothyroidism (which is associated with high TRH) can cause hyperprolactinaemia.[67]

Higher concentrations of prolactin inhibit progesterone, and reduce oestrogen levels by inhibiting the activity of aromatase (the enzyme which catalyses the conversion of androgens to oestrogen), leading to infertility.[68] Symptoms of hyperprolactinaemia include galactorrhoea (due to the effect of prolactin on breast endothelial cells), and amenorrhoea and infertility (due to suppression of GnRH by prolactin). The presence of a pituitary adenoma may also cause visual field defects and headaches. This is usually diagnosed by magnetic resonance imaging (MRI).[69]

Reducing prolactin levels

Orthodox treatment of hyperprolactinaemia is with dopamine agonist medication (such as bromocriptine). Radiation or surgery for prolactinomas is not usually recommended due to the associated risk of hypopituitarism.[70]

Herbal medicines may be used to reduce prolactin levels and improve fertility in patients with hyperprolactinaemia. *Vitex agnus castus* (chaste tree) has been shown to increase conception in infertile women with hyperprolactinaemia and luteal phase dysfunction.[39,71] *Salvia officinalis* (sage) has been traditionally used to decrease production of breast milk.[72] It binds to GABA receptors,[73] and thereby reduces prolactin synthesis and release, and also increases dopamine, which in turn further inhibits prolactin.[74] *Cimicifuga racemosa* (black cohosh) also has a dopaminergic action, which inhibits prolactin release.[75]

Deficiencies of vitamin B6, magnesium, and zinc are associated with low dopamine and raised prolactin.[76] Therefore supplementing these nutrients may help to improve dopamine synthesis[77] and reduce hyperprolactinaemia.

Increasing prostaglandin E1 (PGE1) helps to counteract the effects of higher prolactin levels.[78] Vitamin B6 and zinc are necessary co-factors in the production of series-1 prostaglandins. Vitamin E can also positively influence prostaglandin ratios. Essential fatty acid supplements such as evening primrose or starflower oil contain linolenic and gamma linolenic acid, which increase PGE1.[79]

Finally, since stress affects prolactin levels, stress management and relaxation techniques may be useful for reducing elevated prolactin levels, in conjunction with herbal medicine and nutritional supplements.[80]

Energetics

In Ayurveda, hyperprolactinaemia is associated with excess Kapha. In TCM, hyperprolactinaemia may be due to Yang deficiency, with consequent Qi stagnation and accumulation of Dampness (signified by swollen tender breasts and galactorrhoea). Western herbs commonly used to treat hyperprolactinaemia, such as *Vitex agnus castus* (chaste tree) and *Salvia officinalis* (sage) are warm, dry and pungent, and are therefore suitable for treating both Yang Deficiency and damp patterns, as well as Kapha excess. For more information about "energetic" approaches to understanding and treating infertility, please see Chapter 6.

Ovarian insufficiency and early menopause

Primary ovarian insufficiency (POI) affects about 1% of women. It occurs when the ovaries stop functioning normally before the age of forty. The failure of the ovarian follicles to secrete oestrogen causes pituitary FSH levels to rise, as a result of a lack of negative feedback inhibition by oestrogen. Primary ovarian insufficiency is therefore associated with *low* levels of oestrogen and *elevated* FSH.[81] This is the same process as menopause, which occurs when the ovaries naturally cease to function between the ages of forty-five and fifty-five years, except that it happens early.

Oestrogen levels vary widely in premenopausal women, with normal ranges of oestradiol extending from 45.4 pmol/L to 845 pmol/L during the follicular phase, and 81.9–1251 pmol/L during the luteal phase.[82] Therefore it can be difficult to establish what actually constitutes "low" levels for each individual, based on the level of oestrogen alone. However, a higher level of FSH, and particularly an elevated FSH/LH ratio strongly suggests a decreased ovarian response.[83]

Primary ovarian insufficiency is also associated with low anti-Mullerian hormone (AMH), which is secreted by the ovarian granulosa cells. AMH reflects the number of primary follicles present, which is an indicator of the remaining ovarian reserve.[84] Low AMH levels reflect a lower number of primary follicles, whereas abnormally high AMH suggests a higher number of primary follicles (as occurs in PCOS).[85]

Primary ovarian insufficiency may be due to a low initial number of primordial follicles during foetal development, or accelerated follicle atresia due to chromosomal abnormalities, or autoimmunity.[86] Approximately 20% of women with POI have a coexisting autoimmune disorder, most commonly autoimmune hypothyroidism.[87] Although the cause is often unknown, POI may be hereditary, or it may be associated

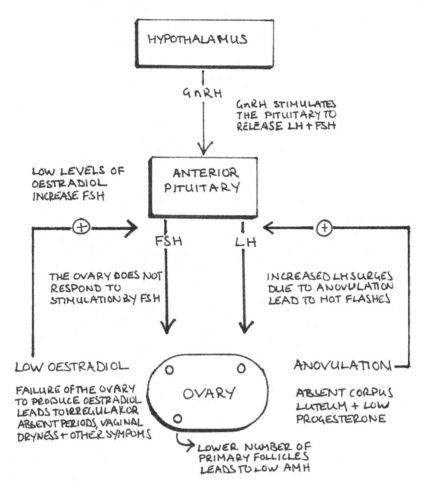

Figure 3: Primary ovarian insufficiency.

with immune system diseases, radiation or chemotherapy treatment,[88] smoking,[89] and viral infections such as mumps and varicella viruses.[90]

Primary ovarian insufficiency may lead to premature menopause, which is permanent and irreversible.[91] However, the early stages of POI are characterised by intermittent ovarian failure, interspersed with periods of normal follicular activity, and women with POI may continue to have occasional periods for several years.[92]

Symptoms of ovarian insufficiency are the same as those often experienced during normal perimenopause, and include irregular or absent periods, hot flushes and night sweats, mood changes, poor concentration, sleep disturbance, reduced libido, vaginal dryness, and changes in skin and hair. Low levels of oestrogen can also predispose to dry eye syndrome, heart disease, osteoporosis, and hypothyroidism.[93]

Improving fertility in women with primary ovarian insufficiency

Orthodox treatment of ovarian insufficiency involves hormone replacement therapy to alleviate symptoms, prevent bone loss, and reduce the risk of cardiovascular disease, while women with POI who wish to conceive are usually advised to consider IVF using donor eggs.[94]

However, in women with low AMH, raised FSH, and/or increased FSH/LH ratio, complete ovarian failure may be delayed by protecting the remaining follicles from atresia by reducing follicle damage (due to oxidative stress, or autoimmune destruction).

Accumulation of reactive oxygen species (ROS) contributes to mitochondrial dysfunction and oxidative stress. This, in turn, leads to oxidative damage to DNA and other cell structures, similar to age-related changes. Therefore, improving mitochondrial function by supplementing antioxidants is important for improving oocye quality and increasing fertility.[95] Coenzyme Q10 is an antioxidant enzyme that has been shown to help improve oocyte quality and embryo development.[96] Supplementation of 750 mg per day of vitamin C has also been shown to reduce the effects of oxidative stress during oocyte maturation, and to increase progesterone levels, and improve fertility.[97]

The hormone DHEA is essential for oestrogen production in the ovary. DHEA supplementation has been shown to significantly improve levels of AMH (which reflects an increased number of developing primary follicles); and to increase the quality of oocytes produced.[98]

DHEA enhances insulin-like growth factor (IGF-I), which is involved in follicular growth. DHEA may also improve ovarian reserve by increasing recruitment of follicles from the dormant primordial follicular pool; and reducing apoptosis (the process by which recruited follicles are destroyed).[99] DHEA supplementation has been shown to significantly improve outcomes in women undergoing in vitro fertilisation (IVF) or intracytoplasmic sperm injection (ICSI).[100] Improving DHEA levels may therefore be very beneficial for women with low ovarian reserve or primary ovarian insufficiency, in order to increase the number of available follicles and improve egg quality.

Withania somnifera has been shown to increase levels of DHEA[101] and may therefore have a beneficial effect on ovarian reserve, egg quality, and pregnancy outcomes, as a result of its ability to improve endogenous DHEA levels. DHEA is produced by the adrenal gland, and less is produced when cortisol is high. Therefore measures to reduce stress and improve adrenal function (discussed later) may help to increase DHEA and thereby improve ovarian function.[102]

Lepidium meyenii (maca) can also help to improve ovarian function in women with premature ovarian insufficiency. It reduces elevated FSH, improves the LH:FSH ratio, increases oestrogen and progesterone levels,[103] and increases production of ACTH and thyroid hormones.[104] Short-term use of maca initially increases secretion of both FSH and LH by the pituitary. This improves ovarian function, and thereby increases production of both oestrogen and progesterone, reducing symptoms associated with low ovarian hormone levels, such as hot flushes, sweating, sleep disturbance, mood changes, joint pains, and heart palpitations. After several months of treatment, improved ovarian hormone levels allow FSH levels to fall due to negative feedback, and the FSH:LH ratio improves.[105]

Constituents of maca include various alkaloids, sterols, glucosinolates, amino acids, fatty acids, and minerals.[106] Maca does not contain phytoestrogens, but is thought to act as an adaptogen, positively affecting pituitary function, and thereby improving ovarian, adrenal, and thyroid activity.[107]

Treating the symptoms of primary ovarian insufficiency

The symptoms of primary ovarian insufficiency, such as hot flushes and night sweats, mood changes, poor concentration, sleep disturbance, reduced libido, and vaginal dryness, can be improved with various herbs and phytoestrogens.

Phytoestrogens are plant-based compounds, which include isoflavones (such as genistein, daidzein, and glycitein), coumestans, lignans, and flavonoids. Soybeans are a particularly rich source of isoflavones, and flaxseeds are a good source of lignans. Phytoestrogens have an affinity for oestrogen receptors, and exert a weak oestrogenic effect in comparison to oestradiol.[108] They can help to reduce symptoms associated with lower oestrogen levels, with limited side effects.[109] Consumption of phytoestrogens is also associated with lower fracture risk.[110]

Dioscorea villosa (wild yam) and *Tribulus terrestris* (puncture vine) contain steroidal saponins such as diosgenin, which compete with endogenous oestrogens for hypothalamic oestrogen receptors. They have a weaker effect on hypothalamic oestrogen receptors than endogenous oestrogen, causing the body to respond as if oestrogen levels are lower than they really are, stimulating the pituitary to increase FSH secretion, which in turn increases oestrogen production.[111] This has a beneficial effect on symptoms of ovarian insufficiency, such as hot flushes, night sweats, depression, insomnia, and reduced libido. Improved levels of FSH also lead to improved ovulation, especially when given on days 5–14.[112]

Cimicifuga racemosa (black cohosh) is also helpful in alleviating symptoms of ovarian insufficiency. It reduces luteinising hormone (LH) levels, which have been linked to hot flushes. Its oestrogenic effects promote proliferation of vaginal epithelium, reducing vaginal dryness and atrophy. It also acts as an agonist at serotonin and dopamine receptors, helping to improve mood disturbances such as depression, anxiety, and irritability.[113] *Humulus lupulus* (hops) also contains phytoestrogens and is traditionally used for the treatment of hot flushes, especially when associated with anxiety and insomnia.[114] A vaginal application of gel containing hops can help to reduce vaginal dryness, and associated inflammation, discomfort, and dyspareunia.[115]

Salvia officinalis (sage) reduces excessive sweating, including hot flushes and night sweating associated with ovarian insufficiency.[116] It also improves cognitive function, memory, mood, and energy levels, which can deteriorate with declining oestrogen levels in women with primary ovarian insufficiency.[117]

Hypericum perforatum (St John's wort) is beneficial in relieving mood disturbances associated with primary ovarian insufficiency. It has been shown to reduce symptoms of mild to moderate depression.[118] It may also have some hormonal effects, since it seems to improve both psychological and psychosomatic symptoms including vasomotor symptoms, and sexual well-being.[119] Cooling, sedative herbs (such as *Passiflora incarnata* and *Lactuca virosa*) are useful for sleep disturbance.

In traditional Chinese medicine, ovarian insufficiency is commonly associated with Blood Deficiency, Kidney Yin Deficiency, and empty heat.[120] These are treated with nourishing herbs, which tonify the Blood and Yin, such as *Angelica sinensis* (Dang Gui), *Paeonia lactiflora* (white paeony), and *Rehmannia glutinosa* (Chinese foxglove).

In Ayurveda, primary ovarian insufficiency is most commonly associated with Vata excess, which may be followed by other Dosha imbalances (such as Pitta aggravation), depending on the individual patient.[121] Vata aggravation also benefits from moist, nourishing herbs, such as those named above, as well as *Asparagus racemosus* (shatavari), *Trigonella foenum graecum* (fenugreek), and *Withania somnifera* (ashwagandha), which are more commonly used in Ayurveda. For more information about "energetic" approaches to understanding and treating infertility, please see Chapter 6.

Case study

Thirty-two-year-old female

Presenting complaint
- Trying to conceive for 18 months. Miscarriage at 8 weeks (6 months ago)
- AMH 12.85 pmol/L (low fertility)
- Very light menses for 6 months, vaginal dryness, low libido
- Follicular blood tests: FSH 10.5 IU/L, LH 4.9 IU/L, Oestradiol 87 pmol/L
- Mid luteal progesterone: 36 nmol/L

Medical history
- High stress levels, no exercise
- Smokes 2–3 cigarettes per day

BP: 120/75

Pulse: 60 bpm, regular, impalpable at third position on right hand

Tongue: Dry, bluish tongue body, red tip

Rx
• *Asparagus racemosus*	(1:1)	20
• *Hypericum perforatum*	(1:3)	30
• *Vitex agnus castus*	(1:3)	15
• *Angelica sinensis*	(1:1)	20
• *Withania somnifera*	(1:1)	20
		105 ml (Sig. 7.5 ml bid)

Rx *Lepidium Meyenii* powder   (Sig. 3 g per day)

Recommendations
- Vitamin and mineral supplement for fertility, vitamin C (1000 mg a day)
- Omega-3 EFAs (3 g a day), coenzyme Q10 (300 mg a day)
- Stop smoking
- Consume phytoestrogen-rich foods

Follow-up
- After 3 months of treatment, luteal progesterone increased to 56
- Follicular FSH 9.1 IU/L, LH 6.2 IU/L, oestradiol 164 pmol/L
- Patient conceived after 6 months of treatment and gave birth to a healthy baby boy

Thyroid hormone imbalance

Thyroid function is regulated by the hypothalamic-pituitary axis, and therefore changes in thyroid function can impact greatly on reproductive hormone function.[122]

Hypothyroidism

Hypothyroidism is associated with weight gain, oedema, intolerance of cold, dry skin and hair, bradycardia, depression, constipation, hoarse voice, and non-pitting pretibial oedema. Primary hypothyroidism may be congenital or autoimmune (Hashimoto's). It may be due to iodine deficiency, or may follow treatment for hyperthyroidism. It is associated with suboptimal levels of T4 and T3, and *elevated* levels of thyroid stimulating hormone (TSH). This is because low levels of thyroid hormones trigger the pituitary gland to increase TSH. Hypothyroidism is also associated with hypercholesterolaemia; low ferritin (due to the effect of thyroid hormones on ferritin synthesis); and low sex hormone binding globulin (due to the effect of hypothyroidism on oestrogen levels).

Secondary hypothyroidism is not due to a problem with the thyroid itself, but to a problem with the pituitary gland or hypothalamus. In this case, suboptimal levels of T3 and T4 are associated with *low* TSH. This is because the thyroid gland receives insufficient stimulation from pituitary thyrotropin hormones, and the hypothalamus or pituitary fails to respond to the resulting low thyroid hormone levels.

In euthyroid sick syndrome (which may be due to any severe, acute illness) free T3 is reduced, but TSH and T4 may be normal. It is therefore essential to measure TSH, T4, *and* T3 in patients with symptoms of underactive thyroid.

In cases of primary hypothyroidism, decreased production of T3 and/or T4 by the thyroid gland results in elevated thyroid releasing hormone (TRH), due to reduced negative feedback on the hypothalamus. The elevated TRH increases prolactin release from the pituitary.[123] Elevated prolactin in turn causes suppression of gonadotropin-releasing hormone (GnRH) by the hypothalamus, as previously described, resulting in low pituitary secretion of follicle stimulating hormone (FSH). The lack of stimulation of ovarian follicles by FSH leads to low levels of oestrogen, and prevents normal follicular growth and maturation, leading to sub-fertility.[124]

Evidence suggests that keeping thyroid stimulating hormone (TSH) levels at the lower end of normal (<2.5 mU/l) in euthyroid women may improve conception rates in subfertile women and reduce early pregnancy loss.[125] There is also increasing evidence for the role of auto-antibodies in subfertility and early pregnancy loss, even in euthyroid women. This may be linked to inflammatory changes in the reproductive tissues.[126]

In cases of secondary hypothyroidism due to damage to the hypothalamus or pituitary gland, associated deficiency of GnRH and/or FSH/LH leads to oligo- or amenorrhoea and infertility as previously described. Again, it is very important to ensure that both pituitary hormones (in this case TSH) *and* target hormones (in this case thyroxine) are tested, since a low target gland hormone level, yet normal or low pituitary hormone level, suggests pituitary disease, rather than target gland failure. Central hypothyroidism may be missed by only measuring levels of stimulating hormone.[127]

Improving thyroid function

Consuming iodine rich foods including seaweeds (such as kelp), and ensuring adequate selenium intake (from nuts such as brazils), and exercising for at least 20–30 minutes a day can help to improve thyroid

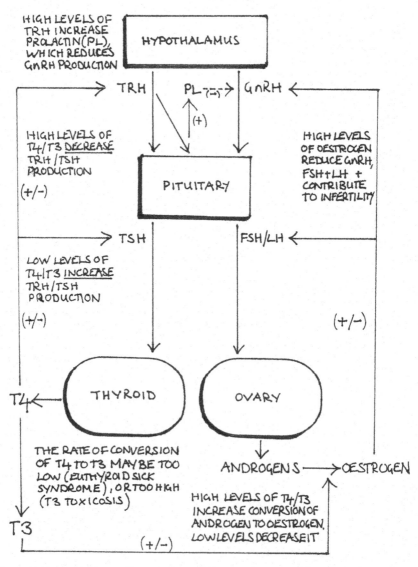

Figure 4: Hypothyroidism and reproductive hormone function.

function in women with low levels of T3 or T4, and/or elevated TSH.[128] Other important nutrients for Thyroxine synthesis include L-tyrosine, and vitamin B complex. Herbal medicines such as *Fucus vesiculosus* (bladderwrack), *Withania somnifera* (ashwagandha), and *Commiphora mukkul* (guggul) can also increase thyroid function.[129] Measures to improve oestrogen may help to improve thyroid function. *Lepidium meyenii* (maca) increases both oestrogen and thyroid hormone levels.[130] *Withania somnifera* and vitamin D can help to reduce autoimmunity.

Energetics

In Ayurveda, hypothyroid conditions are most commonly associated with excess Kapha, which benefits from warm, dry, and pungent foods and herbs, such as *Withania somnifera* (ashwagandha) and *Commiphora mukkul* (guggul). In TCM, hypothyroidism is most commonly associated with Yang Deficiency and accumulation of Dampness and Phlegm, which also requires warm, dry, and pungent foods and herbs.

Hyperthyroidism

Hyperthyroidism on the other hand, is associated with increased appetite, weight loss, heat intolerance, sweating, tachycardia, diarrhoea, restlessness, fine tremor, menstrual disturbance, and exopthalmus. Primary hyperthyroidism may be autoimmune (Graves disease), or due to subacute thyroiditis, toxic adenoma, or multinodular goitre. Amiodorone, which is used to treat cardiac arrhythmia, may also cause hyperthyroidism. In hyperthyroidism, both T4 and T3 levels are usually elevated, but in a small subset of hyperthyroid patients only T3 is elevated (T3 toxicosis).

Secondary hyperthyroidism may be due to pituitary tumours, which secrete high levels of TSH, triggering increased T4 production by the thyroid gland. TSH-secreting tumours do not respond to negative feedback from increasing T4 or T3 levels.

Hyperthyroidism is also associated with high ferritin (due to the effect of thyroid hormones on ferritin synthesis); hypocholesterolaemia; low triglyceride; low folate (due to the increased metabolic state); high blood calcium levels (due to altered bone metabolism); and high sex hormone-binding globulin (SHBG) (due to increased oestrogen levels).

An overactive thyroid increases conversion of testosterone to oestrogen, which may lead to oestrogen excess.[131] Higher levels of oestrogen also inhibit secretion of hypothalamic gonadotropin-releasing hormone (GnRH) and other important reproductive hormones such as follicle stimulating hormone (FSH) and luteinising hormone (LH),[132] thereby contributing to infertility. Abnormalities in thyroid function can therefore have an adverse effect on reproductive health and result in reduced rates of conception and increased early pregnancy loss, and adverse neonatal outcomes.

Reducing thyroid overactivity

For patients with hyperthyroidism, herbs such as *Melissa officinalis* (lemon balm) and *Lycopus virginicus* (gypsywort) reduce thyroid over-activity;[133] *Ganoderma lucidum* (reishi mushroom), *Hemidesmus indicus* (sariva),[134] *Melissa officinalis* (lemon balm), and vitamin D reduce autoimmunity. *Leonurus cardiaca* (motherwort) is useful for reducing cardiovascular symptoms in patients with overactive thyroid. Measures to reduce oestrogen and prolactin can also help to reduce thyroid autoimmunity (discussed in more detail in Chapter 4).

Energetics

In Ayurveda, hyperthyroid conditions are most commonly disturbances of Vata/Pitta,[135] which benefit from calming nervines such as *Melissa officinalis* (lemon balm), *Lycopus virginicus* (gypsywort), and *Leonurus cardiaca* (motherwort).

In traditional Chinese medicine (TCM), hyperthyroidism is considered to be the result of Yin Deficiency.[136] For more information about "energetic" approaches to understanding and treating infertility, see Chapter 6.

Systemic lupus erythematosus

Systemic lupus erythematosus (SLE) is a multi-system, autoimmune condition that can lead to infertility and increase the risk of early pregnancy loss in some women.[137] It causes widespread symptoms such as fever, joint pain and inflammation, skin manifestations (including the classic "butterfly" malar rash), inflammation of mucosal surfaces, photosensitivity, renal disease, nervous system problems, Raynaud's phenomenon, and other cardiovascular complications.[138] The presentation and the course of the disease are highly variable between individuals.

Systemic lupus erythematosus most commonly affects women during their thirties, the age at which they are most likely to want to start a family. Reduced fertility in women with SLE can be due to problems preventing successful fertilisation of oocytes, issues affecting implantation, or difficulty in maintaining pregnancy.[139]

There is no single diagnostic test for SLE. Patients with SLE will nearly always have antinuclear antibodies (ANA) present at least some of the time, but these are not specific to SLE, and ANA tests may be negative in patients who are not experiencing active disease at the time. Other abnormalities that are frequently detected in patients with SLE include leukopenia and thrombocytopenia. The erythrocyte sedimentation rate (ESR), which is a non-specific marker for inflammation, is usually raised in active disease; but unusually, C-reactive protein (CRP), which is elevated in most inflammatory diseases, may be normal or only slightly elevated in patients with SLE.

In women with SLE, episodes of amenorrhoea have been associated with anti-corpus luteum antibodies and raised FSH levels.[140] Autoimmunity can also lead to primary ovarian insufficiency/primary ovarian failure (POI/POF) in some cases.[141] For more information about pathophysiology and improving fertility in women with POI/POF, see Chapter 1.

Thyroid autoimmune diseases including Grave's disease and Hashimoto's thyroiditis are also more common in women with SLE and may cause endocrine disturbances and reduced fertility, due to the presence of thyroid autoantibodies.[142] Pathophysiology and treatment for women with thyroid abnormalities is discussed in more detail in Chapter 1.

Patients with SLE are also more prone to infection, either due to low white blood cells counts, or due to immunosuppressant therapy, and may be more likely to experience infertility as a result.[143] For more information about pathophysiology and treatment of infective causes of infertility, see Chapter 3.

Infertility in women with SLE may be due to the disease process itself, or it may be the result of immunosuppressive treatment, or use of non-steroidal anti-inflammatory drugs (NSAIDs) to reduce pain and inflammation.[144] High doses of steroids used to suppress autoimmune inflammation may induce transient suppression of the hypothalamic-pituitary-ovarian axis, inducing reversible infertility. However, cyclophosphamide, which is used to treat SLE, can cause irreversible infertility as a result of ovarian failure. NSAIDs may cause infertility by interfering with ovulation, implantation, and placental development, due to inhibition of prostaglandin synthesis.[145] Drug induced infertility is discussed in more detail in Chapter 5.

Antibodies in SLE also have a direct effect on trophoblastic cells, reducing implantation, cellular differentiation, and synthesis of hCG (human chorionic gonadotropin).[146] Therefore, women with SLE who manage to conceive are at increased risk of miscarriage, hypertension, and pre-eclampsia, particularly if they have coexisting antiphospholipid syndrome (which is more common in patients with SLE).[147]

In over a third of pregnant women with SLE, the size of the placenta is reduced because of placental vasculitis, thrombosis, and resulting ischaemia. This may compromise the delivery of nutrition and oxygen to the foetus, resulting in delayed growth and increasing the risk of pregnancy loss.[148] For more information about improving blood flow and preventing early pregnancy loss, see Chapter 14.

Oestrogens stimulate release of prolactin, which in turn stimulates T-lymphocyte proliferation, B-lymphocyte maturation, and antibody synthesis. The level of prolactin is positively correlated with disease activity in women with SLE. Therefore, increased oestrogen and prolactin levels (discussed in more detail in Chapter 4) can induce disease flares.[149]

Reducing inflammation in patients with SLE

In addition to addressing the issues described above and discussed in more detail in other parts of this book, herbs such as Ganoderma lucidum (reishi mushroom), and Hemidesmus Indicus (sariva),[150] and supplemental vitamin D may help to reduce autoimmunity. Reducing series 2 (inflammatory) prostaglandins can help to reduce inflammation, and lower the risk of early pregnancy loss in women with SLE.

Reducing consumption of animal fats, and increasing essential fatty acids, selectively decreases dietary precursors of series 2 (inflammatory) prostaglandins, and increases series 1 prostaglandins, which have anti-inflammatory, anti-thrombotic, and anti-spasmodic effects.[151] Omega 3 fatty acids (found in oily fish and flaxseed) reduce the production of inflammatory cytokines.[152] Vitamin E can also positively influence prostaglandin ratios; and vitamin B6 and zinc are necessary co-factors in the production of series 1 prostaglandins.[153] Zingiber officinale (ginger) has also been shown to reduce the production of series 2 prostaglandins.[154]

Case study

Thirty-six-year-old female

Presenting complaint
- Previous unsuccessful cycle of IVF 6 months ago. Intends to try again using frozen embryos
- Regular periods, occasional mastalgia
- Blood tests showed raised TPO, leukocytosis, lymphocytosis, granulocytopenia, thrombopenia, low NK cells, low CD56+, elevated CD57 (results suggest diagnosis of SLE)

Medical history
- Sluggish digestion, irregular bowel movements, bloating
- Currently overweight
- Non-smoker, social alcohol, no current medication
- Exercises for one hour per day (running/walking)

BP: 115/75

Pulse: 68 bpm (regular)

Tongue: Pale, deep centre crack, yellowish coating

Rx
• Vitex agnus castus	(1:3)	15
• Rosmarinus officinalis	(1:3)	25
• Ginkgo biloba	(2:1)	20
• Glycyrrhiza glabra	(1:1)	15
• Viburnum prunifolium	(1:3)	30

105 ml per week   (Sig. 7.5 ml bid)

Rx *Ganoderma lucidum* (extract powder)   (Sig. 4 g per day)

Rx *Rubus idaeus* (dried herb)   25 g
    Melissa offcinalis (dried herb)   15 g
                                          40 g   (Sig. 6 g per day
                                                       as infusion)

Recommendations
- Vitamin B6 (50 mg), vitamin E (200 mg), vitamin D (5,000 iu), omega-3 (3 g)
- Avoid gluten, anti-inflammatory diet, measures to reduce body weight

Follow-up
- After 3 months blood tests were within normal ranges
- Successful IVF transfer carried out 6 months after starting herbal treatment.

Notes

30. Romm, A. (2016). *Botanical Medicine for Women's Health* (2nd edn). London: Churchill Livingstone.
31. Gurdeep, S., Sellars, E. K., & Sidhu, P. S. (2011). The paediatric uterus, ovaries and testes. In: *Clinical Ultrasound* (3rd edn) *Volume 2: 1468–1496*. London: Churchill Livingstone.
32. Master-Hunter, T., & Heiman, D. L. (2006). Amenorrhea: evaluation and treatment. *American Family Physician, 73*(8): 1374–1382.
33. Trickey, R. (2011). *Women, Hormones and the Menstrual Cycle*. Clifton Hill, Victoria, Australia: Melbourne Holistic Health Group.
34. Weiss, J. (2001). *Weiss's Herbal Medicine*. New York: Thieme.
35. Master-Hunter, T., & Heiman, D. L. (2006). Amenorrhea: evaluation and treatment. *American Family Physician, 73*(8): 1374–1382.
36. Romm, A. (2016). *Botanical Medicine for Women's Health* (2nd edn). London: Churchill Livingstone.
37. Klein, D. A., & Poth, M. A. (2016). Amenorrhea: an approach to diagnosis and management. *American Family Physician, 87*(11): 718–788.
38. Marshall, J. C. (2016). Hypothalamic amenorrhea. In: J. L. Jameson, L. J. DeGroot, D. M. de Kretser, L. C. Giudice, A. B. Grossman, S. Melmed, J. T. Potts Jr., & G. C. Weir (Eds.), *Endocrinology: Adult and Pediatric* (7th edn). Philadelphia, PA: Elsevier.
39. De Souza, M. J., & Toombs, R. J. (2010). Amenorrhea. In: N. F. Santoro & G. Neal-Perry (Eds.), *Amenorrhea: A Case-Based, Clinical Guide* (pp. 101–125). Totowa, NJ: Humana Press.
40. Wright, K. P., & Johnson, J. V. (2008). Evaluation of extended and continuous use oral contraceptives. *Therapeutics and Clinical Risk Management, 4*(5): 905–911.
41. Leyendecker, G., Wildt, L., & Hansmann, M. (1983). Induction of ovulation with chronic intermittent (pulsatile) administration of Gn-RH in women with hypothalamic amenorrhoea. *Journal of Reproduction & Fertility, 69*: 397–409.
42. Kaiser, U. B. (2011). Gonadotropin hormones. In: S. Melmed (Ed.), *The Pituitary* (3rd edn). London: Elsevier.
43. Meczekalski, B., Katulski, K., Czyzyk, A., Podfigurna-Stopa, A., & Maciejewska-Jeske, M. (2014). Functional hypothalamic amenorrhea and its influence on women's health. *Journal of Endocrinological Investigation, 37*(11): 1049–1056.

44. Trickey, R. (2011). *Women, Hormones and the Menstrual Cycle.* Clifton Hill, Victoria, Australia: Melbourne Holistic Health Group.
45. Meczekalski, B., Katulski, K, Czyzyk, A., Podfigurna-Stopa, A., & Maciejewska-Jeske, M. (2014). Functional hypothalamic amenorrhea and its influence on women's health. *Journal of Endocrinological Investigation, 37*(11): 1049–1056.
46. Dueck, C. A., Matt, K. S., Manore, M. M., & Skinner, J. S. (1996). Treatment of athletic amenorrhoea with a diet and training intervention program. *International Journal of Sports Nutrition, 6*: 24–40.
47. Marshall, J. C. (2016). Hypothalamic amenorrhea. In: J. L. Jameson, L. J. DeGroot, D. M. de Kretser, L. C. Giudice, A. B. Grossman, S. Melmed, J. T. Potts Jr., & G. C. Weir (Eds.), *Endocrinology: Adult and Pediatric (7th Edition).* Philadelphia, PA: Elsevier.
48. Gordon, C. M., Ackerman, K. E., Berga, S. L., Kaplan, J. R., Mastorakos, G., Misra, M., Murad, M. H., Santoro, N. F., & Warren, M. P. (2017). Functional hypothalamic amenorrhea: An Endocrine Society Clinical Practice Guideline. *Journal of Clinical Endocrinology & Metabolism, 102*(5): 1413–1439.
49. Dueck, C. A., Matt, K. S., Manore, M. M., & Skinner, J. S. (1996). Treatment of athletic amenorrhoea with a diet and training intervention program. *International Journal of Sports Nutrition, 6*: 24–40.
50. Milowicz, A., & Jedrzejuk, D. (2006). Premenstrual syndrome: From etiology to treatment. *Maturitas, 55*(1): s47–s54.
51. Meissner, H. O., Reich-Bilinska, H., Mscisz, A., & Kedzia, B. (2006). Therapeutic effects of pre-gelatinized maca (Lepidium peruvianum chacon) used as a non-hormonal alternative to HRT in perimenopausal women—clinical pilot study. *International Journal of Biomedical Science, 2*(2): 143–159.
52. Trickey, R. (2011). *Women, Hormones and the Menstrual Cycle.* Clifton Hill, Victoria, Australia: Melbourne Holistic Health Group.
53. Brice-Ytsma, H., & McDermott, A. (2020). *Herbal Medicine in Treating Gynaecological Conditions.* London: Aeon.
54. Tabakova, P., Dimitrov, M., & Tashkov, B. (2012). Clinical tudies on Tribulus terrestris protodioscin in women with endocrine infertility or menopausal syndrome. *Herbpharm USA* [online]. Available from http://scicompdf.se/tiggarnot/tabakova-Herb-PharmUSA.pdf (accessed 2 March 2020).
55. Pole, S. (2006). *Ayurvedic Medicine: The Principles of Traditional Practice.* London: Churchill Livingstone.
56. Middlebrooks, Z. (2015). An Ayurvedic approach to the treatment of secondary amenorrhea. *California College of Ayurveda* [online]. Available from https://ayurvedacollege.com/articles/students/Secondary-Amenorrhea (accessed 17 July 2015).
57. Maciocia, G. (2004). *Diagnosis in Chinese Medicine: A Comprehensive Guide.* London: Churchill Livingstone.
58. Maciocia, G. (2012). On blood deficiency. *European Journal of Oriental Medicine, 7*(1): 6–12.
59. Regal, M., Paramo, C., Sierra, S. M., & Garcia-Mayor, R. V. (2001). Prevalence and incidence of hypopituitarism in an adult Caucasian population in North-Western Spain. *Journal of Clinical Endocrinology & Metabolism (Oxford), 55*(6): 753–740.
60. Corenblum, B. (2018). Hypopituitarism (Panhypopituitarism). *Medscape* [online]. Available from https://emedicine.medscape.com/article/122287-overview#a4 (accessed 14 November 2019).

61. Schneider H. J., Aimaretti, G., Kreitschmann-Andermahr, I., Stalla, G.-K., & Ghigo, E. (2007). Hypopituitarism. *Lancet, 369*(9571): 1461–1470.

62. Corenblum, B. (2018). Hypopituitarism (Panhypopituitarism). *Medscape* [online]. Available from https://emedicine.medscape.com/article/122287-overview#a4 (accessed 14 November 2019).

63. Corenblum, B. (2018). Hypopituitarism (Panhypopituitarism). *Medscape* [online]. Available from https://emedicine.medscape.com/article/122287-overview#a4 (accessed 14 November 2019).

64. Shenenberger, D. (2018). Hyperprolactinemia. *Medscape* [online]. Available from https://emedicine.medscape.com/article/121784-overview (accessed 14 November 2019).

65. Longo, D. L., Fauci, A. S., Kasper, D. L., Hauser, S. L., Jameson, J. L., & Loscalzo, J. (2011). *Harrison's Principles of Internal Medicine* (18th edn) (p. 2887). New York: McGraw-Hill Professional.

66. Heffner, L. J., & Schust, D. J. (2014). *The Reproductive System at a Glance*. Oxford: John Wiley & Sons.

67. Shenenberger, D. (2018). Hyperprolactinemia. *Medscape* [online]. Available from https://emedicine.medscape.com/article/121784-overview (accessed 14 November 2019).

68. Brice-Ytsma, H., & McDermott, A. (2020). *Herbal Medicine in Treating Gynaecological Conditions*. London: Aeon.

69. Shenenberger, D. (2018). Hyperprolactinemia. *Medscape* [online]. Available from https://emedicine.medscape.com/article/121784-overview (accessed 14 November 2019).

70. Shenenberger, D. (2018). Hyperprolactinemia. *Medscape* [online]. Available from https://emedicine.medscape.com/article/121784-overview (accessed 14 November 2019).

71. Webster, D. E., Dentali, S. J., Farnsworth, N. R., & Jim Wang, Z. (2008). Chaste tree fruit and premenstrual syndrome (Chapter 12). In: D. Mischoulon & J. F. Rosenbaum (Eds.), *Natural Medications for Psychiatric Disorders: Considering the Alternatives*. Riverwoods, IL: Wolters Kluwer Health.

72. Engels, G. (2010). Sage. *HerbalGram, 89*: 1–4.

73. Kavvadias, D., Monschein, V. S., Sand, P., Riederer, P., & Schreier, P. (2003). Constituents of Sage (*Salvia officinalis*) with in vitro affinity to human brain benzodiazepine receptor. *Planta Medica, 69*: 113–117.

74. Heffner, L. J., & Schust, D. J. (2014). *The Reproductive System at a Glance*. Oxford: John Wiley & Sons.

75. Brice-Ytsma, H., & McDermott, A. (2020). *Herbal Medicine in Treating Gynaecological Conditions*. London: Aeon.

76. Brice-Ytsma, H., & McDermott, A. (2020). *Herbal Medicine in Treating Gynaecological Conditions*. London: Aeon.

77. Trickey, R. (2011). *Women, Hormones and the Menstrual Cycle*. Clifton Hill, Victoria, Australia: Melbourne Holistic Health Group.

78. Brice-Ytsma, H. & McDermott, A. (2020). *Herbal Medicine in Treating Gynaecological Conditions*. London: Aeon.

79. Puolakka, J., Mäkäräinen, L., Viinikka, L., & Ylikorkala, O. (1985). Biochemical and clinical effects of treating the premenstrual syndrome with prostaglandin synthesis precursors. *Journal of Reproductive Medicine, 30*(3): 149–153.

80. Trickey, R. (2011). *Women, Hormones and the Menstrual Cycle.* Clifton Hill, Victoria, Australia: Melbourne Holistic Health Group.

81. Trickey, R. (2011). *Women, Hormones and the Menstrual Cycle.* Clifton Hill, Victoria, Australia: Melbourne Holistic Health Group.

82. MedLab Pathology (Ireland) (2018). *Reference Ranges* [online]. Available from http:// sonichealthcare.ie/test-information/reference-ranges-(1).aspx (accessed 6 December 2019).

83. Shrim, A., Elizur, S. E., Seidman, D. S., Rabinovici, J., Wiser, A., & Dor, J. (2006). Elevated day 3 FSH/LH ratio due to low LH concentrations predicts reduced ovarian response. *Reproductive BioMedicine Online, 12*(4): 418–422.

84. Weenen, C., Laven, J. S. E., Von Bergh, A. R. M., Cranfield, M., Groome, N. P., Visser, J. A., Kramer, P., Fauser, B. C. J. M., & Themmen, P. N. (2004). Anti-Müllerian hormone expression pattern in the human ovary: potential implications for initial and cyclic follicle recruitment. *Molecular Human Reproduction, 10*(2): 77–83.

85. Broer, S. L., Broekman, F. J. M., Laven, J. S. E., & Fauser, B. C. J. M. (2014). Anti-Mullerian hormone: ovarian reserve testing and its potential clinical implications. *Human Reproduction Update, 20*(5): 688–701.

86. Popat, V., & Lucidi, R. S. (2013). Ovarian insufficiency. *Medscape* [online]. Available from http://emedicine.medscape.com/article/271046-overview#a6 (accessed 10 July 2015).

87. Goswami, D., & Conway, G. S. (2005). Premature ovarian failure. *Human Reproduction Update, 11*(4): 394–410.

88. Morgan, S., Anderson, R. A., Gourley, C., Wallace, W. H., & Spears, N. (2012). How do chemotherapeutic agents damage the ovary? *Human Reproduction Update, 18*(5): 525–535.

89. Mattison, D. R., Plowchalk, D. R., Meadows, M. J., Miller, M. M., Malek, A., & London, S.(1989). The effect of smoking on oogenesis, fertilization, and implantation. *Seminars in Reproductive Endocrinology, 7*(4): 291–304.

90. Sharara, F. I., Seifer, D. B., & Flaws, J. A. (1998). Environmental toxicants and female reproduction. *Fertility and Sterility, 70*(4): 613–622.

91. National Institutes of Health (2016). Primary ovarian insufficiency. MedlinePlus [online]. Available from https://medlineplus.gov/primaryovarianinsufficiency.html (accessed 15 November 2019).

92. Kalantaridou, S. N., & Nelson, L. M. (2000). Premature ovarian failure is not premature menopause. *Annals of the New York Academy of Sciences, 900*: 393–402.

93. National Institutes of Health (2016). Primary ovarian insufficiency. MedlinePlus [online]. Available from https://medlineplus.gov/primaryovarianinsufficiency.html (accessed 15 November 2019).

94. Torrialday, S., Kodaman, P., & Pal, L. (2017). Premature ovarian insufficiency—an update on recent advances in understanding and management. *F1000Research, 6*: 2069.

95. Van Blerkom, J. (2011). Mitochondrial function in the human oocyte and embryo and their role in developmental competence. *Mitochondrion*, *11*(5): 797–813.

96. Xu, Y., Nisenblat, V., Lu, C., Li, R., Qiao, J., Zhen, X., & Wang, S. (2018). Pretreatment with coenzyme Q10 improves ovarian response and embryo quality in low-prognosis young women with decreased ovarian reserve: a randomized controlled trial. *Reproductive Biology & Endocrinology*, *16*: 29.

97. Dennehy, C. E. (2006). The use of herbs and dietary supplements in gynecology: an evidence-based review. *Journal of Midwifery & Women's Health*, *51*: 402–409.

98. Gleicher, N., Weghofer, A., & Barad, D. H. (2010). Improvement in diminished ovarian reserve after dehydroepiandrosterone supplementation. *Reproductive BioMedicine Online*, *21*(3): 360–365.

99. Naredi, N., Sandeep, K., Jamwal, V. D. S., Nagraj, N., & Rai, S. (2015). Dehydroepiandrosterone: A panacea for the ageing ovary? *Medical Journal Armed Forces India*, *71*(3): 274–277.

100. Xu, L., Hu, C., Liu, Q., & Li, Y. (2019). The effect of dehydroepiandrosterone (DHEA) supplementation on IVF or ICSI: a meta-analysis of randomized controlled trials. *Geburtshilfe und Frauenheilkunde*, *79*(7): 705–712.

101. Lopresti, A. L., Smith, S. J., Malvi, H., & Kodgule, R. (2019). An investigation into the stress-relieving and pharmacological actions of an ashwagandha (*Withania somnifera*) extract. A randomized, double-blind, placebo-controlled study. *Medicine (Baltimore)*, *98*(37): e17186.

102. Trickey, R. (2011). *Women, Hormones and the Menstrual Cycle*. Clifton Hill, Victoria, Australia: Melbourne Holistic Health Group.

103. Meissner, H. O., Kapczynski, W., Mscisz, A., & Lutomski, J. (2005). Use of gelatinized maca (Lepidium peruvianum) in early postmenopausal women. *International Journal of Biomedical Science*, *1*(1): 33–45.

104. Meissner, H. O., Reich-Bilinska, H., Mscisz, A., & Kedzia, B. (2006). Therapeutic effects of pre-gelatinized maca (Lepidium peruvianum chacon) used as a non-hormonal alternative to HRT in perimenopausal women—clinical pilot study. *International Journal of Biomedical Science*, *2*(2): 143–159.

105. Meissner, H. O., Reich-Bilinska, H., Mscisz, A., & Kedzia, B. (2006). Therapeutic effects of pre-gelatinized maca (Lepidium peruvianum chacon) used as a non-hormonal alternative to HRT in perimenopausal women—clinical pilot study. *International Journal of Biomedical Science*, *2*(2): 143–159.

106. Dini, A., Migliuolo, G., Rastrelli, L., Saturnino, P., & Schettino, O. (1994). Chemical composition of Lepidium meyenii. *Food Chemistry*, *49*(4): 347–349.

107. Meissner, H. O., Reich-Bilinska, H., Mscisz, A., & Kedzia, B. (2006). Therapeutic effects of pre-gelatinized maca (Lepidium peruvianum chacon) used as a non-hormonal alternative to HRT in perimenopausal women—clinical pilot study. *International Journal of Biomedical Science*, *2*(2): 143–159.

108. Dennehy, C. E. (2006). The use of herbs and dietary supplements in gynecology: an evidence-based review. *Journal of Midwifery & Women's Health*, *51*: 402–409.

109. Ye, Y. B., Tang, X. Y., Verbruggen, M. A., & Su, Y. X. (2006). Soy isoflavones attenuate bone loss in early postmenopausal Chinese women: a single-blind randomized, placebo-controlled trial. *European Journal of Nutrition*, *45*(6): 327–334.

110. Zhang, X., Shu, X.-O., Li, H., Yang, G., Li, Q., Gao, Y.-T., & Zheng, W. (2005). Prospective cohort study of soy food consumption and risk of bone fracture among postmenopausal women. *Archives of Internal Medicine, 165*(16): 1890–1895.
111. Brice-Ytsma, H., & McDermott, A. (2020). *Herbal Medicine in Treating Gynaecological Conditions.* London: Aeon.
112. Tabakova, P., Dimitrov, M., & Tashkov, B. (2012). Clinical studies on Tribulus terrestris protodioscin in women with endocrine infertility or menopausal syndrome. *Herbpharm USA* [online]. Available from: http://scicompdf.se/tiggarnot/tabakova-HerbPharmUSA.pdf (accessed 2 March 2020).
113. Dennehy, C. E. (2006). The use of herbs and dietary supplements in gynecology: an evidence-based review. *Journal of Midwifery & Women's Health, 51*: 402–409.
114. Trickey, R. (2011). *Women, Hormones and the Menstrual Cycle.* Clifton Hill, Victoria, Australia: Melbourne Holistic Health Group.
115. Morali, G., Polatti, F., Metelitsa, E. N., Mascarucci, P., Magnani, P., & Marre, G. B. (2006). Open, non-controlled clinical studies to assess the efficacy and safety of a medical device in form of gel topically and intravaginally used in postmenopausal women with genital atrophy. *Arzneimittelforschung, 56*(3): 230–238.
116. Rahte, S., Evans, R., Eugster, P. J., Marcourt, L., Wolfender, J. L., Kortenkamp, A., & Tasdemir, D. (2013). Salvia officinalis for hot flushes: towards determination of mechanism of activity and active principles. *Planta Medica, 79*(9):753–760.
117. Moss, L., Rouse, M., Wesnes, K. A., & Moss, M. (2010). Differential effects of the aromas of Salvia species on memory and mood. *Human Psychopharmacology, 25*(5): 388–396.
118. Dennehy, C. E. (2006). The use of herbs and dietary supplements in gynecology: an evidence-based review. *Journal of Midwifery & Women's Health, 51*: 402–409.
119. Grube, B., Walper, A., & Wheatley, D. (1999). St. John's wort extract: efficacy for menopausal symptoms of psychological origin. *Advances in Therapy, 16*(4): 177–186.
120. Yu, Q. (2018). Traditional Chinese medicine: perspectives on and treatment of menopausal symptoms. *Climacteric, 21*(2): 93–95.
121. Ayare, K., & Waghamare, N. (2017). Premature menopause: a critical review through ayurveda. *International Ayurvedic Medical Journal, 5*(4): 1291–1299.
122. Jefferys, A., Vanderpump, M., &Yasmin, E. (2015). Thyroid dysfunction and reproductive health. *Obstetrician & Gynaecologist, 17*: 39–45.
123. Heffner, L. J., & Schust, D. J. (2014). *The Reproductive System at a Glance.* Oxford: John Wiley & Sons.
124. Kaiser, U. B. (2011). Gonadotropin hormones. In: S. Melmed (Ed.), *The Pituitary* (3rd edn). London: Academic Press.
125. Jefferys, A., Vanderpump, M., & Yasmin, E. (2015). Thyroid dysfunction and reproductive health. *Obstetrician & Gynaecologist, 17*: 39–45.
126. Jefferys, A., Vanderpump, M., &Yasmin, E. (2015). Thyroid dysfunction and reproductive health. *Obstetrician & Gynaecologist, 17*: 39–45.
127. Corenblum, B. (2018). Hypopituitarism (Panhypopituitarism). *Medscape* [online]. Available from https://emedicine.medscape.com/article/122287-overview#a4 (accessed 14 November 2019).
128. Trickey, R. (2011). *Women, Hormones and the Menstrual Cycle.* Clifton Hill, Victoria, Australia: Melbourne Holistic Health Group.

129. Romm, A. (2016). *Botanical Medicine for Women's Health* (2nd edn). London: Churchill Livingstone.
130. Meissner, H. O., Kapczynski, W., Mscisz, A., & Lutomski, J. (2005). Use of gelatinized maca (Lepidium peruvianum) in early postmenopausal women. *International Journal of Biomedical Science*, 1(1): 33–45.
131. Trickey, R. (2011). *Women, Hormones and the Menstrual Cycle*. Clifton Hill, Victoria, Australia: Melbourne Holistic Health Group.
132. Greenstein, B., & Wood, D. F. (2006). *The Endocrine System at a Glance* (2nd edn). Oxford: Blackwell.
133. Holmes, P. (2007). *The Energetics of Western Herbs: A Materia Medica Integrating Western & Chinese Herbal Therapeutics, Volume 2* (4th edn). Santa Rosa, CA: Snow Lotus.
134. Bone, K., & Mills, S. (2013). *Principles and Practice of Phytotherapy: Modern Herbal Medicine*. London: Churchill Livingstone.
135. Aswathy Prakash, C., & Byresh, A. (2015). Understanding hypothyroidism in Ayurveda. *International Ayurvedic Medical Journal*, 3(11): 2349–2357.
136. Dharmananda, S. (1996). Treatments for thyroid diseases with Chinese herbal medicine [online]. Available from http://itmonline.org/arts/thyroid.htm (accessed 8 March 2020).
137. Hickman, R. A., & Gordon, C. (2011). Causes and management of infertility in systemic lupus erythematosus. *Rheumatology*, 50(9): 1551–1558.
138. Bălănescu, A., Donisan, T., & Bălănescu, D. (2017). An ever-challenging relationship: lupus and pregnancy. *Reumatologia*, 55(1): 29–37.
139. Hickman, R. A., & Gordon, C. (2011). Causes and management of infertility in systemic lupus erythematosus. *Rheumatology*, 50(9): 1551–1558.
140. Pasoto, S. G., Viana, V. S., Mendonca, B. B., Yoshinari, N. H., & Bonfa, E. (1999). Anti-corpus luteum antibody: a novel serological marker for ovarian dysfunction in systemic lupus erythematosus? *Journal of Rheumatology*, 26(5): 1087–1093.
141. Hickman, R. A., & Gordon, C. (2011). Causes and management of infertility in systemic lupus erythematosus. *Rheumatology*, 50(9): 1551–1558.
142. Biró, E., Szekanecz, Z., Czirják, L., Danko, K., Kiss, E., Szabo, N. A., Szucs, G., Zeher, M., Bodolay, E., Szegedi, G., & Bakó, G. (2006). Association of systemic and thyroid autoimmune diseases. *Clinical Rheumatology*, 25(2): 240–245.
143. Bălănescu, A., Donisan, T., & Bălănescu, D. (2017). An ever-challenging relationship: lupus and pregnancy. *Reumatologia*, 55(1): 29–37.
144. Hickman, R. A., & Gordon, C. (2011). Causes and management of infertility in systemic lupus erythematosus. *Rheumatology*, 50(9): 1551–1558.
145. Bălănescu, A., Donisan, T., & Bălănescu, D. (2017). An ever-challenging relationship: lupus and pregnancy. *Reumatologia*, 55(1): 29–37.
146. Bălănescu, A., Donisan, T., & Bălănescu, D. (2017). An ever-challenging relationship: lupus and pregnancy. *Reumatologia*, 55(1): 29–37.
147. Bermas, B. L., & Sammaritano, L. R. (2015). Fertility and pregnancy in rheumatoid arthritis and systemic lupus erythematosus. *Fertility Research and Practice*, 1(13) [online]. Available from https://doi.org/10.1186/s40738-015-0004-3 (accessed 29 October 2020).
148. Bălănescu, A., Donisan, T., & Bălănescu, D. (2017). An ever-challenging relationship: lupus and pregnancy. *Reumatologia*, 55(1): 29–37.

149. Bălănescu, A., Donisan, T., & Bălănescu, D. (2017). An ever-challenging relationship: lupus and pregnancy. *Reumatologia, 55*(1): 29–37.

150. Bone, K., & Mills, S. (2013). *Principles and Practice of Phytotherapy: Modern Herbal Medicine.* London: Churchill Livingstone.

151. Puolakka, J., Mäkäräinen, L., Viinikka, L., & Ylikorkala, O. (1985). Biochemical and clinical effects of treating the premenstrual syndrome with prostaglandin synthesis precursors. *Journal of Reproductive Medicine, 30*(3): 149–153.

152. Trickey, R. (2011). *Women, Hormones and the Menstrual Cycle.* Clifton Hill, Victoria, Australia: Melbourne Holistic Health Group.

153. Trickey, R. (2003). *Women, Hormones & the Menstrual Cycle.* Sydney, Australia: Allen & Unwin.

154. Gonlachanvit, S., Chen, Y. H., Hasler, W. L., Sun, W. M., & Owyang, C. (2003). Ginger reduces hyperglycemia-evoked gastric dysrhythmias in healthy humans: possible role of endogenous prostaglandins, *Journal of Pharmacology and Experimental Therapeutics, 307*(3): 1098–1103.

CHAPTER TWO

PCOS, hyperandrogenism, and insulin resistance

Polycystic ovary syndrome

Polycystic ovary syndrome (PCOS) is estimated to affect around 7% of women.[155] It is the most common endocrine disorder in women of reproductive age, and is the most common cause of failure to ovulate.[156] PCOS accounts for 75% of anovulatory infertility. Additionally, if or when pregnancies do occur, the first trimester miscarriage rate is as high as 30% to 50%.[157] Orthodox medicine has little to offer in terms of safe, effective treatments for women with PCOS; particularly those who wish to become pregnant. However, herbal medicine with dietary modification is an effective approach to treatment in many cases.

PCOS is a complex endocrine and metabolic disorder, which causes abnormal ovarian function, and *not* (as is commonly assumed) a syndrome caused by a disorder of the ovaries. It is associated with hormonal abnormalities (including hyperandrogenism), insulin resistance, metabolic syndrome, obesity, oligomenorrhoea or amenorrhoea, ovarian cysts, and failure to ovulate, resulting in infertility. The symptom picture can vary, and individual women may experience all or only some of these signs and symptoms.[158]

Genetic predisposition may contribute to the development of PCOS and it has also been proposed that exposure to high levels of testosterone during foetal development may increase the risk of PCOS in adulthood.[159]

Diagnosis of PCOS

PCOS is diagnosed on the basis of the presence of at least two criteria, including:

- Biochemical or clinical signs of androgen excess
- Ovulatory dysfunction, and/or
- Polycystic ovaries.[160]

Androgens are usually only slightly to moderately raised in PCOS (if at all),[161] but LH levels are often significantly higher than FSH levels,[162] and ovarian oestrogen and progesterone are usually low.[163]

Lower levels of FSH result in insufficient stimulation of ovarian follicles, which prevents normal follicular growth and maturation, and leads to low levels of oestrogen, and reduced endometrial growth. In females, cyclic LH secretion normally causes ovulation and transformation of the ovarian follicle into the corpus luteum, which in turn secretes progesterone. However, in women with PCOS, follicles may not mature, and ovulation may not occur. Anovulation and the consequent absence of a corpus luteum lead to low progesterone levels, and a compensatory rise in LH, giving the classic raised LH/FSH ratio.

The LH/FSH ratio

In women with secondary amenorrhoea, the LH/FSH ratio is a useful diagnostic tool. A raised LH/FSH ratio (where levels of LH are typically two to three times higher than the levels of FSH) suggests a diagnosis of PCOS, whereas a raised FSH/LH ratio (where FSH levels are much higher than LH levels) suggests a diagnosis of premature ovarian insufficiency. Low levels of both FSH and LH with low oestrogen and progesterone are seen in hypothalamic amenorrhoea.

Anti-Mullerian hormone

Anti-Mullerian hormone (AMH), which is usually low in premature ovarian insufficiency, may be abnormally high in PCOS due a higher number

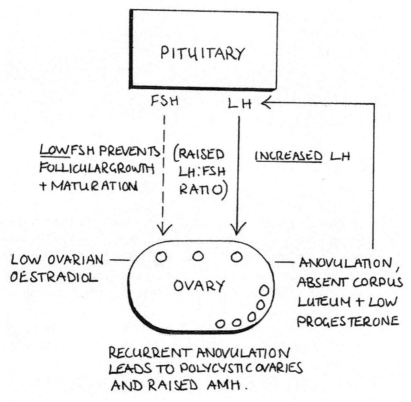

Figure 5: Anovulation in PCOS.

of immature follicles.[164] This does not suggest increased egg quality or improved fertility, but is simply the result of a large number of follicles that progress to the pre-antral or early antral stage, but fail to mature fully and instead form the characteristic pattern of cysts on the ovaries.

Sex hormone-binding globulin

Sex hormone-binding globulin (SHBG) is a glycoprotein that binds to oestradiol, testosterone, and dihydrotestosterone (DHT). SHBG transports these hormones in the blood as biologically inactive forms. Changes in SHBG levels can affect the amount of hormone that is available to be used by the body's tissues. Because of the higher affinity of SHBG for DHT and testosterone, compared to oestrogen, SHBG also has effects on the balance between bioavailable androgens and oestrogens.

Where measurements are for "total" rather than "free" levels of androgens and other hormones, it is essential to measure SHBG. A high SHBG level means that less free hormones are available to the tissues; while a low SHBG level means that more of the total hormone is bioavailable and not bound to SHBG.

Decreased SHBG in women may be associated with symptoms of high androgens (such as male pattern baldness, hirsutism, and acne). SHBG is reduced by low levels of oestrogen, and by high levels of testosterone. Therefore low levels of oestrogen, and higher levels of androgens, which are typical in PCOS, reduce SHBG, and further increase the activity of androgens. This represents one of several self-perpetuating cycles, which are common in PCOS.

Useful blood tests for diagnosis of PCOS include LH, FSH, oestradiol, progesterone, total androgens, free testosterone, SHBG, AMH, lipid profile and HBA1c. Blood values of various hormones may be normal or slightly elevated in PCOS, while grossly elevated hormone levels generally suggest a different disorder. Clinical examinations should include assessment of body mass index (BMI), and waist to hip ratio, which ideally should be <0.8, as increased abdominal fat is associated with metabolic syndrome. Ultrasonography is used to detect polycystic ovaries.

Use of oral contraceptives may mask many of the biochemical and clinical signs of PCOS.[165] In some women, PCOS may be masked by the coexistence of functional hypothalamic amenorrhoea. (Hypothalamic amenorrhoea is associated with absent or deficient hypothalamic secretion of GnRH by the hypothalamus, which essentially "shuts down" the reproductive hormone axis, and results in low FSH.[166] It may be caused by excessive weight loss, exercise, physical illness, or emotional stress,[167] or it may also follow use of oral contraceptives).[168] In such cases, symptoms consistent with PCOS only appear when hypothalamic activity recovers.[169]

Polycystic ovaries

The term "polycystic ovaries" (PCO) refers to the appearance of numerous small cysts on the ovaries, whereas the term "PCOS" refers to a *syndrome*, which is characterised by various signs and symptoms such as hormonal abnormalities, menstrual cycle disturbance, hyperandrogenism, insulin resistance, and obesity.[170]

In cases of polycystic ovaries, folliculogenesis is arrested at 5–10 mm. Failure to ovulate, which may be due to PCOS or another cause (such as hypothalamic amenorrhoea), means that the follicles do not rupture, and instead give rise to numerous fluid filled cysts on the surface of the ovary. Women with PCOS do not always have PCO, and conversely, a finding of PCO does not necessarily mean a woman has PCOS; in fact 20% of women with normal ovulatory cycles are found to have PCO on ultrasound, due to occasional anovulatory cycles.[171]

Hyperandrogenism

PCOS is often (though not always) associated with elevated ovarian and adrenal androgens. Less commonly, hyperandrogenism in women may be due to hyperthecosis, hyperinsulinaemia, Cushing's syndrome, adrenal hyperplasia, or ovarian/adrenal tumours. This gives rise to symptoms such as acne, androgenic alopecia, and hirsutism. Hirsutism is the growth of coarse hair in a male pattern, particularly on the upper lip, chin, chest, upper abdomen, and back, and is distinguished from hypertrichosis, which involves a more uniform distribution of fine hair. However, clinical signs of androgen excess are usually mild, and virilisation (clitoromegaly, deep voice, increased musculature) is not a feature of PCOS.[172]

Elevated insulin directly triggers androgen production by the ovarian theca cells; stimulates LH secretion; and increases adrenal androgen production, due to increased activity of 11ß-hydroxysteroid dehydrogenase (11ß-OHSD), which increases cortisol clearance, and causes a compensatory rise in ACTH, which in turn leads to increased adrenal androgen production.[173]

Genetic abnormalities of the hypothalamus or pituitary gland may be responsible for inappropriate secretion of GnRH and/or LH, leading to an increase in ovarian and adrenal androgen secretion.[174] There is also reduced activity of aromatase (the enzyme which catalyses the conversion of androgens to oestrogen) in ovarian granulosa cells, leading to poor conversion of androgens to oestrogen. The androgens inhibit development of follicles, resulting in anovulation, absence of the corpus luteum, and consequent low progesterone; which in turn leads to elevated LH through lack of negative feedback. The elevated LH further stimulates the ovarian theca cells, producing more ovarian androgens.

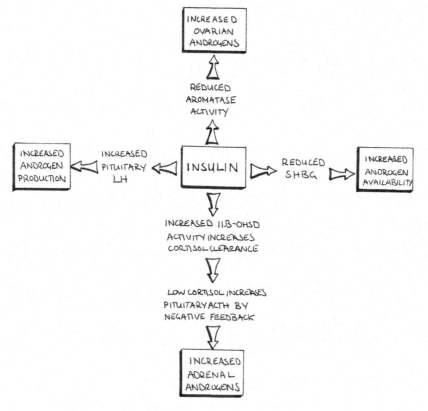

Figure 6: The role of insulin in hyperandrogenism.

Acyclic oestrogens

Anovulation in PCOS leads to a loss of the cyclic variation in oestradiol levels. Oestrone on the other hand is derived from aromatisation of androgens, primarily in adipose tissue. Women with PCOS frequently have high levels of androgen available for conversion to oestrone, and excess stores of adipose tissue where conversion can take place. Higher levels of acyclic oestrone combined with reduced endometrial shedding can lead to increased risk of endometrial hyperplasia and cancer.

Acyclic oestrogens may also cause reduced levels of FSH due to reduced negative feedback. Low FSH reduces the aromatisation of androgens in the ovarian granulosa cells, contributing further to hyperandrogenism.

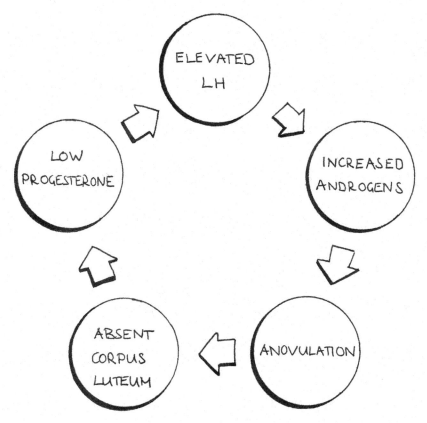

Figure 7: The self-perpetuating cycle of androgen excess.

Insulin resistance

Up to 75% of women with PCOS have some degree of insulin resistance, which is associated with acanthosis nigrans (hyperpigmentation of the axillae, the back of the neck, and/or the breast folds);[175] increased central fat distribution;[176] and elevated fasting glucose, cholesterol, and triglycerides.[177] Insulin resistance triggers a compensatory rise in insulin secretion; this in turn increases storage of fat, leading to obesity, which in turn further increases insulin resistance.[178] This represents another self-perpetuating cycle in cases of PCOS.

Insulin resistance may be caused by various factors that affect the expression of insulin receptors, including a family history of type 2

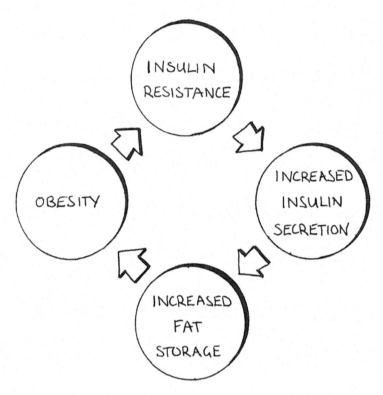

Figure 8: Insulin resistance.

diabetes, smoking, use of certain drugs (such as corticosteroids, and oestrogen-containing contraceptives), and obesity (especially central obesity).[179] Insulin resistance is associated with menstrual cycle disturbance and infertility. PCOS sufferers with insulin resistance have more menstrual cycle disturbance and reduced fertility when compared to those who are insulin sensitive.[180]

As previously described, elevated insulin triggers hyperandrogenism by directly inducing ovarian androgen production, stimulating LH secretion, and increasing adrenal androgen production. The increased adrenal androgen production is the result of elevated insulin causing increased activity of 11ß-hydroxysteroid dehydrogenase (11ß-OHSD), which increases cortisol clearance, with a compensatory rise in ACTH (resulting in increased adrenal androgens).[181] Insulin resistance also reduces SHBG,[182] which reduces the amount of androgens that are bound (and therefore inactivated) by SHBG, and thereby leads to increased androgen activity.

Insulin resistance and PCOS lead to an increased risk of type 2 diabetes, and 40% of women with PCOS experience impaired glucose tolerance or diabetes by the age of forty.[183] Increased risk of cardiovascular disease can also be caused by impaired glucose metabolism: insulin resistance is associated with elevated HBA1c (glycated Hb above 42 mmol/mol), elevated triglycerides, and low HDL cholesterol.[184]

Orthodox treatment

Orthodox treatment of PCOS includes the following drugs:[185]

- Combined oral contraceptives (which reduce androgens by decreasing gonadotropins, regulate menstruation, and decrease the risk of endometrial hyperplasia)
- Anti-androgens (such as spironolactone: an aldosterone antagonist, which also blocks testosterone receptors)
- Insulin-sensitising drugs (such as Metformin) to reduce insulin resistance
- Clomiphene citrate (to improve ovulation and fertility).

Holistic treatment

Dietary modification and increased exercise are essential to reduce insulin resistance and obesity, and to help reduce cardiovascular risk factors.[186] Consuming only low glycaemic load (low GL) carbohydrates, and reducing overall intake of carbohydrates, helps to increase the sensitivity of insulin receptors, improves levels of SHBG (which binds to and inactivates androgens), promotes weight loss, and reduces cardiovascular risk factors.

Improved insulin sensitivity is associated with improved ovulatory function and fertility in women with polycystic ovary syndrome (PCOS).[187] Fertility increases with diets that include a lower intake of high glycaemic index foods, and a higher intake of high-fibre, low-glycaemic index carbohydrates.[188]

Insulin resistance may also be improved by using herbs such as *Cinnamonum zeylonicum* (cinnamon), *Eleutherococcus senticosus* (Siberian ginseng), *Trigonella foenum-graecum* (fenugreek), and/or *Galega officinalis* (goat's rue).[189] Magnesium deficiency predisposes to insulin resistance and increased cardiovascular risk factors, and individuals with PCOS have significantly reduced serum magnesium levels.[190] Therefore supplemental magnesium is recommended for those with PCOS.

Androgen production can be reduced with herbs such as *Paeonia lactiflora* (white paeony), and *Glycyrrhiza glabra* (liquorice), which increase aromatisation of androgens, and reduce 11ß-OHSD respectively.[191] Both of these herbs also reduce levels of 5-alpha reductase (the enzyme which converts testosterone to the more potent dihydrotestosterone),[192] and they both have a strong reputation for the treatment of PCOS when used in combination.

Serenoa repens (saw palmetto), *Ganoderma lucidum* (reishi mushroom), and *Camellia sinensis* (green tea), all reduce 5-alpha reductase, and *Mentha spicata* (spearmint) has also been shown to reduce free testosterone and reduce symptoms of hyperandrogenism in women with PCOS, without reducing DHEA.[193] *Humulus lupulus* (hops) and *Cimicifuga racemosa* (black cohosh) also reduce both LH and androgens.[194]

Tribulus terrestris (puncture vine), *Asparagus racemosus* (shatavari), *Trigonella foenum graecum* (fenugreek), or other steroidal saponin-containing herbs may be given in the early follicular phase (or for the first 10 days of the month if there is associated amenorrhoea). Phytoestrogens (such as dietary beans and pulses) reduce androgens, improve lipid metabolism, and competitively inhibit oestrone at target tissues.

Inositol supplementation improves metabolic and endocrine profiles in women with PCOS. It reduces leptin concentration, plasma triglycerides, and LDL cholesterol, and improves insulin sensitivity. It also reduces prolactin and androgen levels and normalises the LH:FSH ratio, increasing frequency of spontaneous ovulation and enhancing oocyte quality, thereby improving fertility in women with PCOS. Most studies used 1–4 g myo-inositol per day (or myo-inositol in combination with D-chiro-inositol in a ratio of at least 40:1). The same results have not been demonstrated with D-chiro-inositol alone.[195]

Other recommended supplements include omega-3 essential fatty acids (at least 3 g a day to help reduce visceral fat, serum triglycerides, and cardiovascular risk), and biotin (3 g), magnesium (400 mg), and GTF chromium (200 mcg), to improve insulin resistance.[196]

Energetics

From an "energetic" perspective, PCOS is often associated with excess Kapha, which is characterised by excess mucus and a swollen tongue with white coating.[197] Pungent, astringent, and bitter herbs (such as *Cinnamonum zeylonicum*, *Camellia sinensis*, and *Taraxacum officinale* respectively) help to reduce Kapha. Pungent, astringent, and bitter foods also reduce Kapha. It is important to avoid sweet, sour, salty, oily, and damp foods such as dairy products, as they increase Kapha.[198] It is also essential to avoid overeating and to take regular exercise.

In traditional Chinese medicine (TCM), PCOS is often associated with Kidney Yang Deficiency and Dampness,[199] which also benefit from pungent and astringent foods, and from avoiding cold, damp foods. For more information about "energetic" approaches to understanding and treating infertility, see Chapter 6.

Natural treatment of PCOS	
Diet and lifestyle changes	• Measures to reduce BMI if overweight • Avoid high GL carbohydrates and reduce overall carbohydrate intake • Eat high fibre, low GI foods • Increase intake of phytoestrogens • Increase exercise • Supplement omega-3 EFAs (3 g per day)
Improve insulin sensitivity	• *Cinnamonum zeylonicum, Eleutherococcus senticosus, Trigonella foenum-graecum, Galega officinalis* • Inositol (2 g), magnesium (400 mg), GTF chromium (200 mcg), biotin (3 g)
Reduce LH and androgens	• *Humulus lupulus, Cimicifuga racemosa, Mentha spicata*
Increase aromatisation	• *Paeonia lactiflora*
Reduce 11ß-OHSD	• *Glycyrrhiza glabra*
Reduce 5-alpha reductase	• *Paeonia lactiflora, Glycyrrhiza glabra, Serenoa repens, Ganoderma lucidum*, green tea (*Camellia sinensis*)
Reduce acyclic oestrogens	• Vitamin B complex & magnesium supplements • Reduce xenoestrogens • Increase intake of phytoestrogens • Improve oestrogen clearance (see Chapter 4)

Being overweight/underweight

Obesity

Over 28% of obese women suffer from PCOS, compared to less than 6% of women with normal body mass index (BMI).[200] Increasing levels of obesity among the population are likely to increase the prevalence of PCOS and associated problems in the future. Higher levels of LH and androgens, accompanied by anovulatory cycles, are normal during puberty, and it is thought that excessive weight gain during puberty may prolong these features, leading to development of PCOS.[201]

Obese women with PCOS, particularly those with a BMI greater than 30, suffer worse symptoms of PCOS than those with normal BMI. Obesity contributes to metabolic and reproductive abnormalities by reducing sex hormone-binding globulin (thereby increasing availability of androgens), and increasing insulin resistance; and independently further increases the risk of diabetes and cardiovascular disease.[202]

Obesity is also associated with increased production of leptin, and leptin resistance, which has an adverse effect on gonadotropin release and follicle development.[203]

Abdominal visceral fat is more likely to be associated with metabolic and reproductive problems than subcutaneous fat.[204] Women with PCOS who have a normal BMI are more likely to have increased central fat distribution (reduced waist to hip ratio) than those without PCOS.[205] In women with PCOS who are overweight, as little as 5% weight reduction reduces insulin resistance and increases ovulation.[206] In fact, it is theorised that women with PCOS have adapted to remain fertile during food shortages, when others experience reduced fertility.[207]

Insufficient body fat

Fat cells produce oestrogen,[208] via aromatisation of ovarian and adrenal androgens. Excess body fat therefore causes production of excess oestrogen, which reduces fertility. Likewise, insufficient fat stores result in suboptimal oestrogen levels. Excessive weight loss may also lead to hypothalamic amenorrhoea as previously described. Therefore it is advisable for women who wish to conceive to try to maintain an optimal level of body fat, by eating a healthy, balanced diet and taking adequate (but not excessive) exercise.

Notes

155. Grant, P., & Ramasamy, S. (2012). An update on plant derived anti-androgens. *International Journal of Endocrinology & Metabolism, 10*(2): 497–502.
156. Trickey, R. (2011). *Women, Hormones and the Menstrual Cycle.* Clifton Hill, Victoria, Australia: Melbourne Holistic Health Group.
157. Homburg, R., Armar, N. A., Eshel, A., Adams, J., & Jacobs, H. S. (1988). Influence of serum luteinising hormone concentrations on ovulation, conception, and early pregnancy loss in polycystic ovary syndrome. *British Medical Journal, 297*(6655): 1024–1026.
158. Trickey, R. (2011). *Women, Hormones and the Menstrual Cycle.* Clifton Hill, Victoria, Australia: Melbourne Holistic Health Group.
159. Dumesic, D. A., Abbot, D. H., & Padmanhaban, V. (2007). Polycystic ovary syndrome and its developmental origins. *Endocrine & Metabolic Disorders, 8*(2): 127–141.
160. Legro, R. S., Arslanian, S. A., Ehrmann, D. A., Hoeger, K. M., Murad, M. H., Pasquali, R., & Welt, C. K. (2013). Diagnosis and treatment of polycystic ovary syndrome: an Endocrine Society clinical practice guideline. *Journal of Clinical Endocrinology & Metabolism, 98*(12): 4565–4592.
161. Legro, R. S., Arslanian, S. A., Ehrmann, D. A., Hoeger, K. M., Murad, M. H., Pasquali, R., & Welt, C. K. (2013). Diagnosis and treatment of polycystic ovary syndrome: an Endocrine Society clinical practice guideline. *Journal of Clinical Endocrinology and Metabolism, 98*(12): 4565–4592.
162. Bone, K., & Mills, S. (2013). *Principles and Practice of Phytotherapy: Modern Herbal Medicine* (2nd edn). London: Churchill Livingstone.
163. Trickey, R. (2011). *Women, Hormones and the Menstrual Cycle.* Clifton Hill, Victoria, Australia: Melbourne Holistic Health Group.
164. Broer, S. L., Broekman, F. J. M., Laven, J. S. E., & Fauser, B. C. J. M. (2014). Anti-Mullerian hormone: ovarian reserve testing and its potential clinical implications. *Human Reproduction Update, 20*(5): 688–701.
165. Sheehan, M. T. (2004). Polycystic ovarian syndrome: diagnosis and management. *Clinical Medicine & Research, 2*(1): 13–27.
166. Leyendecker, G., Wildt, L., & Hansmann, M. (1983). Induction of ovulation with chronic intermittent (pulsatile) administration of Gn-RH in women with hypothalamic amenorrhoea. *Journal of Reproduction & Fertility, 69*: 397–409.
167. De Souza, M. J., & Toombs, R. J. (2010). Amenorrhea. In: N. F. Santoro & G. Neal-Perry (Eds.), *Amenorrhea: A Case-Based, Clinical Guide* (pp. 101–125). Totowa, NJ: Humana.
168. Wright, K. P., & Johnson, J. V. (2008). Evaluation of extended and continuous use oral contraceptives. *Therapeutics and Clinical Risk Management, 4*(5): 905–911.
169. Wang, J. G., & Lobo, R. A. (2008). The complex relationship between hypothalamic amenorrhoea and polycystic ovary syndrome. *Journal of Clinical Endocrinology and Metabolism, 93*(4): 1394–1397.
170. Trickey, R. (2011). *Women, Hormones and the Menstrual Cycle.* Clifton Hill, Victoria, Australia: Melbourne Holistic Health Group.

171. Clayton, R. N., Ogden, V., Hodgkinson, J., Worswick, L., Rodin, D. A., Dyer, S., & Meade, T. W.s (1992). How common are polycystic ovaries in normal women, and what is their significance for the fertility of the population? *Clinical Endocrinology*, 37(2): 127–134.

172. Sheehan, M. T. (2004). Polycystic ovarian syndrome: diagnosis and management. *Clinical Medicine & Research*, 2(1): 13–27.

173. Trickey, R. (2011). *Women, Hormones and the Menstrual Cycle*. Clifton Hill, Victoria, Australia: Melbourne Holistic Health Group.

174. Barontini, M., Garcia-Rudaz, M. C., & Veldhuis, J. D. (2001). Mechanisms of hypo-thalamic-pituitary-gonadal disruption in polycystic ovarian syndrome. *Archives of Medical Research*, 32(6): 544–552.

175. Trickey, R. (2011). *Women, Hormones and the Menstrual Cycle*. Clifton Hill, Victoria, Australia: Melbourne Holistic Health Group.

176. Kirchengast, S., & Huber, J. (2001). Body composition characteristics and body fat distribution in lean women with polycystic ovary syndrome. *Human Reproduction*, 16(6): 1255–1260.

177. Sheehan, M. T. (2004). Polycystic varian syndrome: diagnosis and management. *Clinical Medicine & Research*, 2(1): 13–27.

178. Trickey, R. (2011). *Women, Hormones and the Menstrual Cycle*. Clifton Hill, Victoria, Australia: Melbourne Holistic Health Group.

179. Venkatesan, A. M., Dunaif, A., & Corbould, A. (2001). Insulin resistance in polycystic ovary syndrome: progress and paradoxes. *Recent Progress in Hormone Research, 56*: 295–308.

180. Trickey, R. (2011). *Women, Hormones and the Menstrual Cycle*. Clifton Hill, Victoria, Australia: Melbourne Holistic Health Group.

181. Trickey, R. (2011). *Women, Hormones and the Menstrual Cycle*. Clifton Hill, Victoria, Australia: Melbourne Holistic Health Group.

182. Sheehan, M. T. (2004). Polycystic ovarian syndrome: diagnosis and management. *Clinical Medicine & Research*, 2(1): 13–27.

183. Kidson, W. (1998). Polycystic ovary syndrome: a new direction in treatment. *Medical Journal of Australia, 169*(10): 537–540.

184. Trickey, R. (2011). *Women, Hormones and the Menstrual Cycle*. Clifton Hill, Victoria, Australia: Melbourne Holistic Health Group.

185. Sheehan, M. T. (2004). Polycystic ovarian syndrome: diagnosis and management. *Clinical Medicine & Research*, 2(1): 13 –27.

186. Norman, R. J., Davies, M. J., Lord, J., & Moran, L. J. (2002). The role of lifestyle modi-fication in polycystic ovary syndrome. *Trends in Endocrinology & Metabolism, 13*(6): 251–257.

187. Chavarro, J. E., Rich-Edwards, J. W., Rosner, B. A., & Willett, W. C. (2009). A prospec-tive study of dietary carbohydrate quantity and quality in relation to risk of ovula-tory infertility. *European Journal of Clinical Nutrition, 63*: 78–86.

188. Chavarro, J. E., Rich-Edwards, J. W., Rosner, B. A., & Willett, W. C. (2007). Diet and Lifestyle in the Prevention of Ovulatory Disorder Infertility. *Obstetrics & Gynecology, 110*(5): 1050–1058.

189. Trickey, R. (2011). *Women, Hormones and the Menstrual Cycle*. Clifton Hill, Victoria, Australia: Melbourne Holistic Health Group.

190. Muneyyirci-Delale, O., Nacharaju, V. L., Dalloul, M., Jalou, S., Rahman, M., Altura, B. M., & Altura, B. T. (2001). Divalent cations in women with PCOS: implications for cardiovascular disease. *Gynecologic Endocrinology, 15*(3): 198–201.

191. Trickey, R. (2011). *Women, Hormones and the Menstrual Cycle.* Clifton Hill, Victoria, Australia: Melbourne Holistic Health Group.

192. Grant, P., & Ramasamy, S. (2012). An update on plant derived anti-androgens. *International Journal of Endocrinology & Metabolism, 10*(2): 497–502.

193. Grant, P., & Ramasamy, S. (2012). An update on plant derived anti-androgens. *International Journal of Endocrinology & Metabolism, 10*(2): 497–502.

194. Trickey, R. (2011). *Women, Hormones and the Menstrual Cycle.* Clifton Hill, Victoria, Australia: Melbourne Holistic Health Group.

195. Unfer, V., Nestler, J. E., Kamenov, Z. A., & Faccinetti, F. (2016). Effects of inositol(s) in women with PCOS: a systematic review of randomized controlled trials. *International Journal of Endocrinology,* 1849162 [online]. Available from https://ncbi.nlm.nih.gov/pmc/articles/PMC5097808/ (accessed 22 December 2019).

196. Trickey, R. (2011). *Women, Hormones and the Menstrual Cycle.* Clifton Hill, Victoria, Australia: Melbourne Holistic Health Group.

197. Lad, V. D. (2006). *Textbook of Ayurveda: A Complete Guide to Clinical Assessment. Volume 2.* Albuquerque, NM: Ayurvedic Press.

198. Tillotson, A. K. (2001). *The One Earth Herbal Sourcebook.* New York: Kensington.

199. Maciocia, G. (2004). *Diagnosis in Chinese Medicine: A Comprehensive Guide.* London: Elsevier.

200. Alvarez-Blasco, F., Botella-Carretero, J. I., San Millan, J. L., & Escobar-Morreale, H. F. (2006). Prevalence and characteristics of the polycystic ovary syndrome in overweight and obese women. *Archives of Internal Medicine, 166*(19): 2081–2086.

201. Pasquali, R., & Gambineri, A. (2006). Polycystic ovary syndrome: a multifaceted disease from adolescence to old age. *Annals of the New York Academy of Sciences, 1092:* 158–174.

202. Trickey, R. (2011). *Women, Hormones and the Menstrual Cycle.* Clifton Hill, Victoria, Australia: Melbourne Holistic Health Group.

203. Trickey, R. (2011). *Women, Hormones and the Menstrual Cycle.* Clifton Hill, Victoria, Australia: Melbourne Holistic Health Group.

204. Zaadstra, B. M., Seidell, J. C., Van Noord, P. A., Te Velde, E. R., Habbema, J. D., Vrieswijk, B., & Karbaart, J. (1993). Fat and female fecundity: Prospective study of effect of body fat distribution on conception rates. *British Medical Journal, 306*(6876): 484–487.

205. Kirchengast, S., & Huber, J. (2001). Body composition characteristics and body fat distribution in lean women with polycystic ovary syndrome. *Human Reproduction, 16*(6): 1255–1260.

206. Franks, S., Kiddy, D., Sharpe, P., Singh, A., Reed, M., Seppala, M., Koistinen, R., & Hamilton-Fairley, D. (1991). Obesity and polycystic ovary syndrome. *Annals of the New York Academy of Sciences, 626:* 201–206.

207. Azziz, R., Dumesic, D. A., & Goodarzi, M. O. (2011). Polycystic ovary syndrome: An ancient disorder? *Fertility and Sterility, 95*(5): 1544–1548.

208. Nelson L. R., & Bulun S. E. (2001). Estrogen production and action. *Journal of the American Academy of Dermatology, 45*(3 Suppl): S116–S124.

CHAPTER THREE

Organic infertility: structural issues

S tructural infertility is due to an abnormality of the reproductive organs, which prevents conception from occurring.[209] Unlike functional problems (which are discussed in Chapter 4), structural problems can usually be readily diagnosed with the help of investigations such as blood tests, ultrasound scans, and laparoscopy.

Fallopian tube damage or blockage

Pelvic inflammatory disease

Pelvic inflammatory disease (PID) most frequently affects young women under the age of twenty-five.[210] It is most commonly caused by sexually transmitted infection, such as gonorrhoea or chlamydia. However, it may also be the result of other infections affecting the vagina or cervix, which spread to the endometrium, fallopian tubes, and other pelvic structures.

The risk of developing PID is increased by anything that involves opening of the cervix, such as childbirth or miscarriage; medical procedures such as endometrial biopsy or dilation and curettage (D&C); and insertion of an intrauterine device (IUD).[211] Symptoms of PID include pelvic pain, fever, vaginal discharge, irregular vaginal bleeding, and dyspareunia. However, symptoms may be very minor or absent in some cases.[212] Pelvic inflammatory disease causes inflammation of the fallopian tubes (salpingitis), and subsequent tubal damage or occlusion. Infertility closely correlates with the extent of tubal damage, and increases dramatically with recurrent episodes of PID.[213]

Tubal blockages may prevent the oocyte from reaching sperm, leading to infertility. In the case of partial tubal blockage, sperm may reach the oocyte, but the fertilised egg may not be able to leave the tube, resulting in an ectopic or tubal pregnancy. Ectopic pregnancy may cause rupture of the fallopian tube and is a life threatening medical emergency. In some cases ectopic pregnancy may be treated with methotrexate to prevent growth of the ectopic mass, or surgical removal of the pregnancy and repair of the affected tube by laparotomy. However, in cases where there is extensive damage to the fallopian tube, it may be necessary to remove it, which further impacts fertility.[214]

Pelvic inflammatory disease requires prompt orthodox treatment with antibiotics to help prevent long-term complications.[215] However, herbal therapies such as castor oil packs, herbal anti-inflammatories and immune stimulants, and anti-inflammatory nutrients, may be used alongside orthodox treatment to help to reduce inflammation and prevent adhesions.

Immune enhancing and antimicrobial herbs such as *Echinacea angustifolia* (purple coneflower), *Astragalus membranaceus* (huang qi), *Andrographis paniculata* (kalamegha), and *Hydrastis canadensis* (goldenseal) are useful adjuncts in cases of chronic infection. Topical treatment to the vagina using antimicrobial and anti-inflammatory herbs also provides a route for treating PID.[216]

Herbal anti-inflammatories include *Zingiber officinalis* (ginger) and *Curcuma longa* (turmeric),[217] while *Centella asiatica* (gotu kola) and *Salvia miltorrhiza* (Dan Shen) are useful for reducing the formation of adhesions.[218] Vitamin E supplementation can help to both reduce inflammation and prevent adhesions.[219]

There are numerous herbs which can help to reduce pelvic pain, not only in cases of pelvic inflammatory disease, but also in other painful, spasmodic, or inflammatory conditions of the reproductive organs and tissues, such as endometriosis, adenomyosis, and vaginismus. They include *Anemone pulsatilla* (pasque flower), *Cimicifuga racemosa* (black cohosh), *Corydalis yanhuoso* (yan huo so), *Eschscholzia californica*

(California poppy), *Piscidia erythrina* (Jamaican dogwood), *Viburnum opulus* (cramp bark), *Viburnum prunifolium* (black haw), and *Zingiber officinale* (ginger).[220,221] In addition, *Cannabis indica* (CBD) possesses significant uterine antispasmodic and analgesic effects,[222] and *Gelsemium sempervirens* (yellow jasmine) is also very effective for pelvic pain.[223]

Energetics

In traditional Chinese medicine (TCM), pelvic inflammatory disease is due to the invasion of Damp Heat. In Ayurveda it is most commonly associated with excess Pitta (inflammation) and Vata (spasm and pain). For more information about "energetic" approaches to understanding and treating infertility, see Chapter 6.

Endometriosis

Endometriosis affects up to 35% of women with infertility,[224] and is the most common cause of chronic pelvic pain in women.[225] Endometrial tissue develops outside the uterus in response to stimulation from oestrogen, affecting the function of the ovaries, uterus, and/or fallopian tubes, and compromising fertility.[226] Endometrial tissue may implant into any of the pelvic peritoneal surfaces, including the rectovaginal space, and ovaries,[227] or into the fallopian tubes, vagina, bladder, or bowel. Implants on the peritoneal surfaces eventually develop into scar tissue and may form adhesions, which reduce motility of the pelvic organs, causing pain.[228]

Endometriosis of the ovary forms cysts known as endometriomas, endometrial cysts, or "chocolate cysts", which are filled with blood, and may rupture and shed their contents into the peritoneal cavity, causing inflammation and pain. Endometriosis of the bladder or bowel may lead to scarring which causes pain and difficulty with urination or defecation.[229]

The endometrial tissue is continually influenced by the cyclical variation of hormones. During the follicular phase, increasing levels of oestrogen cause normal proliferation of the endometrium, but in women with endometriosis, they also stimulate the growth of endometrial tissue located outside the uterus. When menstruation begins, the normal endometrium is shed vaginally, while misplaced endometrial tissue is shed into the pelvic cavity, leading to inflammation and pain.[230]

High levels of aromatase activity (the enzyme which catalyses the conversion of androgens to oestrogen) have been found in the endometrial tissue of women with endometriosis. This results in increased local oestrogen production. Increased oestrogen induces the formation of inflammatory prostaglandins such as PGE2, which mediates pain and inflammation,[231] provokes uterine muscle spasm, and increases blood loss by dilating blood vessels.[232] PGE2 in turn is a potent stimulant of aromatase, which generates more oestrogen.[233]

Endometriosis is also associated with increased levels of other inflammatory markers, such as interleukin-1 (IL-1), interleukin-6 (IL-6), tissue necrosis factor-alpha (TNF-α), and cyclooxygenase-2 (COX-2),[234] as well as transcription factor nuclear factor-κB (NF-κB),[235] which promote cell proliferation, inflammation, and pain.

Women with endometriosis also have an increased number of oestrogen receptors, and fewer progesterone receptors in the endometrial tissue. In healthy endometrial tissue, progesterone favours the conversion of biologically potent oestradiol to the less potent oestrone, by the enzyme 17β-hydroxysteroid dehydrogenase. The lack of progesterone receptors in women with endometriosis therefore further contributes to high oestradiol activity in endometriosis, as well as increasing the risk of embryo implantation failure.

The cell-mediated immune response is responsible for clearing menstrual debris from the peritoneal cavity and preventing implantation of endometrial cells. An abnormal immune response in women with endometriosis leads to residual endometrial cells in the peritoneal cavity, which may implant and form endometriosis.[236]

In the early stages of endometriosis, macrophages (a type of leucocyte) proliferate in the peritoneal fluid in order to remove endometrial debris shed into the peritoneal cavity. However, these cells may also reduce sperm motility, engulf and destroy sperm, and prevent fertilisation, thereby contributing to infertility.[237] They also lead to the formation of adhesions.[238] Macrophages produce various substances that act as growth factors for the implantation and maintenance of endometrial tissue. They also produce PGE2, which mediates pain and inflammation, provokes uterine muscle spasm, and increases blood loss by dilating blood vessels.[239]

Meanwhile the activity of T-lymphocytes and natural killer cells (which are important in the destruction of abnormal cells) is decreased in endometriosis. Low natural killer cell activity is associated with increased levels of oestradiol, and results in persistence of misplaced endometrial tissue.[240]

Many of the processes associated with endometriosis, as detailed above, are the result of inherited genetic abnormalities. However, other factors, such as lack of exercise, use of an intrauterine contraceptive device (IUCD), and caffeine and alcohol consumption can also increase the risk of developing endometriosis.[241] Endometriosis has additionally been linked to exposure to environmental pollutants, particularly dioxin-like compounds, which have an immunosuppressive effect. Dioxin-like compounds can also increase oestrogenic activity, both by direct interaction with oestrogen receptors, and by increasing the activity of aromatase, the enzyme which catalyses the conversion of androgens to oestrogen.[242]

Laparoscopy is the only way to definitively diagnose endometriosis. Symptoms of endometriosis overlap with other diseases, particularly irritable bowel syndrome (IBS) and pelvic inflammatory disease (PID). Symptoms of endometriosis include chronic pelvic pain, severe dysmenorrhoea, dyspareunia, cyclical bowel pain or irregularity, urinary symptoms, and infertility. Symptoms are usually cyclical but can occur at any time throughout the month. They do not always correlate with the severity of the disease and some women with endometriosis are asymptomatic.[243]

Adenomyosis

Adenomyosis is a similar condition to endometriosis, but in adenomyosis, the endometrial cells grow into the uterine muscle, rather than outside the uterus. Adenomyosis may occur due to damage to the uterus, as a result of uterine inflammation or trauma (such as uterine surgery). As in endometriosis, the misplaced endometrial cells proliferate, and are shed in response to cyclical hormone changes, but in this case they proliferate and are shed within the uterine muscle. This leads to inflammation of the uterus, pressure on adjacent structures (such as the bladder and bowel), and similar symptoms to endometriosis. However, adenomyosis is less likely to cause fallopian tube damage or blockage, and therefore less likely to cause infertility, compared to endometriosis. The pathophysiology and treatment of adenomyosis is very similar to that of endometriosis.

Treatment of endometriosis

Orthodox treatment for endometriosis (and adenomyosis) includes gonadotropin-releasing hormone (GnRH) analogues, danazol (an oral androgen which suppresses oestrogen activity), and progestagens. However these treatments are associated with significant side effects. Other interventions include use of a levonorgestrel- releasing intrauterine devise (LNG- IUD), and laparoscopic surgery to remove endometriosis. Non-steroidal anti-inflammatories (NSAIDs) are generally not very effective for pain relief in endometriosis.[244] They are also associated with adverse effects, such as gastrointestinal bleeding, increased risk of cardiovascular thrombosis, and kidney toxicity.[245] Long-term use of NSAIDs has also been linked to infertility.[246]

In terms of improving fertility in women with endometriosis, three months of treatment with a GnRH agonist improves pregnancy rates in women undergoing assisted reproduction. Laparoscopic surgery improves spontaneous pregnancy rates in the nine to twelve months after surgery, and improves live birth and pregnancy rates.[247] However, all orthodox treatments for endometriosis are associated with a high recurrence rate upon discontinuation of therapy.[248]

A comprehensive natural healthcare protocol, including herbal medicine, nutritional therapy, and lifestyle changes, may provide a safe alternative for reducing pain and inflammation, and improving fertility in women with endometriosis;[249] and may help to prevent recurrence of the condition in women who have already undergone orthodox medical treatment. In order to improve fertility in women with endometriosis, it is necessary to address the various aspects of the condition, including oestrogen excess, immune dysfunction, and inflammation.[250] Unlike orthodox treatments, the natural approaches discussed here are not associated with unpleasant side effects.

Natural treatment of endometriosis

Natural treatment of endometriosis includes measures to reduce the effects of excess oestrogen (discussed in more detail in Chapter 4). In addition, *Vitex agnus castus* (chaste tree) may be prescribed at up to 5 ml a day of 1:1 fluid extract to regulate reproductive hormone function in women with endometriosis.[251]

N-acetyl cysteine (up to 600 mg 3 times daily, for 3 consecutive days per week), targets the various molecular and biochemical pathways involved in the initiation and maintenance of the disease. It reduces cell proliferation, down-regulates inflammatory cytokines, and has been shown to reduce endometrial cysts and relieve pain in women with endometriosis, without causing side effects.[252] A dose of 60 mg a day of Pycnogenol, an extract of maritime pine bark, which contains antioxidant and anti-inflammatory oligomeric proanthocyanidins (OPCs), also significantly reduces symptoms in women with endometriosis.[253]

The cell-mediated immune response is responsible for clearing menstrual debris from the peritoneal cavity and preventing implantation of endometrial cells.[254] Therefore immune modulating herbs such as *Echinacea* spp. (purple coneflower), and lymphatics such as *Phytolcacca decandra* (poke root) and *Calendula officinalis* (marigold), may help to prevent and resolve endometrial cysts.[255]

Omega-3 fatty acids (found in oily fish) reduce the production of inflammatory cytokines. A fish oil supplement containing a total of 400–600 mg EPA and 200–300 mg DHA per day is recommended for women with endometriosis.[256] Increasing intake of oily fish and supplementing with evening primrose oil can also help to reduce inflammatory markers.[257]

Vitamin E supplementation can help to both reduce inflammation and prevent adhesions. Herbal anti-inflammatories include *Zingiber officinalis* (ginger) and *Curcuma longa* (turmeric),[258] while *Centella asiatica* (gotu kola) and *Salvia miltorrhiza* (Dan Shen) are useful for reducing the formation of adhesions.[259]

There are numerous herbs which can help to reduce pelvic pain, not only in cases of endometriosis, but also in other painful, spasmodic, or inflammatory conditions of the reproductive organs and tissues. They include *Anemone pulsatilla* (pasque flower), *Cimicifuga racemosa* (black cohosh), *Corydalis yanhuoso* (Yan Huo So), *Eschscholzia californica* (California poppy), *Piscidia erythrina* (Jamaican dogwood), *Viburnum opulus* (cramp bark), *Viburnum prunifolium* (black haw), and *Zingiber officinale* (ginger).[260,261]

Cannabis indica (CBD) is very useful for reducing cell proliferation, inflammation, pelvic pain, dysmenorrhoea, and dyspareunia in women with endometriosis, due to its effects on the endocannabinoid system.[262] *Gelsemium sempervirens* (yellow jasmine) is also very effective for pelvic pain.[263]

Energetics

In traditional Chinese medicine (TCM) endometriosis is most commonly considered to be due to Blood Stasis, which is discussed in more detail in Chapter 4. In Ayurveda, endometriosis may be associated with disturbances in all three doshas: Kapha (chronic cellular proliferation), Pitta (inflammation and heavy bleeding), and Vata (misplacement of cells outside the uterus, and pain). For more information about "energetic" approaches to understanding and treating infertility, see Chapter 6.

Case study

Thirty-seven-year-old female

Presenting complaint
- Endometriosis. Finished progestagen treatment 12 months ago, symptoms returned 2 months ago. Regular cycle 10/28
- Pelvic pain, premenstrual mastalgia and fluid retention, mid-cycle bleeding, dysmenorrhoea, menorrhagia, and migraine on day 1
- Recurrent vaginal candida before and during menstruation
- Constant fatigue and low mood. Insomnia during period

Medical history
- Currently overweight, very little exercise, high stress levels
- Non-smoker, social alcohol, no current medication

BP: 120/80

Pulse: 68 bpm (regular) spleen and kidney pulses impalpable, wiry liver pulse

Tongue: Pale/blue colour, swollen

Rx
- *Vitex agnus castus*   (1:1)   15
- *Schisandra chinensis*   (1:3)   30
- *Echinacea purpurea* (rad)   (1:3)   30
- *Anemone pulsatilla*   (1:3)   10
- *Trillium erectum*   (1:3)   10
- *Tanacetum parthenium*   (1:3)   10

- *Zingiber officinalis*   (1:2)   5
- *Hypericum perforatum*   (1:3)   25
- *Gelsemium sempervirens* (1:10)   5

                              140 ml per week   (Sig. 10 ml bid)

Rx   *Pycnogenol* 50 mg tablets   (Sig. 2 tabs od.)

Recommendations
- Vitamin B6 (50 mg), vitamin E (200 mg), magnesium (300 mg), zinc (20 mg), omega-3 (3 g), probiotics
- Avoid red meat, dairy products, high GL foods, non organic foods
- Linseed, brassica vegetables, dark berries, green tea, phytoestrogens

Follow-up
- All symptoms resolved within 3 months of treatment

Uterine or cervical or vaginal abnormalities

Dyspareunia and vaginismus

Dyspareunia (pain during intercourse) and vaginismus (involuntary spasm of pelvic muscles that makes penetration impossible), may be caused by structural abnormalities; pelvic tumours; endometriosis; atrophic vaginitis; chronic infection (such as urinary tract infection, bacterial vaginosis, candida, or pelvic inflammatory disease); or psychogenic causes (such as religious beliefs, trauma during childbirth, history of rape or abuse, or anxiety).[264]

Treatment of dyspareunia and vaginismus involves addressing the underlying problem. Psychotherapy, increasing lubrication, pelvic floor exercises to regain control of the muscles, and progressive desensitisation (using vaginal dilators or fingers, starting with one finger and gradually increasing to three) may help to reduce spasm and pain.[265]

It is also important to maintain the health of the vagina and lactic-acid-producing commensal bacteria, and to provide topical treatments for any underlying infection (such as reducing candida with apple cider vinegar, *Calendula officinalis*, *Aloe vera*, and coconut oil). Oestrogen promoting herbs such as *Dioscorea villosa* (wild yam) may be indicated for low oestrogen, and *Viburnum opulus* (cramp bark) is useful for reducing spasm.[266]

In women with dyspareunia and/or vaginismus due to vaginal atrophy, vaginal pessaries containing phytoestrogens, such as genistein, which is found in *Trifolium pratense* (red clover), reduce symptoms and improve the health of the local tissues.[267] A vaginal application of gel containing *Humulus lupulus* (hops) can also reduce vaginal dryness and associated inflammation, discomfort, and dyspareunia.[268]

There are numerous herbs that can help to reduce spasm and pain, such as *Anemone pulsatilla* (pasque flower), *Cimicifuga racemosa* (black cohosh), *Corydalis yanhuoso* (Yan Huo So), *Eschscholzia californica* (California poppy), *Piscidia erythrina* (Jamaican dogwood), *Viburnum opulus* (cramp bark), *Viburnum prunifolium* (black haw), and *Zingiber officinale* (ginger).[269,270] *Gelsemium sempervirens* (yellow jasmine) is also very effective for spasmodic pain.[271]

Withania somnifera (ashwagandha) is a relaxing nervine, which has been shown to improve sexual function and diminish sexual distress in women with dyspareunia and/or vaginismus due to psychogenic causes.[272] *Cannabis indica* (CBD) is particularly useful for dyspareunia. It possesses significant antispasmodic and analgesic effects.[273] It can also help with pain that is caused or exaggerated by social, cultural, or psychological factors.[274]

Congenital vaginal obstruction

Transverse septum, imperforate hymen, or longitudinal vaginal septum can cause infertility, but may be corrected surgically.[275] Herbal medicines and other complementary and alternative approaches may be used to promote healing, or address other aspects of fertility, depending on the needs of the individual patient.

Cervical factor infertility

Cervical factors account for 5–10% of cases of infertility. Cervical stenosis (problems with the opening of the cervix) may cause infertility by blocking the passage of sperm into the uterine cavity. It may be congenital, or may be caused by trauma, surgical procedures (such as colposcopy), radiation, repeated vaginal infections, adhesions, or cervical atrophy as a result of low oestrogen levels.[276]

Cervical stenosis may be treated by cervical dilation or surgery. However the rate of recurrence is very high.[277] Herbal medicine may be used to help prevent recurrence, by addressing the underlying causes, such as adhesions, recurrent vaginal infections, or low oestrogen levels.

Vitamin E supplementation can help to both reduce inflammation and prevent adhesions.[278] Immune enhancing and antimicrobial herbs such as *Echinacea* spp. (purple coneflower) *and Hydrastis canadensis* (goldenseal) are useful adjuncts in cases of chronic infection. Topical treatments (such as reducing candida with *Calendula* and *Aloe vera*, apple cider vinegar, and coconut oil) are also indicated in cases of chronic or recurrent infection. Oestrogen promoting herbs such as *Dioscorea villosa* (wild yam) and *Asparagus racemosus* (shatavari) are useful for cervical atrophy due to low oestrogen levels. It is also important to maintain the health of the vagina and lactic-acid-producing commensal bacteria.[279]

Cervical mucus may be non-receptive due to low oestrogen levels or may contain anti-sperm antibodies.[280] The latter are detected by the post-coital test.[281] The receptivity of cervical mucus may be improved by consuming a diet that is low in protein, and high in fruit and vegetables, and by oestrogen-promoting herbs (such as *Dioscorea villosa* and *Asparagus racemosus*) to stabilise vaginal flora. Immune regulating herbs such as *Echinacea* spp. (purple coneflower) are useful for reducing anti-sperm antibodies.[282]

Energetics

In Ayurvedic medicine, vaginal and cervical problems affecting fertility, such as dyspareunia, vaginismus, and cervical stenosis, especially where associated with symptoms such as anxiety, tissue dryness, and/or muscle spasm are often thought to be due to excess Vata. In traditional Chinese medicine, these conditions are associated with either Qi and Blood Stasis, or Wind Cold. For more information about "energetic" patterns of disharmony, see Chapter 6.

Uterine abnormalities

Abnormalities in the shape of the uterus are responsible for up to 5% of cases of infertility. Uterine abnormalities may be congenital (such as septate, unicornate, or bicornate uterus), or result from adhesions due to pelvic inflammatory disease, or prior surgery such as dilation and curettage (D&C).[283]

Asherman's syndrome is a condition in which fibrotic tissue or adhesions develop in the uterine cavity as a result of trauma, most commonly due to curettage.[284] Uterine abnormalities may cause infertility or pregnancy loss, but can often be corrected by hysteroscopic or laparoscopic surgery.

Uterine fibroids

Uterine fibroids (also known as *myoma* or *leiomyoma*) are benign tumours arising from the smooth muscle of the uterus. They are most commonly intramural (located within the wall of the uterus), but may also be subserosal (located beneath the serosa, the membrane which lines the outer surface of the uterus), submucosal (located in the uterine cavity beneath the inner lining of the uterus), or pedunculated (attached to the inner or outer surface of the uterus by a stalk of tissue). Uterine fibroids are estimated to affect up to 80% of women by the age of fifty, and up to 25% of women have significant growths.[285] They are more common in women of African descent compared to Caucasian.[286]

Fibroids are often asymptomatic. However, depending on their size and location, they can cause severe pelvic pain, metrorrhagia and menorrhagia, which may lead to anaemia.[287] Larger fibroids may also cause pressure on surrounding structures, leading to bowel dysfunction, and bladder symptoms, such as urinary frequency and urgency.[288]

Fibroids may sometimes cause infertility by blocking the fallopian tubes, distorting the uterine cavity, compromising blood supply, or interfering with implantation of the fertilised egg.[289] During pregnancy, fibroids may increase in size and cause pain and increased incidence of complications, including pregnancy loss.[290]

The tendency to develop uterine fibroids is genetically inherited, but the growth of fibroids is dependent on steroid hormones, particularly oestrogen.[291] Risk factors include obesity, early menarche, nulliparity, and early use of oral contraceptives,[292] all of which are associated with increased exposure to oestrogens. Fibroids tend to naturally reduce in size when oestrogen levels fall after menopause.[293]

Fibroid tissue has elevated levels of oestrogen receptors, and exhibits significant alterations in oestrogen metabolism, such as increased activity of aromatase (the enzyme which catalyses the conversion of androgens to oestrogen), which further increases local oestrogen levels.[294] Oestradiol is a potent oestrogen, which upregulates oestrogen receptor alpha (ER-α), increasing the sensitivity of fibroid tissue to the effects of oestrogen. Oestradiol also induces the production of progesterone receptors, which increases the response of fibroid tissue to progesterone, further promoting fibroid growth, by increasing cell proliferation and survival, and enhancing extracellular matrix formation.[295]

High oestrogen levels in women with fibroids can increase series 2 prostaglandins such as PGE2,[296] which is associated with dysmenorrhoea.[297] Prostaglandin E2 (PGE2) causes inflammation,[298] increased uterine muscle spasm, and uterine ischaemia.[299]

Hypoxia (which can be the result of previous infection or injury to the local tissues) may be involved in the development of uterine fibroids.[300] Hypertension also increases the risk of developing fibroids, due to damage to blood vessels, resulting in local hypoxia and/or smooth muscle injury similar to that found in atherosclerosis.[301,302]

Heavy bleeding in women with uterine fibroids is due to growth factors such as insulin-like growth factor one and two (IGF1/IGF2), and prolactin, which not only promote the development of fibroids, but also increase angiogenesis (blood vessel formation).[303]

Orthodox diagnosis and treatment of fibroids

Diagnosis of uterine fibroids is most commonly made using ultrasonography or magnetic resonance imaging (MRI).[304] Orthodox treatment of fibroids is generally only necessary where they are causing infertility, pain, heavy bleeding, bladder or bowel dysfunction, or other symptoms.

Surgical interventions

Hysterectomy is generally considered to be the most effective treatment for symptomatic uterine fibroids in women who do not wish to conceive,[305] and fibroids are the most common reason for women to have a hysterectomy. However, for many women, this is a last resort, and it is obviously not an option for women who wish to conceive. For women with symptomatic uterine fibroids who are planning to conceive, or who wish to retain their uterus, myomectomy (surgical removal of fibroids) is an option. However, this is associated with a 15% recurrence rate.[306] The procedure may also cause uterine scarring which can affect fertility.[307]

Uterine artery embolisation consists of injecting an occluding agent into one or both uterine arteries, to reduce the blood supply to the fibroids. It is effective for shrinking fibroids. However, due to the impact on the uterine circulation, it may reduce fertility and lead to complications in pregnancy, including increased risk of miscarriage.[308,309]

Other treatments for fibroids include focused energy delivery systems, which involve ablation of fibroid tissue using cryotherapy, laser, magnetic resonance-guided focused ultrasound (MRg-FUS), or an electrical current (radiofrequency ablation). However, these procedures may be associated with a risk of infection and scarring which may reduce fertility, and lack long-term data on possible risks and benefits.[310]

Medical treatments

Medical treatments for women with symptomatic uterine fibroids cannot be used for those who are actively trying to become pregnant, but may be used to shrink fibroids prior to trying to conceive. They include gonadotropin-releasing hormone analogues, which inhibit oestrogen and progesterone production, and result in shrinking of fibroids by up to 50% within three months of therapy. GnRH analogues cause unpleasant menopausal-type symptoms, such as hot flushes, vaginal dryness, reduced libido, mood changes, joint and muscle aches, and reduced bone density. Regrowth of fibroids usually occurs within twelve weeks of cessation of therapy. However, GnRH analogues may be used in advance of myomectomy to shrink fibroids and make surgical removal easier.[311]

Selective progesterone receptor modulators (such as mifepristone), antagonise progesterone (which along with oestrogen, promotes fibroid growth, by increasing cell proliferation and survival). They may be prescribed for three to six months to reduce the size of uterine fibroids and alleviate symptoms such as pain and heavy bleeding. They are associated with side effects such as hot flushes and endometrial thickening, however there is insufficient evidence to indicate that mifepristone treatment leads to endometrial atypical hyperplasia.[312]

Other medical treatments for fibroids, such as aromatase inhibitors and danazol (a synthetic androgen), reduce fibroid volume by lowering oestrogen levels. However, they are both associated with significant side effects, and there is insufficient evidence that their benefits outweigh the risks in treating uterine fibroids.[313,314]

Oral contraceptives and progestins (including the levonorgestrel intrauterine device) reduce menstrual bleeding in women with menorrhagia due to fibroids, but do not reduce the size of fibroids, and cannot be used for women who are trying to conceive.[315]

Natural treatment of fibroids

Fibroids are associated with excess oestrogen, and therefore measures to reduce oestrogen can help to reduce fibroids. For more information about reducing oestrogen excess see Chapter 4.

It is also important to reduce prolactin, which promotes the development of fibroids, and increases angiogenesis.[316] *Vitex agnus-castus* (chaste tree) reduces prolactin levels, and doses of 5 ml per day of a 1:1 fluid extract are recommended for treatment of fibroids.[317] Deficiencies of vitamin B6, magnesium, and zinc are also associated with low dopamine and raised prolactin.[318] Therefore supplementing these nutrients may help to improve dopamine synthesis,[319] and thereby reduce hyperprolactinaemia. (For more information about reducing prolactin levels see Chapter 4).

Reducing series 2 prostaglandins, which are elevated in women with fibroids, can help to reduce inflammation, uterine muscle spasm, and uterine ischaemia. Reducing consumption of animal fats, and increasing essential fatty acids (found in fish oils, flax oil, and evening primrose or starflower oil), selectively decreases dietary precursors of series 2 prostaglandins, and increases series 1 prostaglandins, which have anti-inflammatory, anti-thrombotic, and anti-spasmodic effects.[320] Vitamin E can also positively influence prostaglandin ratios; and vitamin B6 and zinc are necessary co-factors in the production of series 1 prostaglandins.[321] *Zingiber officinale* has also been shown to reduce the production of series 2 prostaglandins.[322] (For more information about reducing inflammatory prostaglandins excess see Chapter 4).

Measures to improve uterine circulation should be introduced to prevent local hypoxia. *Ginkgo biloba* (maidenhair tree) may help to improve uterine circulation and thereby relieve pain due to fibroids.[323] Warming herbs (such as *Rosmarinus officinalis* and *Zingiber officinale*) may also be used to promote healthy blood flow.[324] Nutrients that help to improve uterine circulation include: niacin (vitamin B3), vitamin C, vitamin E, and omega-3 fatty acids.[325] Increasing exercise may also help to improve healthy blood flow.[326] (For more information about improving uterine circulation, see the section on abnormal blood flow in Chapter 4).

Serum vitamin D levels have been shown to correlate with fibroid size. Vitamin D deficiency is associated with larger fibroids, whereas women with uterine myoma who had higher levels of serum vitamin D had the smallest fibroids.[327] Therefore women with fibroids should be advised to check their vitamin D levels, and to take supplemental vitamin D where this is found to be suboptimal.

Green tea has been shown to significantly reduce the volume of uterine fibroids and improve symptoms of blood loss and anaemia.[328] This is partly due to the inhibitory action of epigallocatechin-3-gallate (EGCG) on catechol-O-methyltransferase (COMT), an enzyme that is elevated in uterine fibroids and involved in their pathogenesis.[329]

In terms of nutrition, the incidence of uterine fibroids is greater in women who consume more meat[330] and less fruits and vegetables.[331] This is probably due to the effects of increased meat consumption and insufficient fruit and vegetable intake on levels of oestrogen and inflammatory prostaglandins. Women with fibroids should therefore be encouraged to avoid red meat and consume more oily fish, beans, pulses, fruits, and vegetables.[332]

Women who drink one unit of alcohol per day or more increase the risk of developing uterine fibroids by more than 50%.[333] Therefore, women with fibroids should be encouraged to reduce their consumption of alcohol.

Herbs such as *Echinacea* spp. (purple coneflower), *Thuja occidentalis* (arborvitae), and *Chelidonium majus* (greater celandine) are traditionally used to control benign growths,[334] and dysfunctional uterine bleeding associated with fibroids responds well to uterine astringent and haemostatic herbs such as *Achillea millefolium* (yarrow), *Alchemilla vulgaris* (lady's mantle), *Capsella bursa-pastoris* (shepherd's purse), and *Trillium erectum* (beth root or birth root).[335]

Increased exercise, weight loss, reduced intake of carbohydrates, and intermittent fasting all help to reduce insulin, and insulin-like growth factor, which are responsible for promoting cell proliferation.[336] Weight loss also helps to reduce hypertension and atherosclerosis, both of which predispose to fibroid development.[337]

Chronic stress, and its consequences (such as overconsumption of unhealthy foods, weight gain, and hypertension), increases the incidence of uterine fibroids.[338] Elevated cortisol levels, which occur in response to stress, may eventually cause insulin resistance, which in turn may result in the development of obesity, hypertension, and atherosclerosis, all of which are implicated in fibroid growth.[339] Therefore strategies to reduce stress may help to reduce fibroids.

In conjunction with stress management techniques, nervine tonics, nervine sedatives, and adaptogens help to reduce the adverse effects of stress.[340] *Hypericum perforatum* is thought to inhibit monoamine oxidase (MAO).[341] Therefore, in addition to reducing the effects of stress, it may also help to reduce oestrogen excess, since monoamine oxidase activity is positively correlated with the progesterone to oestradiol ratio.[342] Nervine sedatives include *Anemone pulsatilla*, *Leonurus cardiaca*, and *Melissa officinalis*, while herbal adaptogens include *Schisandra chinensis* and *Withania somnifera*. B vitamins and magnesium also help to reduce tension and to improve sleep patterns.[343] (For more information about reducing stress levels, see Chapter 4).

Energetics

In Ayurvedic medicine, uterine fibroids are often thought to be due to excess Kapha, which benefits from dry and pungent foods and herbs, such as *Myristica fragrans* (nutmeg), *Cinnamonum zeylonicum* (cinnamon), *Capsella bursa-pastoris* (shepherd's purse), and *Trillium erectum* (beth root). Similarly, in TCM, fibroids are considered to be due to an accumulation of Damp Phlegm. For more information about "energetic" patterns of disharmony, and treating Kapha disturbance, see Chapter 6.

Case study

Thirty-one-year-old female

Presenting complaint
- Trying to conceive for 18 months
- Multiple uterine fibroids diagnosed on ultrasound. Largest fibroid is 5 cm
- Regular periods 10/30, menorrhagia, dysmenorrhoea, premenstrual mastalgia, and mood swings. Continuous white vaginal discharge
- Exhaustion from 7 days before until 7 days after menstruation. Shortness of breath on exertion

Medical history
- Jaundice age 15
- Drinks 3–4 units of alcohol most days (especially premenstrually)

BP: 130/85

Pulse: 60 bpm (regular) deep, slippery pulse

Rx

• Vitex agnus castus	(1:1)	15
• Rosmarinus officinalis	(1:3)	20
• Ginkgo biloba	(2:1)	10
• Achillea millefolium	(1:3)	30
• Capsella bursa pastoris	(1:3)	30
• Zingiber officinalis	(1:2)	5
• Hypericum perforatum	(1:3)	30

140 ml per week   (Sig. 10 ml bid)

Recommendations

- Vitamin B complex, vitamin C (1,000 mg), Vitamin D (5,000 iu), vitamin E (200 mg), magnesium (300 mg), zinc (20 mg), omega-3 (3,000 mg), probiotics
- Avoid red meat, dairy products, high GL foods, non organic foods
- Linseed, brassica vegetables, dark berries, green tea, phytoestrogens
- Reduce alcohol consumption

Follow-up

- Symptoms improved after 3 months of treatment. Patient conceived after 8 months of treatment and went on to have 4 healthy children

Notes

209. Liu, W., & Gong, C. (2009). Opening the blockage to reproduction: infertility. *Traditional Chinese Medicine Information Page* [online]. Available from http://tcmpage.com/hpinfertility.html (accessed 4 July 2011).

210. Trickey, R. (2011). *Women, Hormones and the Menstrual Cycle.* Clifton Hill, Victoria, Australia: Melbourne Holistic Health Group.

211. Rose-Wilson, D., & Brazier, Y. (2017). What is pelvic inflammatory disease? *Medical News Today* [online]. Available from https://medicalnewstoday.com/articles/177923.php (accessed 26 December 2019).

212. Trickey, R. (2011). *Women, Hormones and the Menstrual Cycle.* Clifton Hill, Victoria, Australia: Melbourne Holistic Health Group.

213. Pavletic, A. J., Wolner-Hanssen, P., Paavonen, J., Hawes, S. E., & Eschenbach, D. A. (1999). Infertility following pelvic inflammatory disease. *Infectious Diseases in Obstetrics and Gynecology, 7*(3): 145–152.

214. Rose-Wilson, D., & Selner, M. (2018). What is an ectopic pregnancy? *Healthline* [online]. Available from https://healthline.com/health/pregnancy/ectopic-pregnancy (accessed 26 December 2019).

215. University of Maryland Medical Center (2014). *Pelvic Inflammatory Disease* [online]. Available from http://umm.edu/health/medical/altmed/condition/pelvic-inflammatory-disease (accessed 18 July 2015).

216. Bone, K., & Mills, S. (2013). *Principles and Practice of Phytotherapy: Modern Herbal Medicine*. London: Churchill Livingstone.

217. Trickey, R. (2011). *Women, Hormones and the Menstrual Cycle*. Clifton Hill, Victoria, Australia: Melbourne Holistic Health Group.

218. Bone, K., & Mills, S. (2013). *Principles and Practice of Phytotherapy: Modern Herbal Medicine*. London: Churchill Livingstone.

219. Trickey, R. (2011). *Women, Hormones and the Menstrual Cycle*. Clifton Hill, Victoria, Australia: Melbourne Holistic Health Group.

220. Bone, K., & Mills, S. (2013). *Principles and Practice of Phytotherapy: Modern Herbal Medicine*. London: Churchill Livingstone.

221. Romm, A. (2016). *Botanical Medicine for Women's Health* (2nd edn). London: Churchill Livingstone.

222. Romm, A. (2016). *Botanical Medicine for Women's Health* (2nd edn). London: Churchill Livingstone.

223. Ellingwood, F. (1919) *The American Materia Medica* [online]. Available from http://henriettesherbal.com/eclectic/ellingwood/index.html (accessed 3 May 2020).

224. Cramer, D. W., Wilson, E., Stillman, R. J., Berger, M. J., Belisle, S., Schiff, I., Albrecht, B., Gibson, M., Stadel, B. V., & Schoenbaum, S. C. (1986). The relationship of endometriosis to menstrual characteristics, smoking and exercise. *Journal of the American Medical Association, 255*(14): 1904–1908.

225. Bulun, S. E., Gurates, B., & Fang, Z. (2002). Mechanisms of excessive estrogen formation in endometriosis. *Journal of Reproductive Immunology, 55*(1–2): 21–33.

226. Wang, W., Li, W., Maitituoheti, M., Yang, R., Wu, Z., Wang, T., Ma, D., & Wang, S. (2013). Association of an oestrogen receptor gene polymorphism in Chinese Han women with endometriosis and endometriosis-related infertility. *Reproductive BioMedicine Online, 26*(1): 93–98.

227. Bulun, S. E., Gurates, B., & Fang, Z. (2002). Mechanisms of excessive estrogen formation in endometriosis. *Journal of Reproductive Immunology, 55*(1–2): 21–33.

228. Trickey, R. (2011). *Women, Hormones and the Menstrual Cycle*. Clifton Hill, Victoria, Australia: Melbourne Holistic Health Group.

229. Trickey, R. (2011). *Women, Hormones and the Menstrual Cycle*. Clifton Hill, Victoria, Australia: Melbourne Holistic Health Group.

230. Trickey, R. (2011). *Women, Hormones and the Menstrual Cycle*. Clifton Hill, Victoria, Australia: Melbourne Holistic Health Group.

231. Bulun, S. E., Gurates, B., & Fang, Z. (2002). Mechanisms of excessive estrogen formation in endometriosis. *Journal of Reproductive Immunology, 55*(1–2): 21–33.

232. Trickey, R. (2011). *Women, Hormones and the Menstrual Cycle*. Clifton Hill, Victoria, Australia: Melbourne Holistic Health Group.

233. Bone, K., & Mills, S. (2013). *Principles and Practice of Phytotherapy: Modern Herbal Medicine*. London: Churchill Livingstone.

234. Weiss, G., Goldsmith, L. T., Taylor, R. N., Bellet, D., & Taylor, H. S. (2009). Inflammation in reproductive disorders. *Reproductive Sciences, 16*(2): 216–229.

235. González-Ramos, R., Van Langendonckt, A., Defrere, S., Lousse, J.-C., Colette, S., Devoto, L., & Donnez, J. (2010). Involvement of the nuclear factor-κB pathway in the pathogenesis of endometriosis. *Fertility and Sterility*, *94*(6): 1985–1994.

236. Lebovic, D. I., Mueller, M. D., & Taylor, R. N. (2001). Immunobiology of endometriosis. *Fertility and Sterility*, *75*(1): 1–10.

237. Dunselman, G. A., Hendrix, M. G., Bouckaert, P. X., & Evers, J. L. (1988). Functional aspects of peritoneal macrophages in endometriosis of women. *Journal of Reproduction & Fertility*, *82*(2): 707–710.

238. Halme, J., Becker, S., & Wing, R. (1984). Accentuated cyclic activation of peritoneal macrophages in patients with endometriosis. *American Journal of Obstetrics & Gynecology*, *148*(1): 85–90.

239. Ramey, J. W., & Archer, D. F. (1993). Peritoneal fluid: its relevance to the development of endometriosis. *Fertility and Sterility*, *60*(1): 1–14.

240. Garzetti, G. G., Ciavattini, A., Provinciali, M., Fabris, N., Cignitti, M., & Romanini, C. (1993). Natural killer cell activity in endometriosis: correlation between serum estradiol levels and cytotoxicity. *Obstetrics & Gynecology*, *81*(5[pt 1]): 665–668.

241. Trickey, R. (2011). *Women, Hormones and the Menstrual Cycle*. Clifton Hill, Victoria, Australia: Melbourne Holistic Health Group.

242. Simsa, P., Mihalyi, A., Schoeters, G., Koppen, G., Kyama, C. M., Den Hond, E. M., Fülöp, V., & D'Hooghe, T. M. (2010). Increased exposure to dioxin-like compounds is associated with endometriosis in a case-control study in women. *Reproductive Biomedicine Online*, *20*(5): 681–688.

243. National Institute for Health and Care Excellence (UK) 2017. Endometriosis: diagnosis and management. *Nice Guideline*, No. 73.

244. Brown, J., & Farquhar, C. (2014). Endometriosis: an overview of Cochrane Reviews. *Cochrane Database of Systematic Reviews* [online]. Available from https://cochranelibrary.com/cdsr/doi/10.1002/14651858.CD009590.pub2/full (accessed 30 December 2019).

245. Moore, N., Pollack, C., & Butkerait, P. (2015). Adverse drug reactions and drug–drug interactions with over-the-counter NSAIDs. *Therapeutics and Clinical Risk Management*, *11*: 1061–1075.

246. Mendonça, L. L. F., Khamashta, M. A., Nelson-Piercy, C., Hunt, B. J., & Hughes, G. R. (2000). Non-steroidal anti-inflammatory drugs as a possible cause for reversible infertility. *Rheumatology*, *39*(8): 880–882.

247. Brown, J., & Farquhar, C. (2014). Endometriosis: an overview of Cochrane Reviews. *Cochrane Database of Systematic Reviews* (online). Available from https://cochranelibrary.com/cdsr/doi/10.1002/14651858.CD009590.pub2/full (accessed 30 December 2019).

248. Romm, A. (2016). *Botanical Medicine for Women's Health* (2nd edn). London: Churchill Livingstone.

249. Romm, A. (2016). *Botanical Medicine for Women's Health* (2nd edn). London: Churchill Livingstone.

250. Mahmood, T. A., & Templeton, A. (1990). Pathophysiology of mild endometriosis: review of literature. *Human Reproduction*, *5*(7): 765–784.

251. Bone, K., & Mills, S. (2013). *Principles and Practice of Phytotherapy: Modern Herbal Medicine*. London: Churchill Livingstone.

252. Grazia Porpora, M., Brunelli, R., Costa, G., Imperiale, L., Krasnowska, E. K., Lundeberg, T., Nofroni, I., Piccioni, M. G., Pittaluga, E., Ticino, A., & Parasissi, T. (2013). A promise in the treatment of endometriosis: an observational cohort study on ovarian endometrioma reduction by N-acetylcysteine. *Evidence Based Complementary Alternative Medicine* [online]. Available from https://ncbi.nlm.nih.gov/pmc/articles/PMC3662115/ (accessed 1 January 2020).

253. Kohama, T., Herai, K., & Inoue, M. (2007). Effect of French maritime pine bark extract on endometriosis as compared with leuprorelin acetate. *Journal of Reproductive Medicine*, 52(8): 703–708.

254. Lebovic, D. I., Mueller, M. D., & Taylor, R. N. (2001). Immunobiology of endometriosis. *Fertility and Sterility*, 75(1): 1–10.

255. Bone, K., & Mills, S. (2013). *Principles and Practice of Phytotherapy: Modern Herbal Medicine.* London: Churchill Livingstone.

256. Trickey, R. (2011). *Women, Hormones and the Menstrual Cycle.* Clifton Hill, Victoria, Australia: Melbourne Holistic Health Group.

257. Romm, A. (2016). *Botanical Medicine for Women's Health* (2nd edn). London: Churchill Livingstone.

258. Trickey, R. (2011). *Women, Hormones and the Menstrual Cycle.* Clifton Hill, Victoria, Australia: Melbourne Holistic Health Group.

259. Bone, K., & Mills, S. (2013). *Principles and Practice of Phytotherapy: Modern Herbal Medicine.* London: Churchill Livingstone.

260. Bone, K., & Mills, S. (2013). *Principles and Practice of Phytotherapy: Modern Herbal Medicine.* London: Churchill Livingstone.

261. Romm, A. (2016). *Botanical Medicine for Women's Health* (2nd edn). London: Churchill Livingstone.

262. Bouaziz, J., Bar On, A., Seidman, D. S., & Soriano, D. (2017). The clinical significance of endocannabinoids in endometriosis pain management. *Cannabis and Cannabinoid Research*, 2(1): 72–80.

263. Ellingwood, F. (1919). *The American Materia Medica* [online]. Available from http://henriettesherbal.com/eclectic/ellingwood/index.html (accessed 3 May 2020).

264. Heffner, L. J., & Schust, D. J. (2014). *The Reproductive System at a Glance.* Oxford: John Wiley & Sons.

265. Rosenfeld, J. A. (2004). *Handbook of Women's Health: An Evidence Based Approach.* Cambridge: Cambridge University Press.

266. Bone, K., & Mills, S. (2013). *Principles and Practice of Phytotherapy: Modern Herbal Medicine.* London: Churchill Livingstone.

267. Le Donne, M., Caruso, C., Mancuso, A., Costa, G., Iemmo, R., Pizzimenti, G., & Cavallari, V. (2011). The effect of vaginally administered genistein in comparison with hyaluronic acid on atrophic epithelium in postmenopause. *Archives of Gynecology and Obstetrics*, 283(6): 1319–1323.

268. Morali, G., Polatti, F., Metelitsa, E. N., Mascarucci, P., Magnani, P., & Marrè, G. B. (2006). Open, non-controlled clinical studies to assess the efficacy and safety of a medical device in form of gel topically and intravaginally used in postmenopausal women with genital atrophy. *Arzneimittelforschung*, 56(3): 230–238.

269. Bone, K., & Mills, S. (2013). *Principles and Practice of Phytotherapy: Modern Herbal Medicine.* London: Churchill Livingstone.

270. Romm, A. (2016). *Botanical Medicine for Women's Health* (2nd edn). London: Churchill Livingstone.

271. Ellingwood, F. (1919). *The American Materia Medica* [online]. Available from http://henriettesherbal.com/eclectic/ellingwood/index.html (accessed 3 May 2020).

272. Dongre, S., Langade, D., & Bhattacharyya, S. (2015). Efficacy and Safety of Ashwagandha (Withania somnifera) Root Extract in Improving Sexual Function in Women: A Pilot Study. *BioMed Research Interntional, 284154.*

273. Romm, A. (2016). *Botanical Medicine for Women's Health* (2nd edn). London: Churchill Livingstone.

274. Bouaziz, J., Bar On, A., Seidman, D. S., & Soriano, D. (2017). The clinical significance of endocannabinoids in endometriosis pain management. *Cannabis and Cannabinoid Research,* 2(1): 72–80.

275. Joki-Erkkila, M. M., & Heinonen, P. K. (2003). Presenting and long-term clinical implications and fecundity in females with obstructing vaginal malformations. *Journal of Pediatric and Adolescent Gynecology,* 16(5): 307–12.

276. Puscheck, E., & Lucidi, R. S. (2015). Infertility. *Medscape* [online]. Available from http://emedicine.medscape.com/article/274143-overview#a3 (accessed 10 July 2015).

277. Baldauff, J. J., Dreyfus, M., Wertz, J. P., Cuénin, C., Ritter, J., & Philippe, E. (1997). Consequences and treatment of cervical stenoses after laser conization or loop electrosurgical excision. *Journal de Gynecologie, Obstetrique et Biologie de la Reproduction,* 26(1): 64–70.

278. Trickey, R. (2011). *Women, Hormones and the Menstrual Cycle.* Clifton Hill, Victoria, Australia: Melbourne Holistic Health Group.

279. Bone, K., & Mills, S. (2013). *Principles and Practice of Phytotherapy: Modern Herbal Medicine.* London: Churchill Livingstone.

280. Puscheck, E., & Lucidi, R. S. (2015). Infertility. *Medscape* [online]. Available from http://emedicine.medscape.com/article/274143-overview#a3 (accessed 10 July 2015).

281. Overstreet, J. W. (1986). Evaluation of sperm-cervical mucus interaction. *Fertility and Sterility,* 45(3): 324–326.

282. Bone, K., & Mills, S. (2013). *Principles and Practice of Phytotherapy: Modern Herbal Medicine.* London: Churchill Livingstone.

283. Trickey, R. (2003). *Women, Hormones & the Menstrual Cycle.* Sydney, Australia: Allen & Unwin.

284. Trickey, R. (2003). *Women, Hormones & the Menstrual Cycle.* Sydney, Australia: Allen & Unwin.

285. Walker, C. L., & Stewart, E. A. (2005). Uterine fibroids: the elephant in the room. *Science,* 308(5728): 1589–1592.

286. Sohn, G. S., Cho, S. H., Kim, Y. M., Cho, C.-H., Kim, M.-R., Lee, S. R., & Working Group of Society of Uterine Leiomyoma (2018). Current medical treatment of uterine fibroids. *Obstetrics & Gynecology Science,* 61(2): 192–201.

287. Walker, C. L., & Stewart, E. A. (2005). Uterine fibroids: the elephant in the room. *Science,* 308(5728): 1589–1592.

288. Lumsden, M. A., & Wallace, E. M. (1998). Clinical presentation of uterine fibroids. *Baillières Clinical Obstetrics and Gynaecology,* 12(2): 177–195.

289. Puscheck, E., & Lucidi, R. S. (2015). Infertility. *Medscape* [online]. Available from http://emedicine.medscape.com/article/274143-overview#a3 (accessed 10 July 2015).

290. Ouyang, D. W., Economy, K. E., & Norwitz, E. R. (2006). Obstetric complications of fibroids. *Obstetrics and Gynecology Clinics of North America, 33*(1): 153–169.

291. Sohn, G. S., Cho, S. H., Kim, Y. M., Cho, C.-H., Kim, M.-R., Lee, S. R., & Working Group of Society of Uterine Leiomyoma (2018). Current medical treatment of uterine fibroids. *Obstetrics & Gynecology Science, 61*(2): 192–201.

292. Sohn, G. S., Cho, S. H., Kim, Y. M., Cho, C.-H., Kim, M.-R., Lee, S. R., & Working Group of Society of Uterine Leiomyoma (2018). Current medical treatment of uterine fibroids. *Obstetrics & Gynecology Science, 61*(2): 192–201.

293. Bulun, S. E. (2013). Uterine fibroids. *New England Journal of Medicine, 369*(14): 1344–1355.

294. Walker, C. L., & Stewart, E. A. (2005). Uterine fibroids: the elephant in the room. *Science, 308*(5728): 1589–1592.

295. Bulun, S. E. (2013). Uterine fibroids. *New England Journal of Medicine, 369*(14): 1344–1355.

296. Trickey, R. (2003). *Women, Hormones & the Menstrual Cycle*. Sydney, Australia: Allen & Unwin.

297. Lumsden, M. A., Kelly, R. W., & Baird, D. T. (2005). Primary dysmenorrhoea: the importance of both prostaglandins E2 and F2α. *British Journal of Obstetrics and Gynaecology, 90*(12): 1135–1140.

298. Curtis-Prior, P. B. (Ed.) (2004). *The Eicosanoids*. New York: John Wiley & Sons.

299. Benedetto, C. (1989). Eicosanoids in primary dysmenorrhea, endometriosis and menstrual migraine. *Gynecological Endocrinology, 3*(1): 71–94.

300. Walker, C. L., & Stewart, E. A. (2005). Uterine fibroids: the elephant in the room. *Science, 308*(5728): 1589–1592.

301. Boynton-Jarrett, R., Rich-Edwards, J., Malspeis, S., Missmer, S. A., & Wright, R. (2005). A prospective study of hypertension and risk of uterine leiomyomata. *American Journal of Epidemiology, 161*(7): 628–638.

302. Faerstein, E., Szklo, M., & Rosenshein, N. B. (2001). Risk factors for uterine leiomyoma: a practice-based case-control study. II. Atherogenic risk factors and potential sources of uterine irritation. *American Journal of Epidemiology, 153*(1): 11–19.

303. Walker, C. L., & Stewart, E. A. (2005). Uterine fibroids: the elephant in the room. *Science, 308*(5728): 1589–1592.

304. Vilos, G. A., Allaire, C., Laberge, P.-Y., Leyland, N., & special contributors (2015). The management of uterine leiomyomas. *Journal of Obstetrics and Gynaecology Canada, 37*(2): 157–178.

305. Weber, A. M., Mitchinson, A. R., Gidwani, G. P., Mascha, E., & Walters, M. D. (1997). Uterine myomas and factors associated with hysterectomy in premenopausal women. *American Journal of Obstetrics and Gynecology, 176*: 1213–1217.

306. Garcia, C. R. (1993). Management of the symptomatic fibroid in women older than 40 years of age: hysterectomy or myomectomy? *Obstetrics and Gynecology Clinics of North America, 20*(2): 337–348.

307. Riquelme, J. (2003). Uterine fibroids (leiomyomata). In: D. Rakel (Ed.), *Integrative Medicine* (pp. 389–392). Philadelphia, PA: W. B. Saunders.

308. Vilos, G. A., Allaire, C., Laberge, P.-Y., Leyland, N., & special contributors (2015). The management of uterine leiomyomas. *Journal of Obstetrics and Gynaecology Canada, 37*(2): 157–178.

309. Mara, M., & Kubinova, K. (2014). Embolization of uterine fibroids from the point of view of the gynecologist: pros and cons. *International Journal of Women's Health, 6*: 623–629.

310. Vilos, G. A., Allaire, C., Laberge, P.-Y., Leyland, N., & special contributors (2015). The management of uterine leiomyomas. *Journal of Obstetrics and Gynaecology Canada*, 37(2): 157–178.

311. Vilos, G. A., Allaire, C., Laberge, P.-Y., Leyland, N., & special contributors (2015). The management of uterine leiomyomas. *Journal of Obstetrics and Gynaecology Canada*, 37(2): 157–178.

312. Shem, Q., Hua, Y., Jiang, W., Zhang, W., Chen, M., & Zhu, X. (2013). Effects of mifepristone on uterine leiomyoma in premenopausal women: a meta-analysis. *Fertility and Sterility*, 100(6): 1722–1726.

313. Ke, L., Yang, K., Li, C.-M., & Li, J. (2009). Danazol for treatment of women with symptoms caused by uterine fibroids. *Cochrane Database of Systematic Reviews* [online] Available from https://cochranelibrary.com/cdsr/doi/10.1002/14651858. CD007692.pub2/full (accessed 27 January 2020).

314. Song, H., Lu, D., Navaratnam, K., & Shi, G. (2013). Aromatase inhibitors for uterine fibroids. *Cochrane Database of Systematic Reviews* [online]. Available from https://ncbi.nlm.nih.gov/pubmed/24151065 (accessed 27 January 2020).

315. Vilos, G. A., Allaire, C., Laberge, P.-Y., Leyland, N., & special contributors (2015). The management of uterine leiomyomas. *Journal of Obstetrics and Gynaecology Canada*, 37(2): 157–178.

316. Walker, C. L., & Stewart, E. A. (2005). Uterine fibroids: the elephant in the room. *Science*, 308(5728): 1589–1592.

317. Bone, K., & Mills, S. (2013). *Principles and Practice of Phytotherapy: Modern Herbal Medicine*. London: Churchill Livingstone.

318. Brice-Ytsma, H., & McDermott, A. (2020). *Herbal Medicine in Treating Gynaecological Conditions*. London: Aeon.

319. Trickey, R. (2011). *Women, Hormones and the Menstrual Cycle*. Clifton Hill, Victoria, Australia: Melbourne Holistic Health Group.

320. Puolakka, J., Mäkäräinen, L., Viinikka, L., & Ylikorkala, O. (1985). Biochemical and clinical effects of treating the premenstrual syndrome with prostaglandin synthesis precursors. *Journal of Reproductive Medicine*, 30(3): 149–153.

321. Trickey, R. (2003). *Women, Hormones & the Menstrual Cycle*. Sydney, Australia: Allen & Unwin.

322. Gonlachanvit, S., Chen, Y. H., Hasler, W. L., Sun, W. M., & Owyang, C. (2003). Ginger reduces hyperglycemia-evoked gastric dysrhythmias in healthy humans: possible role of endogenous prostaglandins, *Journal of Pharmacology & Experimental Therapeutics*, 307(3): 1098–1103.

323. Bone, K., & Mills, S. (2013). *Principles and Practice of Phytotherapy: Modern Herbal Medicine*. London: Churchill Livingstone.

324. Holmes, P. (2007) *The Energetics of Western Herbs: A Materia Medica Integrating Western & Chinese Herbal Therapeutics, Volume 1* (4th edn). Santa Rosa, CA: Snow Lotus.

325. Weiss, R. F. (1988). *Herbal Medicine*.Gothenburg, Sweden: Arcanum.

326. Timonen, S., & Procopé, B. J. (1971). Premenstrual syndrome and physical exercise. *Acta Obstetricia et Gynecologica Scandinavica*, 50(4): 331–337.

327. Sabry, M., Halder, S. K., Allah, A. S. A., Roshdy, E., Rajaratnam, V., & Al-Hendy, A. (2013). Serum vitamin D3 level inversely correlates with uterine fibroid volume in different ethnic groups: a cross-sectional observational study. *International Journal of Women's Health*, 5: 93–100.

328. Roshdy, E., Rajaratnam, V., Maitra, S., Sabry, M., Ait Allah, A. S., & Al-Hendy, A. (2013) Treatment of symptomatic uterine fibroids with green tea extract: a pilot randomized controlled clinical study. *International Journal of Women's Health, 5*: 477–486.

329. Al-Hendy, A., & Salama, S. A. (2006). Catechol-O-methyltransferase polymorphism is associated with increased uterine leiomyoma risk in different ethnic groups. *Journal of the Society for Gynecologic Investigation, 13*(2): 136–144.

330. Wise, L. A., Palmer, J. R., Harlow, B. L., Spiegelman, D., Stewart, E. A., Adams-Campbell, L. L., & Rosenberg, L. (2004). Risk of uterine leiomyomata in relation to tobacco, alcohol and caffeine consumption in the Black Women's Health Study. *Human Reproduction, 19*: 1746–1754.

331. Wise, L. A., Radin, R. G., Palmer, J. R., Kumanyika, S. K., Boggs, D. A., & Rosenberg, L. (2011). Intake of fruit, vegetables, and carotenoids in relation to risk of uterine leiomyomata. *American Journal of Clinical Nutrition, 94*(6): 1620–1631.

332. Dalton-Brewer, N. (2016). The role of complementary and alternative medicine for the management of fibroids and associated symptomatology. *Current Obstetrics and Gynecology Reports, 5*: 110–118.

333. Wise, L. A., Palmer, J. R., Harlow, B. L., Spiegelman, D., Stewart, E. A., Adams-Campbell, L. L., & Rosenberg, L. (2004). Risk of uterine leiomyomata in relation to tobacco, alcohol and caffeine consumption in the Black Women's Health Study. *Human Reproduction, 19*: 1746–1754.

334. Bone, K., & Mills, S. (2013). *Principles and Practice of Phytotherapy: Modern Herbal Medicine.* London: Churchill Livingstone.

335. Romm, A. (2016). *Botanical Medicine for Women's Health* (2nd edn). London: Churchill Livingstone.

336. Klement, R. J. (2016). Dietary and pharmacological modification of the insulin/IGF-1 system: exploiting the full repertoire against cancer. *Oncogenesis, 5*: e193.

337. Dalton-Brewer, N. (2016). The role of complementary and alternative medicine for the management of fibroids and associated symptomatology. *Current Obstetrics and Gynecology Reports, 5*: 110–118.

338. Vines, A. I., Ta, M., & Esserman, D. A. (2010). The association between self-reported major life events and the presence of uterine fibroids. *Women's Health Issues, 20*: 294–298.

339. Dalton-Brewer, N. (2016). The role of complementary and alternative medicine for the management of fibroids and associated symptomatology. *Current Obstetrics and Gynecology Reports, 5*: 110–118.

340. Trickey, R. (2003). *Women, Hormones & the Menstrual Cycle.* Sydney, Australia: Allen & Unwin.

341. Linde, K., Ramirez, G., Mulrow, C. D., Pauls, A., Weidenhammer, W., & Melchart, D. (1996). St John's wort for depression: an overview and meta-analysis of randomised clinical trials. *British Medical Journal, 313*(7052): 253–258.

342. Briggs, M., & Briggs, M. (1972). Relationship between monoamine oxidase activity and sex hormone concentration in human blood plasma. *Journal of Reproduction and Fertility, 29*: 447–450.

343. Trickey, R. (2003). *Women, Hormones & the Menstrual Cycle.* Sydney, Australia: Allen & Unwin.

CHAPTER FOUR

Functional problems

Good diagnosis is a vital part of herbal medicine, and using scientific diagnostic techniques such as blood tests and ultrasonography can be extremely useful for choosing the correct treatment protocol.[344] However, scientific diagnostic techniques cannot always provide an explanation for the problems being encountered by the patient.

A functional disorder is one in which an organ, tissue, or body system does not function normally, even though no structural changes can be detected, and routine tests may remain within the normal ranges.[345] A diagnosis of functional or unexplained infertility is made when no clear organic cause has been found for the inability to conceive.[346] It can be an extremely frustrating diagnosis for couples that are trying to conceive, since it is difficult to decide on an appropriate treatment plan without a definitive diagnosis.

Although careful case-taking frequently reveals symptoms such as menstrual irregularities and abnormal menstrual flow,[347] and there may be a slight hormonal imbalance in some instances,[348] these symptoms are difficult to classify conventionally since they do not fall into any specific disease category.[349] However, the significance of these symptoms may be better understood using a more holistic perspective; and by incorporating traditional or "energetic" approaches to diagnosis, one may find possible causal factors for the infertility where orthodox medicine has failed to do so.

Functional problems that may contribute to reproductive health issues and infertility include: abnormal blood flow, functional hormone problems, stress, and prostaglandin imbalance.

Abnormal blood flow

In traditional Chinese medicine (TCM), Blood Stasis is one of a number of different patterns of disharmony, which may contribute to infertility. Blood Stasis is indicated by a blue or purple tongue-body colour, and various symptoms such as poor peripheral circulation and dysmenorrhoea with clotty menstrual flow.[350]

Poor peripheral circulation

Poor peripheral circulation is a common complaint among women with a history of reproductive problems.[351] It is possible, therefore, that women with poor peripheral circulation may also be suffering from poor pelvic circulation, which impairs nourishment of uterus and ovaries.[352]

Dysmenorrhoea

Dysmenorrhoea may also suggest reduced uterine circulatory capacity.[353] The physiomedicalist tradition describes different "tissue states" such as *constriction* which may arise from stress.[354] Spasmodic dysmenorrhoea (with cramping pains during menstruation) is a constrictive condition caused by a hypertonic uterus, which restricts blood flow. Conversely, congestive dysmenorrhoea, which is signified by a dull, dragging sensation before the onset of menstruation, is due to pelvic blood congestion.[355] It is associated with *torpor* or *atonicity* of the tissues, which leads to stagnation.[356]

Endometrial perfusion, thrombophilia, and ovarian blood flow

Adequate endometrial blood supply is required for implantation to occur, and women with unexplained subfertility demonstrate a significant reduction in endometrial and subendometrial perfusion during the mid–late follicular phase. This is likely to be due to dynamic vascular changes such as vasoconstriction or reduced vasodilation, rather than variation in vessel number.[357]

Thrombophilia is another cause of poor uterine perfusion and may be a factor in subfertility.[358] Poor uterine perfusion may also be due to decreased uterine receptivity to endogenous hormones.[359,360]

Furthermore, poor ovarian blood flow is associated with luteal phase defect, which results in low progesterone levels during the mid-luteal phase. Improving ovarian blood flow therefore improves both luteal function and endometrial growth.[361]

Improving blood flow

Circulatory stimulants

Warming herbs such as *Rosmarinus officinalis*, *Cinnamonum zeylonicum*, and *Zingiber officinale* may be used to stimulate the peripheral circulation, and may also help to promote healthy circulation to the reproductive organs.[362]

Uterine spasmolytics

In cases of spasmodic dysmenorrhoea, uterine spasmolytics such as *Paeonia lactiflora*, *Viburnum opulus*, and *Viburnum prunifolium*, and measures to decrease prostaglandins (described later in this chapter), may be useful to improve uterine blood flow. Magnesium may also help to decrease uterine cramping.[363] It is found in foods such as soya products, whole-grain cereals, seeds, and green leafy vegetables.[364]

Uterine tonics

In cases of pelvic blood congestion, uterine tonics such as *Rubus idaeus* may be more useful, as they are thought to encourage more effective uterine contractions.[365] *Achillea millefolium* also reduces pelvic congestion, possibly due to an anti-thrombotic effect,[366] as well as relaxation of the veins, which allows congestion to move out of the capillaries.[367]

Amphoteric herbs

There are numerous herbs, such as *Leonurus cardiaca*, which seem to possess the apparently contradictory effects of both stimulating uterine

activity and relieving spasm. This combination of actions helps to regulate uterine function by encouraging more orderly and effective contractions, which are then followed by an adequate rest period so that
blood can circulate through the uterine muscle again.[368]

Angelica sinensis is a uterine tonic and antispasmodic herb, which
is widely used to treat dysmenorrhoea,[369] and is traditionally used to
treat blood stasis in TCM.[370] It is also thought to regulate prostaglandin
synthesis,[371] and to act as a circulatory stimulant.[372] In Ayurveda, nutmeg (*Myristica fragrans*) is a warming herb, which is used to relieve pain
and heavy menstrual bleeding.[373]

Other measures

Nutrients which help to reduce blood stagnation include: niacin
(vitamin B3), found in whole grains and sprouted legumes; vitamin C,
found in fresh fruit and vegetables; vitamin E, found in whole grains,
nuts, and seeds and leafy green vegetables; and omega-3 fatty acids,
found in oily fish and seeds such as chia and flax.[374]

Increasing exercise helps to improve pelvic circulatory capacity,[375]
and other approaches such as sitz baths may also be used to increase
the pelvic circulation and reduce congestion.[376]

Functional hormonal imbalance

Functional imbalance of various reproductive hormones may be contributing factors to subfertility in many cases. The function of various
hormones in the body depends on numerous factors, such as: hormone
receptor expression; levels of specific hormone metabolites (some of
which may be more or less active than others); the balance between
different hormones; and the degree to which hormones are bound to
binding globulins. Therefore, when blood tests to measure the levels of
various hormones show them to be within normal ranges, they may still
not be functioning optimally.

Oestrogen

Before menopause, oestradiol, the most potent form of oestrogen, is produced in the ovaries in response to follicle stimulating hormone (FSH)
from the pituitary gland. Oestrone is a less potent form of oestrogen

that is produced by aromatisation of androgens, predominantly in fat cells. Oestrogen is responsible for the development of secondary sexual characteristics in women, lubrication of the vagina, growth of uterine muscle, and thickening of the endometrium in preparation for pregnancy. Both low levels of oestrogen and oestrogen excess can lead to reproductive health problems and reduced fertility.

Low oestrogen levels

In women with low oestrogen levels due to primary ovarian insufficiency, the ovaries do not function normally, leading to a reduction in ovarian oestrogen production.[377] The low oestrogen levels trigger the pituitary gland to increase the secretion of FSH. In women with hypothalamic amenorrhoea, the picture is different. In this case, it is not the ovaries themselves that cause the reduced oestrogen levels, but deficient secretion of gonadotropin-releasing hormone (GnRH) by the hypothalamus, which results in low pituitary secretion of follicle stimulating hormone (FSH), that in turn leads to reduced ovarian oestrogen production.[378] In cases of hypothalamic amenorrhoea, the ovaries themselves are usually healthy, but simply not receiving adequate stimulation.

Symptoms of low oestrogen levels may include irregular or absent periods, hot flushes and night sweats, mood changes, poor concentration, sleep disturbance, reduced libido, vaginal dryness, dry eye syndrome, and changes in skin and hair. In the longer term, low levels of oestrogen can also predispose to cardiovascular disease, osteoporosis, and hypothyroidism.[379]

Improving oestrogen levels

Dioscorea villosa (wild yam), *Tribulus terrestris* (puncture vine), *Asparagus racemosus* (shatavari), and *Trigonella foenum graecum* (fenugreek) contain steroidal saponins such as diosgenin, which compete with endogenous oestrogens for hypothalamic oestrogen receptors. They have a weaker effect on hypothalamic oestrogen receptors than endogenous oestrogen, causing the body to respond as if oestrogen levels are lower than they really are, thus stimulating the pituitary to increase FSH secretion, which in turn increases oestrogen production.[380] Improved levels of FSH also lead to improved ovulation, especially when given on days 5–14.[381]

Lepidium meyenii (maca) can also help to improve ovarian function in women with low oestrogen. Short-term use of maca initially increases secretion of both FSH and LH by the pituitary. This improves ovarian function, and thereby increases production of both oestrogen and progesterone, reducing symptoms associated with low ovarian hormone levels, such as hot flushes, sweating, sleep disturbance, mood changes, joint pains, and heart palpitations.[382] With medium- to longer-term use, the increased oestrogen and progesterone levels lead to a reduction in elevated FSH levels, and an improved LH:FSH ratio.[383]

Adaptogens and adrenal tonics, such as *Withania somnifera* (ashwagandha) improve adrenal function,[384] and may thereby help to increase adrenal reproductive hormone production. *Withania somnifera* has also been shown to increase levels of DHEA, which is essential for oestrogen production in the ovary.[385]

Phytoestrogens are plant based compounds, which include isoflavones (such as genistein, daidzein, and glycitein), coumestans, lignans, and flavonoids. Soybeans are a particularly rich source of isoflavones, and flaxseeds are a good source of lignans. Phytoestrogens have an affinity for oestrogen receptors, and exert a weak oestrogenic effect in comparison to oestradiol.[386] They can help to reduce associated with lower oestrogen levels, with limited side effects.[387] Consumption of phytoestrogens is also associated with lower fracture risk.[388]

Oestrogen excess

Women with conditions such as menorrhagia, endometriosis, fibroids, and oestrogen-dependent cancers, are very likely to have a relative excess of oestrogen, since this is the hormone that is responsible for processes involving cell proliferation. An overactive thyroid also increases conversion of testosterone to oestrogen, which may lead to oestrogen excess.[389]

While these are identifiable medical conditions that are known to be associated with relative oestrogen excess, and may cause infertility, blood tests will still not always show elevated levels of oestrogen. There may be high or high normal levels of oestrogen and/or relatively low levels of FSH due to increased negative feedback, but this is not always the case. The relative activity of oestrogen in the body depends on many factors such as: the levels of specific oestrogen metabolites (some of which may be more or less active than others); the balance between

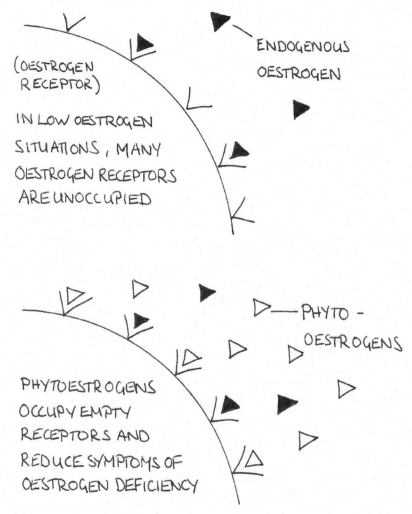

Figure 9: Phytoestrogens in low oestrogen situations.

oestrogen and other hormones (such as FSH and progesterone); the expression of oestrogen receptors; and the degree to which oestrogens are bound to sex hormone-binding globulin.

Sex hormone-binding globulin (SHBG) is a glycoprotein that binds to oestradiol, testosterone, and dihydrotestosterone; and transports these hormones in the blood as biologically inactive forms. Changes in SHBG levels can affect the amount of hormone that is available to be used by the body's tissues. Because of the higher affinity of SHBG for DHT and testosterone, compared to oestrogen, SHBG also affects the balance between bioavailable androgens and oestrogens.

Where blood test results show measurements for "total" rather than "free" levels of other hormones, it is essential to measure SHBG. A high SHBG level means that less free hormones are available to the tissues; whereas a low SHBG level means that more of the total hormone is bioavailable and not bound to SHBG. *SHBG is increased by:* high levels of oestrogen, low levels of testosterone, and nutrient deficiency. Therefore, increased SHBG levels may be seen in:

- Oestrogen dependent conditions (e.g., endometriosis): the increase in SHBG in response to high levels of oestrogen may be designed to help reduce the proliferative effects of oestrogen excess. However, the protective effect of SHBG may be negated by: stress hormones (such as cortisol), growth hormones (such as those found in meat and dairy products), obesity, and insulin resistance.
- Exposure to exogenous oestrogens, such as hormone replacement therapy (HRT), oral contraceptive pills (OCP), and xenoestrogens.
- Hyperthyroidism (which drives oestrogen production), and
- Liver disease (which is associated with higher levels of oestrogen due to decreased conjugation of oestrogen in the liver)

Increased SHBG in women may suggest oestrogen excess, even where total oestrogen levels are within the normal ranges.

Not all women with relative oestrogen excess have an identifiable oestrogen dependent medical condition. Increased exposure to oestrogen is also associated with early menarche, nulliparity, early use of oral contraceptives,[390] larger breast size,[391] and abdominal obesity (characterised by an increased waist to hip ratio).[392] Therefore women are often diagnosed with relative oestrogen excess based on their clinical presentation, even where blood test results do not show elevated levels of oestrogen.

Functional hormone imbalance may also be suggested by symptoms associated with premenstrual syndrome (PMS).[393] The oestrogen/progesterone ratio imbalance theory proposes that in women with PMS, oestrogen levels are too high in relation to the level of progesterone.[394]

Relative oestrogen excess may increase feelings of irritability, aggressiveness, and anxiety by increasing the availability of noradrenaline in the brain.[395] Oestrogen is also involved in the regulation of monoamine oxidase (MAO), the enzyme that breaks down neurotransmitters such as serotonin and dopamine.[396] Oestrogens are also known to increase the renin-angiotensin-aldosterone system and thereby cause fluid retention.[397] Therefore, women with premenstrual mood disturbances and fluid retention who are having difficulty conceiving are likely to have a relative excess of oestrogen.

High levels of oestrogen inhibit secretion of hypothalamic gonadotropin-releasing hormone (GnRH) and other important reproductive hormones such as follicle stimulating hormone (FSH) and luteinising hormone (LH), which are responsible for follicle development and egg release,[398] thereby contributing to infertility. The anti-oestrogenic drug clomiphene citrate (Clomid) is used in orthodox medicine to increase the release of FSH.[399] This suggests that therapeutic measures, which reduce relative oestrogen excess, may be beneficial in the treatment of infertility in women with symptoms of oestrogen dominance.

Reducing relative oestrogen excess

Reduce activity of aromatase

High levels of aromatase activity (the enzyme which catalyses the conversion of androgens to oestrogen) result in increased local oestrogen production.[400] Increased oestrogen induces formation of prostaglandin E2 (PGE2).[401] PGE2 in turn is a potent stimulant of aromatase, which generates more oestrogen.[402] Excessive adipose tissue and high insulin levels (both associated with obesity) are associated with increased aromatase activity.[403] Therefore measures to address obesity and reduce insulin resistance (as discussed in Chapter 1), reduce PGE2 (discussed at the end of this chapter), and directly reduce aromatase activity, can all help to reduce excess oestrogen production.

Linum usitatissimum (linseed) and *Serenoa serrulata* (saw palmetto) are considered to be aromatase inhibitors.[404] Various other foods and herbs have been shown to inhibit aromatase, including: *Camellia sinensis* (green tea), *Curcuma longa* (turmeric), *Tanacetum parthenium* (feverfew), *Taraxacum officinale* (dandelion leaves), *Trifolium pratense* (red clover), *Viscum album* (mistletoe), *Vitis* spp. (grape seed extract), asparagus, bell peppers, broccoli, collard greens, kale, celery, endive, escarole, chanterelle, portobello, shiitake, and white button mushrooms, onion, citrus fruits (such as oranges) and their juices, and strawberries.[405]

Reduce exposure to environmental xenoestrogens

Environmental oestrogen-like chemicals (xenoestrogens), which are found in food contaminants (such as pesticides and plastic residues), may have an oestrogenic effect, and are increasingly implicated in cases of infertility.[406] Non-organic meat and dairy products can also contain high levels of xenoestrogens.[407] Patients are advised to avoid eating food that has been stored or heated in plastic packaging, to avoid using pesticides in the garden, to buy organic produce where possible, and to peel or scrub any non-organic fruit and vegetables. It is also advisable to take a vitamin B complex supplement, since vitamin B deficiency seems to increase susceptibility to the effects of excess oestrogen.[408]

Improve hepatic metabolism of oestrogen

Oestradiol is metabolised by the liver in two phases. Phase 1 (hydroxylation) is catalysed by cytochrome P450 enzymes. The addition of a hydroxyl (-OH) leads to the formation of hydroxyoestrone metabolites, *2-hydroxyoestrone*, *4-hydroxyoestrone*, and *16-α-hydroxyoestrone*. *2-hydroxyoestrone* has low binding affinity for oestrogen receptors and is associated with normal cell differentiation, decreased cell proliferation, and apoptosis (and therefore has a protective effect in oestrogen-dependent conditions), whereas *4-hydroxyoestrone* causes oxidative damage, and has been implicated in the development of oestrogen-dependent conditions, including cancer.[409]

16-α-hydroxyoestrone is another potent form of oestrogen, which increases endometrial thickness and promotes growth of fibroids. Women with breast cancer have increased levels of 16-α-hydroxyoestrone, and lower levels of 2-hydroxyoestrone.[410,411]

Inducers of phase 1 liver metabolism of oestrogen (hydroxylation) include *Curcuma longa* (turmeric), *Hypericum perforatum* (St John's wort), and *Schisandra chinensis* (schisandra berry). Resveratrol (from berries, grapes, and red wine), cruciferous (brassica) vegetables, green tea, and soya are phase 1 inducers which tend to favour metabolism of oestradiol to form the more protective *2-hydroxyoestrone*, rather than more harmful *16-α-hydroxyoestrone*. 10–25 mg a day of linseed has also been shown to significantly reduce relative formation of 16-α-hydroxyoestrone. Conversely, environmental xenoestrogens are more likely to be metabolised to form the more harmful *16-α-hydroxyoestrone*.[412,413]

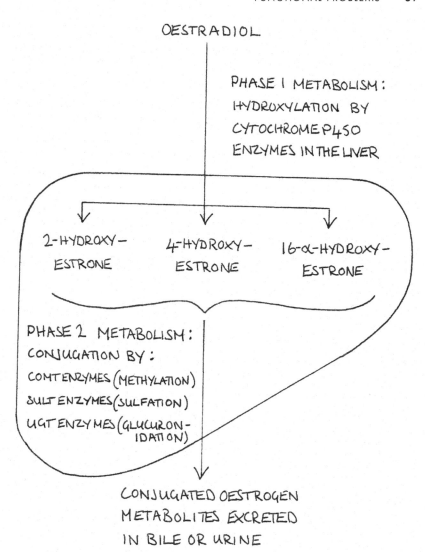

OESTRADIOL

PHASE 1 METABOLISM:
HYDROXYLATION BY
CYTOCHROME P450
ENZYMES IN THE LIVER

2-HYDROXY-
ESTRONE

4-HYDROXY-
ESTRONE

16-α-HYDROXY-
ESTRONE

PHASE 2 METABOLISM:
CONJUGATION BY:
COMT ENZYMES (METHYLATION)
SULT ENZYMES (SULFATION)
UGT ENZYMES (GLUCURON-
                    IDATION)

CONJUGATED OESTROGEN
METABOLITES EXCRETED
IN BILE OR URINE

Figure 10: Hepatic metabolism of oestrogen.

During Phase 2 liver metabolism (conjugation), hydroxyestrone intermediates are detoxified by the addition of methyl groups (methylation), sulphate groups (sulfation), or glucuronides (glucuronidation). Phase 2 metabolites are water soluble and inactive, and may be excreted in the bile or urine. However, effective phase 2 metabolism of oestrogen may be inhibited by gene mutations affecting the enzymes that catalyse conjugation reactions, such as catechol-O-methyltransferase (COMT). Phase 2 metabolism may also be inhibited by lack of co-factors necessary for conjugation of oestrogen (such as vitamins B2, B6, B12, magnesium, zinc); or excess use of methyl-depleting nutrients (such as niacin).

Foods high in methionine (such as beans, pulses, onions, and garlic) assist with methylation of oestrogen in the liver, the process by which oestradiol is converted into the less potent oestriol. B complex vitamins are also necessary for the hepatic metabolism of oestrogens.[414] In addition, phase 2 metabolism and elimination of oestrogen is improved by consumption of cruciferous vegetables (such as cabbage, broccoli, and kale),[415] resveratrol (from berries, grapes and red wine), *Rosmarinus officinalis* (rosemary) and *Schisandra chinensis* (schisandra berry).[416]

Entero-hepatic recirculation of oestrogen

Once oestrogen has been excreted in the bile into the intestine, it may be excreted from the body. However, the story does not always end there. Beta-glucuronidase enzymes, which are produced by intestinal bacteria, may deconjugate oestrogen, allowing it to be reabsorbed into the bloodstream. This is known as entero-hepatic recirculation. Consumption of saturated animal fats encourages the growth of beta-glucuronidase-producing bacteria, while probiotic bacteria such as *Lactobacillus acidophilus* reduce it.[417] Probiotic bacteria are found in foods such as sauerkraut, or may be taken as a supplement.[418]

Constipation also contributes to entero-hepatic recirculation of oestrogen, by allowing more time for bacterial deconjugation and reabsorption. Adequate fluid intake and fibre contained in whole grains, fruit, and vegetables reduces excess oestrogen levels, by reducing constipation and preventing oestrogens that have been excreted in the bile from being reabsorbed. Women who eat more fibre consequently have a lower risk of infertility.[419]

Phytoestrogens

Phytoestrogens, found in soybean products, and to a lesser extent, other beans and pulses, whole-grain cereals, nuts, and seeds, are plant compounds such as isoflavones (such as geniestein and daidzein, mainly found in legumes) and lignans (mainly found in flax and other seeds), which are structurally and functionally similar to human oestrogens.

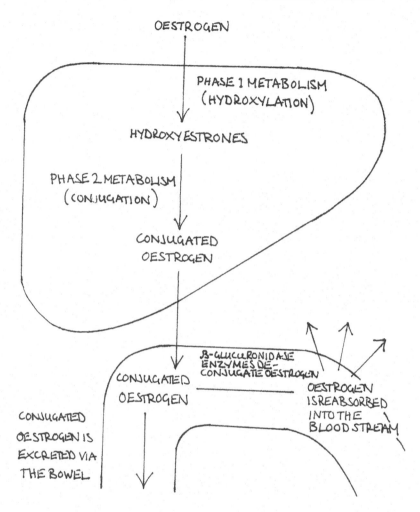

Figure 11: Enterohepatic recirculation of oestrogen.

They bind weakly to oestrogen receptors, competing with endogenous oestrogens and preventing them from exerting stronger oestrogenic effects.[420]

Phytoestrogens may also reduce aromatisation of androstenedione to oestrone in fat cells, and stimulate liver production of sex hormone-binding globulin (SHBG), which binds to excess oestrogen, reducing its ability to bind to hormone-sensitive tissues.[421] In order to be absorbed from the digestive system, isoflavones must first undergo hydrolysis

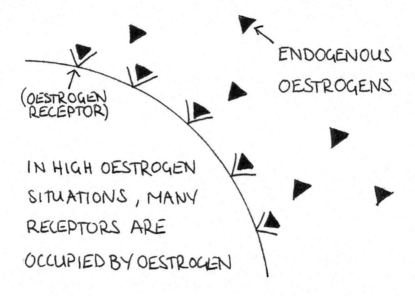

ENDOGENOUS OESTROGENS

(OESTROGEN RECEPTOR)

IN HIGH OESTROGEN
SITUATIONS, MANY
RECEPTORS ARE
OCCUPIED BY OESTROGEN

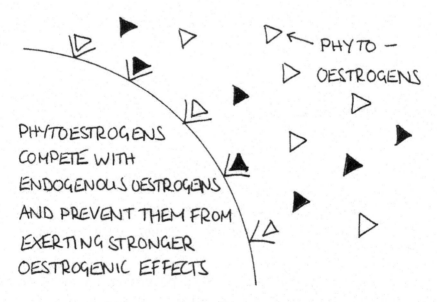

PHYTO – OESTROGENS

PHYTOESTROGENS
COMPETE WITH
ENDOGENOUS OESTROGENS
AND PREVENT THEM FROM
EXERTING STRONGER
OESTROGENIC EFFECTS

Figure 12: Phytoestrogens in high oestrogen situations.

of the sugar moiety by ß-glucosidase enzymes,[422] which are produced by bifidobacteria in the intestine. Therefore, the efficacy of dietary phytoestrogens varies between different individuals depending on their gut flora. Consuming fermented soya products or taking a probiotic supplement may help to enhance the bioavailability of isoflavones.[423]

In summary, excess oestrogen levels may be reduced by using foods, herbs, and supplements which assist its metabolism and excretion,

Reducing oestrogen excess

Reduce exposure to xenoestrogens	• Avoid pesticides and plastic residues • Avoid consumption of non-organic meat and dairy products
Reduce aromatase activity	• Improve insulin sensitivity (low GI diet) • Reduce body fat • Reduce PGE2 (reduce animal fats and increase fish oils, starflower oil) • Linseeds • *Serenoa serrulata*
Improve 2:16-α-hydroxyoestrone ratio during phase 1 hepatic metabolism of oestrogen	• Brassica vegetables • Resveratrol • Green tea • Soya • Avoid xenoestrogens
Improve phase 2 metabolism (conjugation of oestrogen)	• Methionine-containing foods (beans, pulses, alliums) • Indole-3-carbinol—containing foods (cruciferous vegetables) • Resveratrol (grapes, berries) • *Rosmarinus officinalis, Schisandra chinensis* • Vitamin B complex • Magnesium, zinc
Prevent entero-hepatic recirculation of oestrogen	• Reduce consumption of animal fats • Prebiotics and probiotics • Reduce constipation (increase dietary fibre and fluid intake)
Inhibit endogenous oestrogens	• Dietary phytoestrogens

by increasing consumption of organic vegetables, beans, pulses, seeds, and wholegrain cereals, and by avoiding consumption of meat and dairy products. Indeed, women who eat a vegetarian diet excrete more oestrogen than women who eat meat and have a lower risk of infertility.[424]

Progesterone

Progesterone is predominantly produced by the corpus luteum after ovulation, in response to stimulation by LH from the pituitary gland. Its main function is to prepare the endometrium for fertilisation; and if this occurs, to maintain the endometrium during early pregnancy and inhibit uterine contractions that would otherwise result in pregnancy loss. It also stimulates glandular changes in breast tissue in preparation for lactation, and helps to counterbalance the effects of high levels of oestrogen by down-regulating the expression of oestrogen receptors.[425]

Any condition that results in anovulation will lead to low progesterone levels. In women who have no underlying medical condition, and who are ovulating, the corpus luteum may not produce sufficient levels of progesterone, or may not produce it for long enough, leading to a shortened luteal phase. Progesterone is readily converted to other hormones, including stress hormones. Therefore, stress can significantly reduce progesterone levels by favouring production of stress hormones.[426] Progesterone deficiency causes inadequate development of the endometrium leading to infertility and increasing the risk of early pregnancy loss.[427] The duration of progesterone secretion and the maximum serum progesterone concentration during the luteal phase have been shown to be significantly less in patients with unexplained infertility than in fertile controls.[428,429]

Blood tests to measure progesterone should be performed approximately 7 days before the next expected period. This would be day 21 for a woman with a 28-day cycle, but the timing should be adjusted for women who experience shorter or longer cycles. Very low levels of progesterone (<3 nmol/L) suggest anovulation, and levels below 30 nmol/L are generally insufficient for successful implantation or to sustain a pregnancy. However, even where blood test results show adequate levels of progesterone, factors such as the ratio of various progesterone metabolites and receptor sensitivity may affect fertility.[430] Symptoms such as dysfunctional uterine bleeding, cyclic breast disorders, and premenstrual mood changes may suggest progesterone deficiency.[431]

The ratio of progesterone and its derivatives to other hormones is often lower than usual in PMS sufferers.[432] PMS patients have been shown to have an increased number of LH pulses, together with a reduced amplitude and duration, which may suggest inefficient pituitary stimulation of progesterone secretion.[433]

Some studies have found higher levels of progesterone, or both oestradiol and progesterone in women with PMS.[434,435] In this case, premenstrual syndrome may be due to the progesterone receptors, which do not transport sufficient progesterone into the cell, rather than with the actual progesterone concentration.[436] It is also possible that symptoms may be due to altered progesterone metabolism, rather than total progesterone levels.[437]

For example, progesterone is a precursor of aldosterone, which causes retention of sodium and water.[438] Increased conversion of progesterone

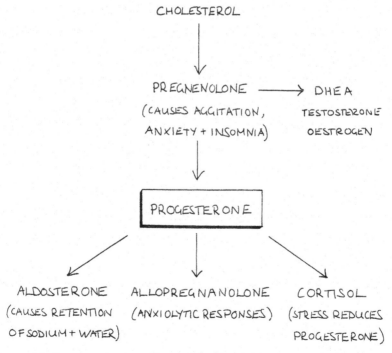

Figure 13: Progesterone and its metabolites.

to aldosterone may therefore result in fluid retention. Allopregnanolone is another important metabolite of progesterone, which is responsible for GABA(A)-mediated anxiolytic responses in stressful conditions. Several studies have demonstrated reduced levels of allopregnanolone in the luteal phase in PMS patients.[439,440] Conversely, women with PMS may have increased levels of pregnenolone (a precursor of progesterone), which acts as a GABA receptor antagonist and leads to agitation, anxiety, and insomnia.[441] Pregnenolone is also a precursor of DHEA, testosterone, and oestradiol.[442]

Since decreased progesterone levels may in turn lead to retarded endometrial development, therapeutic measures that improve progesterone function and metabolism may be beneficial in the treatment of infertility.

Improving progesterone function

Vitex agnus castus addresses a wide range of problems such as premenstrual mood disturbance, fluid retention, and mastalgia due to poor progesterone function and hyperprolactinaemia.[443,444,445] It is thought to inhibit prolactin release from the anterior pituitary, which leads to an increase in luteinising hormone (LH), promoting corpus luteum development in the luteal phase, and thereby increasing levels of progesterone.[446] Other herbs that are thought to improve progesterone function include *Achillea millefolium, Alchemilla vulgaris*,[447] and *Paeonia lactiflora*. In fact, *Paeonia lactiflora* is thought to have a regulating effect on a variety of hormones including oestrogen, androgens, progesterone, and prolactin.[448]

Lepidium meyenii (maca) increases secretion of both FSH and LH by the pituitary. This improves ovarian function, and thereby increases production of both oestrogen and progesterone.[449] Adaptogens and adrenal tonics, such as *Withania somnifera*, improve adrenal function,[450] and may thereby help to increase adrenal production of progesterone and its metabolites.

Vitamin E supplements may correct an abnormal progesterone/oestradiol ratio.[451] Vitamin E is also found in whole grains, green leafy vegetables, nuts, and seeds.[452]

Magnesium helps to decrease conversion of progesterone to aldosterone. It is found in soya products, whole-grain cereals, seeds, and leafy green vegetables. Adaptogens and adrenal tonics improve adrenal function,[453] and may thereby help to increase adrenal production of progesterone and its metabolites. They include herbs such as *Eleuthero-coccus senticosus*, *Withania somnifera*, and *Glycyrrhiza glabra*.

Cortisol

In stressful situations, the hypothalamus secretes corticotropin-releasing hormone (CRH). CRH then triggers release of adrenocortico-tropic hormone (ACTH) from the pituitary, which in turn stimulates release of cortisol from the adrenal glands.

High levels of cortisol

High levels of cortisol may be caused by stress, steroid use, high levels of oestrogen, or by tumours of the pituitary or adrenal glands (Cushing's syndrome). Signs and symptoms of high cortisol levels include cogni-tive difficulties, mood changes, and raised blood pressure. Chronically raised cortisol levels lead to central obesity, a rounded face, fat pad on the upper back, acne, hirsutism, thin or fragile skin that bruises easily, striae on the skin, and bone loss.

Raised cortisol levels are associated with high neutrophils, low eosinophils, and increased plasma fasting glucose. High cortisol also leads to decreases in sex hormone-binding globulin (SHBG), which binds to reproductive hormones and renders them inactive. Therefore, high cortisol levels can worsen problems caused by oestrogen excess. (Note higher levels of oestrogen can lead to raised cortisol, and in turn, raised cortisol can worsen oestrogen dependent conditions by reducing SHBG, leading to a vicious circle effect.)

Low cortisol levels

Low cortisol levels may be caused by pituitary or adrenal insufficiency (Addison's disease). Signs and symptoms of low cortisol levels include low blood pressure, depression, fatigue, allergies, loss of body hair, and hyperpigmentation. Cortisol activity is also thought to be low in women with depression and fatigue.[454]

Low cortisol levels are associated with high eosinophils and low fasting glucose. Low glucose levels (*hypoglycaemia*) in turn may be associated with symptoms such as palpitations, sweating, anxiety, and fainting (due to increased epinephrine levels) or lethargy, confusion, slurred speech, and convulsions (due to neuroglycopaenia).

"Adrenal fatigue" is a term often used by alternative healthcare practitioners to describe patients who present with exhaustion and other symptoms similar to those associated with low cortisol levels, following a period of high stress. Persistent stress and associated chronically raised cortisol levels are thought to result in exhaustion and atrophy of the adrenal glands. This theory, known as the general adaptation syndrome, was first described by Hans Seyle in 1950.[455]

However, in more recent research, patients with symptoms of "adrenal fatigue" have not been found to have low cortisol levels or adrenal gland atrophy.[456] So how do we reconcile the research evidence that shows that "adrenal fatigue" does not exist, with the reality that patients who have experienced a prolonged period of high stress often present with exhaustion and other symptoms similar to those associated with low cortisol levels?

One possible explanation is that rather than leading to adrenal atrophy and low cortisol levels, chronic stress (which is associated with persistent cortisol secretion), over time may lead to *cortisol resistance*; in much the same way as frequent consumption of high glycaemic load foods (associated with persistent insulin secretion), over time leads to insulin resistance.

Low cortisol levels result in an increase in CRH as a result of reduced negative feedback, which in turn inhibits hypothalamic gonadotropin-releasing hormone secretion,[457] and may therefore contribute to infertility. It is possible that cortisol resistance would have the same effect.

Treating raised cortisol and cortisol resistance

Herbal treatment for cortisol resistance includes nervine tonics such as *Hypericum perforatum*, and relaxing nervines such *Anemone pulsatilla*, *Matricaria recutita*, and *Melissa officinalis* to decrease levels of stress. Adrenal adaptogens such as *Eleutherococcus senticosus* and *Withania somnifera* increase the individual's ability to adapt to various environmental factors, and to avoid the damage they may cause.[458] *Glycyrrhiza glabra* is an adrenal tonic, which is thought to increase production of steroid hormones by the adrenal gland, mimic the activity of cortisol, and prolong its activity by reducing its breakdown.[459]

Cortisol is required for the conversion of glycogen to glucose. When cortisol activity is low, insufficient glucose may be released, leading to hypoglycaemia.[460] It is therefore important to eat small frequent meals in order to maintain stable blood sugar levels and avoid further stress. It is also important to avoid consumption of coffee, which increases the rate at which energy is consumed, leading to increased demands on the adrenal glands.[461]

Prolactin

Hyperprolactinaemia refers to elevated levels of prolactin, the pituitary hormone responsible for breast development and lactation.[462] Hyperprolactinaemia may be caused by pituitary trauma, chest wall trauma, stress, various medications (especially those affecting dopamine levels),[463] hypoglycaemia,[464] autoimmune disease, and low thyroid function.[465]

Prolactin levels are frequently higher in women with functional infertility,[466] even where they may not necessarily exceed the normal reference range. Higher concentrations of prolactin inhibit progesterone and reduce oestrogen levels by inhibiting the activity of aromatase (the enzyme which catalyses the conversion of androgens to oestrogen).[467]

Prolactin is thought to contribute to some of the symptoms of PMS, particularly mastalgia and fluid retention.[468,469] Some studies have also identified increased anger and aggression in women with higher levels of prolactin.[470] In women whose prolactin levels fall within reference ranges, symptoms are thought to be due to an excessive sensitivity to normal prolactin levels, or "latent hyperprolactinaemia".[471] Several studies have shown relief from both premenstrual symptoms and infertility using prolactin antagonists such as bromocriptine.[472]

Reducing prolactin levels

Therapeutic measures that reduce prolactin may also help to improve fertility. For example, *Vitex agnus castus* has been shown to increase conception in infertile women with hyperprolactinaemia and luteal phase dysfunction.[473,474] It increases dopamine, which lowers levels of prolactin.[475]

Salvia officinalis has been traditionally used to decrease production of breast milk.[476] It binds to GABA receptors,[477] increases dopamine, and inhibits prolactin synthesis and release.[478] *Cimicifuga racemosa* also has a dopaminergic action, which inhibits prolactin release.[479]

Deficiencies of vitamin B6, magnesium, and zinc are associated with low dopamine and raised prolactin.[480] Therefore supplementing these nutrients may help to improve dopamine synthesis,[481] and thereby reduce hyperprolactinaemia.

Increasing prostaglandin E1 (PGE1) helps to counteract the effects of higher prolactin levels.[482] Vitamin B6 and zinc are necessary co-factors in the production of series-1 prostaglandins. Vitamin E can also positively influence prostaglandin ratios. Essential fatty acid supplements such as evening primrose or starflower oil contain linolenic and gamma linolenic acid, which increase PGE1.[483]

Since stress affects prolactin levels, stress management and relaxation techniques may be useful for reducing elevated prolactin levels in conjunction with herbal medicine and nutritional supplements.[484]

Stress

In stressful situations, the hypothalamus secretes corticotropin-releasing hormone (CRH). CRH then triggers release of adrenocorticotropic hormone (ACTH) from the pituitary, which in turn stimulates release cortisol from the adrenal glands. High cortisol leads to decreases in sex hormone-binding globulin (SHBG), which binds to reproductive hormones and renders them inactive. Therefore, high cortisol levels can worsen problems caused by oestrogen excess.

Stress also causes the body to increase production of epinephrine (adrenalin), which causes blood to be drawn away from the uterus,[485] and prevents the uptake of progesterone by progesterone receptors.[486] When adrenaline is continuously elevated, production of both oestrogen and thyroid hormones are reduced.[487] There is also considerable evidence that stress alters prolactin levels. All of these effects on various reproductive hormones can lead to infertility.[488] According to TCM theory, stress may be indicated by a rapid, tense, or wiry pulse, a red tongue tip and/or a swelling along centre crack of the tongue.[489]

Aside from stresses caused by work, relationship issues, trauma, or other physical, mental, or emotional challenges, the stress associated with trying to conceive may itself also negatively affect fertility.[490] When a couple experiences stress when trying to conceive, lovemaking can lose its spontaneity. However, research has shown that the more enjoyable the lovemaking, the more likely the woman will be to retain the sperm, especially if she has an orgasm. The contractions caused by the orgasm draw in more sperm, and it is thought that arousal may make the vagina less acidic, increasing the rate of sperm survival.[491]

Reducing the effects of stress

In conjunction with stress management techniques, the herbal and dietary management of stress involves reducing the adverse effects of stress with nervine tonics and sedatives, as well as improving the body's capacity to adapt to stress with herbal adaptogens.[492] *Hypericum perforatum* is a nervine tonic, which is thought to inhibit monoamine oxidase (MAO).[493] In addition to reducing the effects of stress it may also help to reduce oestrogen excess, since monoamine oxidase activity is positively correlated with the progesterone to oestradiol ratio.[494] Nervine sedatives include *Anemone pulsatilla*, *Leonurus cardiaca*, *Matricaria recutita*, and *Melissa officinalis*, while herbal adaptogens include *Eleutherococcus senticosus* and *Withania somnifera*. B vitamins and magnesium also help to reduce tension and to improve sleep patterns.[495]

Relaxation or stress management techniques may also be useful for reducing the effects of stress.[496] Other types of stress management could include meditation or yoga.[497] Social activities, such as dancing and relaxing with friends may be useful if the idea of meditating is unappealing.[498] Acupuncture also significantly alleviates depression, anxiety, and stress, by modulating both specific and non-specific neurological signalling and affecting stress hormones such as cortisol, prolactin, and epinephrine and beta endorphin.[499]

Prostaglandin imbalance

Prostaglandin E2 (PGE2) causes inflammation,[500] increased uterine muscle spasm, and uterine ischaemia;[501] and significantly higher concentrations of PGE2 are found in the endometrium and menstrual fluid of women with dysmenorrhoea.[502] Abnormal response to prostaglandins may also lead to premenstrual aches and pains (hyperalgesia) and menstrual migraine.[503] High oestrogen levels can increase series 2 prostaglandins such as PGE2, while low progesterone levels decrease resistance to prostaglandin-induced uterine spasm.[504]

An aberrant uterine response to PGE2 has been demonstrated in women with functional infertility. In fertile women, PGE2 inhibits uterine motility, whereas in women with functional infertility, it causes marked uterine stimulation.[505] It is possible that the aberrant response to PGE2 may be responsible for failure of implantation due to uterine stimulation. Therefore therapeutic measures to reduce PGE2 synthesis and uterine stimulation may improve the chance of conception in women with symptoms of hyperalgesia.

Nutrition and supplements to reduce PGE2

Prostaglandin E2 (PGE2) is synthesised from arachiodonic acid found in animal fats.[506] Therefore, reducing consumption of animal fats and increasing intake of raw vegetable and seed oils selectively decreases dietary precursors of series 2 prostaglandins, and increases series 1 prostaglandins, which have anti-inflammatory, anti-thrombotic, and anti-spasmodic effects.

Essential fatty acid supplements such as evening primrose or starflower oil contain linolenic and gamma linolenic acid, which increase PGE1.[507] Vitamin E can also positively influence prostaglandin ratios; and vitamin B6 and zinc are necessary co-factors in the production of series 1 prostaglandins. Reducing oestrogen excess (as discussed above) can also reduce series 2 prostaglandins.[508]

Herbs that regulate prostaglandin synthesis and reduce uterine stimulation

Zingiber officinale has been shown to reduce the production of prostaglandin E, and thereby reduce excessive uterine contractions.[509] *Angelica sinensis* is also thought to regulate prostaglandin synthesis.[510]

Uterine spasmolytics such as *Anemone pulsatilla*, *Paeonia lactiflora*, *Viburnum prunifolium*, and *Viburnum opulus* may be useful for dysmenorrhoea with intermittent cramping pains. Magnesium may also help to decrease uterine cramping.[511] It is found in foods such as soya products, whole-grain cereals, seeds, and green leafy vegetables.[512] Herbs which are warming, such as *Zingiber officinale* and *Cinnamonum zeylonicum* improve the action of the antispasmodic herbs, especially when the period pain is aggravated by cold, relieved by warmth, or the woman has a tendency to "feel the cold" easily.

The uterine tonics, such as *Angelica sinensis* and *Rubus idaeus* are also used to treat dysmenorrhoea because they are believed to regulate the activity of the uterus and help initiate contractions which are regular, rhythmic, and more orderly, as previously discussed in the section on blood flow.

Summary of functional diagnoses and treatment

Diagnosis	Symptoms	Examples of herbs used	Other recommendations
Poor circulation	Poor peripheral circulation and dysmenorrhoea	*Achillea millefolium, Angelica sinensis, Cinnamomum zeylonicum, Rosmarinus officinalis, Viburnum* spp. *Zingiber officinale*	Magnesium, vitamin B3, C, E, omega-3. Increase consumption of wholegrains, nuts, seeds, and leafy green vegetables. Increase exercise
Oestrogen deficiency	Amenorrhoea/oligo-menorrhoea, hot flushes, night sweats, mood changes, sleep disturbance, vaginal dryness	*Asparagus racemosus, Dioscorea villosa, Lepidium meyenii, Tribulus terrestris, Trigonella foenum graecum*	Dietary phytoestrogens (soya products, wholegrains, nuts, seeds, and beans)
Oestrogen dominance and progesterone insufficiency	PMS, endometriosis, fibroids, larger breast size, abdominal obesity	*Achillea millefolium, Alchemilla vulgaris, Paeonia lactiflora, Rosmarinus officinalis, Schisandra chinensis, Serenoa serrulata, Vitex agnus-castus, Withania somnifera*	Take probiotics, B vitamins, vitamin E, magnesium, zinc & green tea. Eat green leafy vegetables, oily fish, phytoestrogens. Avoid meat & dairy products, & xenoestrogens
Raised cortisol and cortisol resistance	Depression and fatigue	*Hypericum perforatum, Anemone pulsatilla, Melissa officinalis, Eleutherococcus senticosus, Withania somnifera, Glycyrrhiza glabra*	Measures to reduce stress. Avoid coffee and refined sugar. Eat small regular meals to balance blood sugar levels

(Continued)

Summary of functional diagnoses and treatment (Continued)

Diagnosis	Symptoms	Examples of herbs used	Other recommendations
Latent hyperprolactin-aemia	PMS, mastalgia, and fluid retention	*Comicifuga racemosa, Salvia officinalis, Vitex agnus-castus*	Reduce stress levels. Supplement vitamin B6, E, magnesium, zinc, EFAs
Stress	Overwork, feeling stressed, sleep disturbance, loss of appetite or overeating, swelling along centre crack of the tongue	*Anemone pulsatilla, Hypericum perforatum, Leonurus cardiaca, Matricaria recutita, Melissa officinalis, Eleutherococcus senticosus, Withania somnifera*	Magnesium and B vitamins. Take measures to reduce stress levels such as meditation, yoga, or enjoyable social activities
Abnormal response to prostaglandins	Aches and pains; dysmenorrhoea; headaches and migraines.	*Zingiber officinalis, Angelica sinensis, Viburnum* spp. *Anemone pulsatilla, Paeonia lactiflora*	Avoid animal fats and increase consumption of omega-3 oils from nuts and seeds

Notes

344. Tillotson, A. K. (2001). *The One Earth Herbal Sourcebook*. New York: Kensington.

345. Trickey, R. (2003). *Women, Hormones & the Menstrual Cycle*. Sydney, Australia: Allen & Unwin.

346. Sbaragli, C., Morgante, G., Goracci, A., Hofkens, T., De Leo, V., & Castrogiovanni, P. (2008). Infertility and psychiatric morbidity. *Fertility and Sterility*, 90(6): 2107–2111.

347. Gascoigne, S. (2001). *The Clinical Medicine Guide: A Holistic Perspective*. Clonakilty, Ireland: Jigme.

348. Hoffman, D. (2009). Infertility. [Online]. Available from http://healthy.net/scr/Article.asp?id=1182 (accessed 28 January 2009).

349. Gascoigne, S. (2001). *The Clinical Medicine Guide: A Holistic Perspective*. Clonakilty, Ireland: Jigme.

350. Xiufen, W. (Ed.) (2003). *Traditional Chinese Diagnostics*. Beijing: People's Medical Publishing House.

351. Ward, N. (1995). How successful is the environmental approach to infertility? Foresight Figures [letter]. *Journal of Nutritional & Environmental Medicine*, 5: 205.

352. Zhao, L. Q. (2011). TCM treatment of premature ovarian failure and infertility. *Journal of the Association of Traditional Chinese Medicine (UK)*, 18(1): 22–26.

353. Timonen, S., & Procopé, B. J. (1971). Premenstrual syndrome and physical exercise. *Acta Obstetricia et Gynecologica Scandinavica*, 50(4): 331–337.

354. Wood, M. (2004). *The Practice of Traditional Western Herbalism: Basic Doctrine, Energetics and Classification*. Berkeley, CA: North Atlantic.

355. Trickey, R. (2003). *Women, Hormones & the Menstrual Cycle*. Sydney, Australia: Allen & Unwin.

356. Wood, M. (2004). *The Practice of Traditional Western Herbalism: Basic Doctrine, Energetics and Classification*. Berkeley, CA: North Atlantic.

357. Raine-Fenning, N. J., Campbell, B. K., Kendall, N. R., Clewes, J. S., & Johnson, I. R. (2004). Endometrial and subendometrial perfusion are impaired in women with unexplained infertility. *Human Reproduction*, 19(11): 2605–2614.

358. Bick, R. L., & Hoppensteadt, D. (2005). Recurrent miscarriage syndrome and infertility due to blood coagulation protein/platelet defects: a review and update. *Clinical and Applied Thrombosis/Hemostasis*, 11(1): 1–13.

359. Goswamy, R. K., Williams, G., & Steptoe, P. C. (1988). Decreased uterine perfusion – a cause of infertility. *Human Reproduction*, 3(8): 955–959.

360. Kurjak, A., Kupesic-Urek, S., Schulman, H., & Zalud, I. (1991). Transvaginal color flow Doppler in the assessment of ovarian and uterine blood flow in infertile women. *Fertility and Sterility*, 56(5): 870–873.

361. Takasaki, T., Tamura, H., Taniguchi, K., Asada, H., Taketani, T., Matsuoka, A., Yamagata, Y., Shimamura, K., Morioka, H., & Sugino, N. (2009). Luteal blood flow and luteal function. *Journal of Ovarian Research* [online]. Available from http://ovarianresearch.com/content/2/1/1 (accessed 24 January 2009).

362. Holmes, P. (2007). *The Energetics of Western Herbs: A Materia Medica Integrating Western & Chinese Herbal Therapeutics, Volume 1* (4th edn). Santa Rosa, CA: Snow Lotus.

363. Trickey, R. (2003). *Women, Hormones & the Menstrual Cycle*. Sydney, Australia: Allen & Unwin.

364. Pitchford, P. (2002). *Healing With Whole Foods* (3rd edn). Berkeley, CA: North Atlantic.

365. Trickey, R. (2003). *Women, Hormones & the Menstrual Cycle*. Sydney, Australia: Allen & Unwin.

366. Weiss, R. F. (1988). *Herbal Medicine*. Gothenburg, Sweden: Arcanum.

367. Wood, M. (2004). *The Practice of Traditional Western Herbalism: Basic Doctrine, Energetics and Classification*. Berkeley, CA: North Atlantic.

368. Trickey, R. (2003). *Women, Hormones & the Menstrual Cycle*. Sydney, Australia: Allen & Unwin.

369. Bartram, T. (1995). *Encyclopedia of Herbal Medicine*. Christchurch, UK: Grace.

370. Liu, W., & Gong, C. (2009). Opening the blockage to reproduction: infertility. *Traditional Chinese Medicine Information Page* [online]. Available from http://tcmpage.com/hpinfertility.html (accessed 4 July 2011).

371. Trickey, R. (2003). *Women, Hormones & the Menstrual Cycle*. Sydney, Australia: Allen & Unwin.

372. Liu, W., & Gong, C. (2009). Opening the blockage to reproduction: infertility. *Traditional Chinese Medicine Information Page* [online]. Available from http://tcmpage.com/hpinfertility.html (accessed 4 July 2011).

373. Pole, S. (2006). *Ayurvedic Medicine: The Principles of Traditional Practice*. London: Churchill Livingstone.

374. Weiss, R. F. (1988). *Herbal Medicine*. Gothenburg, Sweden: Arcanum.

375. Timonen, S., & Procopé, B. J. (1971). Premenstrual syndrome and physical exercise. *Acta Obstetricia et Gynecologica Scandinavica, 50*(4): 331–337.

376. Hassan, I. (2010). Abzan (sitz bath): a regime in unani system of medicine. *Articlesbase* [online]. Available from http://articlesbase.com/alternative-medicine-articles/abzan-sitz-bath-a-regime-in-unani-system-of-medicine-2749047.html (accessed 27 March 2012).

377. Trickey, R. (2011). *Women, Hormones and the Menstrual Cycle*. Clifton Hill, Victoria, Australia: Melbourne Holistic Health Group.

378. Leyendecker, G., Wildt, L., & Hansmann, M. (1983). Induction of ovulation with chronic intermittent (pulsatile) administration of Gn-RH in women with hypothalamic amenorrhoea. *Journal of Reproduction and Fertility, 69*: 397–409.

379. National Institutes of Health (2016). Primary ovarian insufficiency. *MedlinePlus* [online]. Available from: https://medlineplus.gov/primaryovarianinsufficiency.html (accessed 15 November 2019).

380. Brice-Ytsma, H., & McDermott, A. (2020). *Herbal Medicine in Treating Gynaecological Conditions*. London: Aeon.

381. Tabakova, P., Dimitrov, M., & Tashkov, B. (2012). Clinical studies on Tribulus terrestris protodioscin in women with endocrine infertility or menopausal syndrome. *Herbpharm USA* [online]. Available from http://scicompdf.se/tiggarnot/tabakova-HerbPharmUSA.pdf (accessed 2 March 2020).

382. Meissner, H. O., Reich-Bilinska, H., Mscisz, A., & Kedzia, B. (2006). Therapeutic effects of pre-gelatinized maca (Lepidium peruvianum chacon) used as a non-hormonal alternative to HRT in perimenopausal women – clinical pilot study. *International Journal of Biomedical Science, 2*(2): 143–159.

383. Meissner, H. O., Kapczynski, W., Mscisz, A., & Lutomski, J. (2005). Use of gelatinized maca (Lepidium peruvianum) in early postmenopausal women. *International Journal of Biomedical Science, 1*(1): 33–45.

384. Tillotson, A. K. (2009). Female infertility. [Online] Available from http://oneearth-herbs.squarespace.com/diseases/female-infertility.html (accessed on 28 January 2009).

385. Lopresti, A. L., Smith, S. J., Malvi, H., & Kodgule, R. (2019). An investigation into the stress-relieving and pharmacological actions of an ashwagandha (*Withania somnifera*) extract. A randomized, double-blind, placebo-controlled study. *Medicine (Baltimore)*, *98*(37): e17186.

386. Dennehy, C. E. (2006). The use of herbs and dietary supplements in gynecology: an evidence-based review. *Journal of Midwifery & Women's Health*, *51*: 402–409.

387. Ye, Y. B., Tang, X. Y., Verbruggen, M. A., & Su, Y. X. (2006). Soy isoflavones attenuate bone loss in early postmenopausal Chinese women: a single-blind randomized, placebo-controlled trial. *European Journal of Nutrition*, *45*: 327–334.

388. Zhang, X., Shu, X.-O., Li, H., Yang, G., Li, Q., Gao, Y.-T., & Zheng, W. (2005). Prospective cohort study of soy food consumption and risk of bone fracture among postmenopausal women. *Archives of Internal Medicine*, *165*(16): 1890–1895.

389. Trickey, R. (2011). *Women, Hormones and the Menstrual Cycle*. Clifton Hill, Victoria, Australia: Melbourne Holistic Health Group.

390. Sohn, G. S., Cho, S. H., Kim, Y. M., Cho, C.-H., Kim, M.-R., Lee, S. R., & Working Group of Society of Uterine Leiomyoma (2018). Current medical treatment of uterine fibroids. *Obstetrics & Gynecology Science*, *61*(2): 192–201.

391. Jemström, H. (1997). Breast size in relation to endogenous hormone levels, body constitution and oral contraceptive use in healthy nulligravid women aged 19–25 years. *American Journal of Epidemiology*, *145*(7): 571–580.

392. Paxton, R. H., King, D. W., Garcia-Prieto, C., Connors, S. K., Hernandez, M., Gor, B. J., & Jones, L. A. (2013). Associations between body size and serum estradiol and sex hormone-binding globulin levels in premenopausal African American women. *Journal of Clinical Endocrinology and Metabolism*, *98*(3): E485–E490.

393. Benedek-Jaszmann, L. J., & Hearn-Sturtevant, M. D. (1976). Premenstrual tension and functional infertility: aetiology and treatment. *The Lancet*, *307*(7969): 1095–1098.

394. Bäckström, T., & Carstensen, H. (1974). Estrogen and progesterone in plasma in relation to premenstrual tension. *Journal of Steroid Biochemistry*, *5*(3): 257–260.

395. Munday, M. R., Brush, M. G., & Taylor, R. W. (1981). Correlations between progesterone, oestradiol and aldosterone levels in the premenstrual syndrome. *Clinical Endocriology*, *14*(1): 1–9.

396. Briggs, M., & Briggs, M. (1972). Relationship between monoamine oxidase activity and sex hormone concentration in human blood plasma. *Journal of Reproduction and Fertility*, *29*: 447–450.

397. Davidson, B. J., Rea, C. D., & Valenzuela, G. J. (1988). Atrial natriuretic peptide, plasma renin activity, and aldosterone in women on estrogen therapy and with premenstrual syndrome *Fertility and Sterility*, *50*(5): 743–746.

398. Greenstein, B., & Wood, D. F. (2006). *The Endocrine System at a Glance* (2nd edn). Oxford: Blackwell.

399. Hughes, E., Brown, J., Collins, J. J., & Vanderkerchove, P. (2000). Clomiphene citrate for unexplained subfertility in women. *Cochrane Database of Systematic Reviews* [online]. Available from http://cochrane.org/reviews/en/ab000057.html (accessed 27 January 2009).

400. Bulun, S. E., Gurates, B., & Fang, Z. (2002). Mechanisms of excessive estrogen forma-
     tion in endometriosis. *Journal of Reproductive Immunology*, *55*(1–2): 21–33.
401. Bulun, S. E., Gurates, B., & Fang, Z. (2002). Mechanisms of excessive estrogen forma-
     tion in endometriosis. *Journal of Reproductive Immunology*, *55*(1–2): 21–33.
402. Bone, K., & Mills, S. (2013). *Principles and Practice of Phytotherapy: Modern Herbal Med-
     icine*. London: Churchill Livingstone.
403. Bone, K., & Mills, S. (2013). *Principles and Practice of Phytotherapy: Modern Herbal Med-
     icine*. London: Churchill Livingstone.
404. Bone, K., & Mills, S. (2013). *Principles and Practice of Phytotherapy: Modern Herbal Med-
     icine*. London: Churchill Livingstone.
405. Balunas, M. J., Su, B., Brueggemeier, R. W., & Kinghorn, A. D. (2011). Natural prod-
     ucts as aromatase inhibitors. *Anti-Cancer Agents in Medicinal Chemistry*, *8*(6): 646–682.
406. Hudson, T. (2008). *Women's Encyclopedia of Natural Medicine*. New York: McGraw Hill.
407. Wetherbee, K. (2004). Infertility: improving the odds. *Herbs for Health* [online]. Avail-
     able from http://cms.herbalgram.org/herbclip/278/review44159.html (accessed
     28 January 2009).
408. Bell, E. (1980). The excretion of a vitamin B6 metabolite and the probability of recur-
     rence of early breast cancer. *European Journal of Cancer*, *16*(2): 297–298.
409. Brice-Ytsma, H., & McDermott, A. (2020). *Herbal Medicine in Treating Gynaecological
     Conditions*. London: Aeon.
410. Bone, K., & Mills, S. (2013). *Principles and Practice of Phytotherapy: Modern Herbal Med-
     icine*. London: Churchill Livingstone.
411. Brice-Ytsma, H., & McDermott, A. (2020). *Herbal Medicine in Treating Gynaecological
     Conditions*. London: Aeon.
412. Bone, K., & Mills, S. (2013). *Principles and Practice of Phytotherapy: Modern Herbal Med-
     icine*. London: Churchill Livingstone.
413. Brice-Ytsma, H., & McDermott, A. (2020). *Herbal Medicine in Treating Gynaecological
     Conditions*. London: Aeon.
414. Trickey, R. (2003). *Women, Hormones & the Menstrual Cycle*. Sydney, Australia: Allen
     & Unwin.
415. Michnocicz, J. J., & Bradlow, H. L. (1991). Altered estrogen metabolism and excretion
     in humans following consumption of indole-3-carbinol. *Nutrition and Cancer*, *16*(1):
     59–66.
416. Bone, K., & Mills, S. (2013). *Principles and Practice of Phytotherapy: Modern Herbal Med-
     icine*. London: Churchill Livingstone.
417. Trickey, R. (2003). *Women, Hormones & the Menstrual Cycle*. Sydney, Australia: Allen
     & Unwin.
418. Pitchford, P. (2002). *Healing with Whole Foods* (3rd edn). Berkeley, CA: North Atlantic.
419. Chavarro, J. E., Rich-Edwards, J. W., Rosner, B. A., & Willett, W. C. (2007). Diet and
     lifestyle in the prevention of ovulatory disorder infertility. *Obstetrics & Gynecology*,
     110(5): 1050–1058.
420. Verheus, M., van Gils, C. H., Keinan-Boker, L., Grace, P. B., Bingham, S. A., & Peeters,
     P. H. M. (2007). Plasma phytoestrogens and subsequent breast cancer risk. *Journal of
     Clinical Oncology*, *25*(6): 648–655.
421. Trickey, R. (2003). *Women, Hormones & the Menstrual Cycle*. Sydney, Australia: Allen
     & Unwin.

422. Setchell, K. D. R., Brown, N. M., Zimmer-Nechemias, L., Brashear, W. T., Wolfe, B. E., Kirschner, A. S., & Heubi, J. E. (2002). Evidence for the lack of absorption of soy iso-flavone glycosides in humans, supporting the crucial role of intestinal metabolism for bioavailability. *American Journal of Clinical Nutrition, 76*(2): 447–453.

423. Tsangalis, D., Wilcox, G., Shah, N. P., & Stojanovska, L. (2005). Bioavailability of iso-flavone phytoestrogens in postmenopausal women consuming soya milk fermented with probiotic bifidobacteria. *British Journal of Nutrition, 93*(6): 867–877.

424. Chavarro, J. E., Rich-Edwards, J. W., Rosner, B. A., & Willett, W. C. (2007). Diet and lifestyle in the prevention of ovulatory disorder infertility. *Obstetrics & Gynecology, 110*(5): 1050–1058.

425. Brice-Ytsma, H., & McDermott, A. (2020). *Herbal Medicine in Treating Gynaecological Conditions.* London: Aeon.

426. Brice-Ytsma, H., & McDermott, A. (2020). *Herbal Medicine in Treating Gynaecological Conditions.* London: Aeon.

427. Li, T. C., Lenton, E. A., Dockery, P., & Cooke, I. D. (1990). A comparison of some clini-cal and endocrinological features between cycles with normal and defective luteal phases in women with unexplained infertility. *Human Reproduction, 5*(7): 805–810.

428. Benedek-Jaszmann L. J., & Hearn-Sturtevant, M. D. (1976). Premenstrual tension and functional infertility: aetiology and treatment. *The Lancet, 307*(7969): 1095–1098.

429. Driessen, F., Kremer, J., Alsbach, G. P. J., & deKroon, R. A. (2005). Serum proges-terone and oestradiol concentrations in women with unexplained infertility. *BJOG: International Journal of Obstetrics and Gynaecology, 87*(7): 619–623.

430. Li, T. C., Lenton, E. A., Dockery, P., & Cooke, I. D. (1990). A comparison of some clini-cal and endocrinological features between cycles with normal and defective luteal phases in women with unexplained infertility. *Human Reproduction, 5*(7): 805–810.

431. Ford, O., Mol, B., & Roberts, H. (2006). Progesterone for premenstrual syndrome. *The Cochrane Library* [online]. Available from http://onlinelibrary.wiley.com/doi/10.1002/14651858.CD003415/full (accessed 2 January 2012).

432. Ford, O., Mol, B., & Roberts, H. (2006). Progesterone for premenstrual syndrome. *The Cochrane Library* [online]. Available from http://onlinelibrary.wiley.com/doi/10.1002/14651858.CD003415/full (accessed 2 January 2012).

433. Facchinetti, F., Genazzani, A. D., Martignoni, E., Fioroni, L., Sances, G., & Genazzani A. R. (1990). Neuroendocrine correlates of premenstrual syndrome: changes in the pulsatile pattern of plasma LH. *Psychoneuroendocrinology, 15*(4): 269–277.

434. O'Brien, P. M. S., Selby, C., & Symonds, E. M. (1980) Progesterone, fluid, and electro-lytes in premenstrual syndrome. *British Medical Journal, 280*(6224): 1161–1163.

435. Redei, E., & Freeman, E. W. (1995). Daily plasma oestradiol and progesterone levels over the menstrual cycle and their relation to premenstrual symptoms. *Psychoneuro-endocrinology, 20*(3): 259–267.

436. Dalton, K. (1990). The aetiology of premenstrual syndrome is with the progesterone receptors. *Medical Hypotheses, 31*(4): 323–327.

437. Beers, M. H., & Berkow, R. (1999). *The Merck Manual of Diagnosis and Therapy.* Kenilworth, NJ: Merck.

438. Munday, M. R., Brush, M. G., & Taylor, R. W. (1981) Correlations between proges-terone, oestradiol and aldosterone levels in the premenstrual syndrome. *Clinical Endocriology, 14*(1): 1–9.

439. Lombardi, I., Luisi, S., Quirici, B., Monteleone, P., Bernardi, F., Liut, M., Casaresa, E., Palumbo, M., Petraglia, F., & Genazzini, A. R. (2004). Adrenal response to adrenocorticotropic hormone stimulation in patients with premenstrual syndrome. *Gynecological Endocrinology, 18*(2): 79–87.

440. Monteleone, P., Luisi, S., Tonetti, A., Bernardi, F., Genazzini, A. D., Luisi, M., Petraglia, F., & Genazzini, A. R. (2000). Allopregnanolone concentrations and premenstrual syndrome. *European Journal of Endocrinology, 142*(3): 269–273.

441. Meleran, S. E., Reus, V. I., Webster, R., Shafton, R., & Wolkowitz, O. M. (2003). Chronic pregnenolone effects in normal humans: attenuation of benzodiazepine-induced sedation. *Psychoneuroendocrinology, 29*(4): 486–500.

442. Greenstein, B., & Wood, D. F. (2006). *The Endocrine System at a Glance* (2nd edn). Oxford: Blackwell.

443. Berger, D., Schaffner, W., Schrader, E., Meier, B., &Brattström, A. (2000). Efficacy of Vitex agnus castus L. extract Ze 440 in patients with pre-menstrual syndrome (PMS). *Archives of Gynecology and Obstetrics, 264*(3): 150–153.

444. Gardiner, P. (2000). Chasteberry (*Vitex agnus castus*). *The Longwood Herbal Taskforce* [online]. Available from http://longwoodherbal.org/vitex/vitex.pdf (accessed 28 February 2012).

445. Schellenberg, R. (2001). Treatment for the premenstrual syndrome with agnus castus fruit extract: prospective, randomised, placebo controlled study. *British Medical Journal, 322*(7279): 134–137.

446. Milowicz, A., & Jedrzejuk, D. (2006). Premenstrual syndrome: from etiology to treatment. *Maturitas, 55*(1): s47–s54.

447. Lapraz, J. C. (2008). *Clinical Phytotherapy and Osteoporosis*. London: British Endobiogenic Medicine Society.

448. Trickey, R. (2003). *Women, Hormones & the Menstrual Cycle*. Sydney, Australia: Allen & Unwin.

449. Meissner, H. O., Reich-Bilinska, H., Mscisz, A., & Kedzia, B. (2006). Therapeutic effects of pre-gelatinized maca (Lepidium peruvianum chacon) used as a non-hormonal alternative to HRT in perimenopausal women – clinical pilot study. *International Journal of Biomedical Science, 2*(2): 143–159.

450. Tillotson, A. K. (2009). Female infertility. [Online] Available from http://oneearth-herbs.squarespace.com/diseases/female-infertility.html (accessed 28 January 2009).

451. London, R. S., Sundaram, G. S., Schultz, M., & Nair, P. P. (1981). Endocrine parameters and alpha-tocopherol therapy of patients with mammary dysplasia. *Cancer Research, 41*(9, Pt 2): 3811–3813.

452. Pitchford, P. (2002). *Healing with Whole Foods* (3rd edn). Berkeley, CA: North Atlantic.

453. Tillotson, A. K. (2009). Female infertility. [Online] Available from http://oneearth-herbs.squarespace.com/diseases/female-infertility.html (accessed 28 January 2009).

454. Odber, J., Cawood, E. H., & Bancroft, J. (1998). Salivary cortisol in women with and without perimenstrual mood changes. *Journal of Psychosomatic Research, 45*(6): 557–568.

455. Seyle, H. (1950). Stress and the general adaptation syndrome. *British Medical Journal, 1*(4667): 1383–1392.

456. Cadegiani, F. A., & Kater, C. E. (2016). Adrenal fatigue does not exist: a systematic review. *BMC Endocrine Disorders, 16*(1): 48.

457. Chrousos, G. P., Torpy, D. J., & Gold, P. W. (1998). Interactions between the hypothalamic-pituitary-adrenal axis and the female reproductive system: clinical implications. *Annals of Internal Medicine, 129*(3): 229–240.

458. Panossian, A., & Wagner, H. (2005). Stimulating effect of adaptogens: an overview with particular reference to their efficacy following single dose administration. *Phytotherapy Resources, 19*(10): 819–838.

459. Mills, S. (1991). *The Essential Book of Herbal Medicine*. London: Pengiun Arkana.

460. Dalvi, S. (2003). *Adrenal Fatigue, A Desk Reference*. Sandy, UK: Authors Online.

461. Barker, J., & Meletis, C. (2005). The naturopathic approach to adrenal dysfunction. *Townsend Letter for Doctors & Patients* [online]. Available from http://www.encognitive.com (accessed 24 March 2012).

462. Shenenberger, D. (2018). Hyperprolactinemia. *Medscape* [online]. Available from https://emedicine.medscape.com/article/121784-overview (accessed 14 November 2019).

463. Longo, D. L., Fauci, A. S., Kasper, D. L., Hauser, S. L., Jameson, J. L., & Loscalzo, J. (2011). *Harrison's Principles of Internal Medicine* (18th edn) (p. 2887). New York: McGraw-Hill Professional.

464. Heffner, L. J., & Schust, D. J. (2014). *The Reproductive System at a Glance*. Oxford: John Wiley & Sons.

465. Brice-Ytsma, H., & McDermott, A. (2020). *Herbal Medicine in Treating Gynaecological Conditions*. London: Aeon.

466. Benedek-Jaszmann, L. J., & Hearn-Sturtevant, M. D. (1976). Premenstrual tension and functional infertility: aetiology and treatment. *The Lancet, 307*(7969): 1095–1098.

467. Brice-Ytsma, H., & McDermott, A. (2020). *Herbal Medicine in Treating Gynaecological Conditions*. London: Aeon.

468. Benedek-Jaszmann, L. J., & Hearn-Sturtevant, M. D. (1976). Premenstrual tension and functional infertility: aetiology and treatment. *The Lancet, 307*(7969): 1095–1098.

469. Sharma, P., Kulshreshtha, S., Mohan, G., Singh, S., & Bhagoliwal, A. (2007). Role of bromocriptine and pyridoxine in premenstrual tension syndrome. *Indian Journal of Physiology & Pharmacology, 51*(4): 368–374.

470. Kellner, R., Buckman, M. T., Fava, M., Fava, G. A., & Mastrogiacomo, I. (1984). Prolactin, aggression and hostility: a discussion of recent studies. *Psychiatric Developments, 2*(2): 131–138.

471. Trickey, R. (2003). *Women, Hormones & the Menstrual Cycle*. Sydney, Australia: Allen & Unwin.

472. Benedek-Jaszmann, L. J., & Hearn-Sturtevant, M. D. (1976). Premenstrual tension and functional infertility: aetiology and treatment. *The Lancet, 307*(7969): 1095–1098.

473. Gardiner, P. (2000). Chasteberry (*Vitex agnus castus*). *The Longwood Herbal Taskforce* [online]. Available from http://longwoodherbal.org/vitex/vitex.pdf (accessed 28 February 2012).

474. Webster, D. E., Dentali, S. J., Farnsworth, N. R., & Jim Wang, Z. (2008). Chaste tree fruit and premenstrual syndrome (Chapter 12). In: D. Mischoulon & J. F. Rosenbaum (Eds.), *Natural Medications for Psychiatric Disorders: Considering the Alternatives*. Riverwoods, IL: Wolters Kluwer Health.

475. Trickey, R. (2003). *Women, Hormones & the Menstrual Cycle*. Sydney, Australia: Allen & Unwin.

476. Engels, G. (2010). Sage. *HerbalGram, 89*: 1–4.
477. Kavvadias, D., Monschein, V. S., Sand, P., Riederer, P., & Schreier, P. (2003). Constituents of sage (*Salvia officinalis*) with in vitro affinity to human brain benzodiazepine receptor. *Planta Medica, 69*(2): 113–117.
478. Heffner, L. J., & Schust, D. J. (2014). *The Reproductive System at a Glance.* Oxford: John Wiley & Sons.
479. Brice-Ytsma, H., & McDermott, A. (2020). *Herbal Medicine in Treating Gynaecological Conditions.* London: Aeon.
480. Brice-Ytsma, H., & McDermott, A. (2020). *Herbal Medicine in Treating Gynaecological Conditions.* London: Aeon.
481. Trickey, R. (2011). *Women, Hormones and the Menstrual Cycle.* Clifton Hill, Victoria, Australia: Melbourne Holistic Health Group.
482. Brice-Ytsma, H., & McDermott, A. (2020). *Herbal Medicine in Treating Gynaecological Conditions.* London: Aeon.
483. Puolakka, J., Mäkäräinen, L., Viinikka, L., & Ylikorkala, O. (1985). Biochemical and clinical effects of treating the premenstrual syndrome with prostaglandin synthesis precursors. *Journal of Reproductive Medicine, 30*(3): 149–153.
484. Trickey, R. (2011). *Women, Hormones and the Menstrual Cycle.* Clifton Hill, Victoria, Australia: Melbourne Holistic Health Group.
485. Boyle, M. (2002). *Emergencies around Childbirth: A Handbook for Midwives.* Milton Keynes, UK: Radcliffe.
486. Dalton, K. (1990). The aetiology of premenstrual syndrome is with the progesterone receptors. *Medical Hypotheses, 31*(4): 323–327.
487. Brice-Ytsma, H., & McDermott, A. (2020). *Herbal Medicine in Treating Gynaecological Conditions.* London: Aeon.
488. Harper, R., & Lenton, E. A. (1985). Prolactin and subjective reports of stress in women attending an infertility clinic. *Journal of Reproductive and Infant Psychology, 3*(1): 3–8.
489. Maciocia, G. (2004). *Diagnosis in Chinese Medicine: A Comprehensive Guide.* London: Churchill Livingstone.
490. Louis, G. M. B., Lum, K. J., Sundaram, R., Chen, Z., Kim, S., Lynch, C. D., Schisterman, E. F., & Pyper, C. (2011). Stress reduces conception probabilities across the fertile window: evidence in support of relaxation. *Fertility and Sterility, 95*(7): 2184–2189.
491. Glenville, M. (2000). *Natural Solutions to Infertility.* London: Piatkus.
492. Trickey, R. (2003). *Women, Hormones & the Menstrual Cycle.* Sydney, Australia: Allen & Unwin.
493. Linde, K., Ramirez, G., Mulrow, C. D., Pauls, A., Weidenhammer, W., & Melchart, D. (1996). St John's wort for depression: an overview and meta-analysis of randomised clinical trials. *British Medical Journal, 313*(7052): 253–258.
494. Briggs, M., & Briggs, M (1972). Relationship between monoamine oxidase activity and sex hormone concentration in human blood plasma. *Journal of Reproduction and Fertility, 29*: 447–450.
495. Trickey, R. (2003). *Women, Hormones & the Menstrual Cycle.* Sydney, Australia: Allen & Unwin.
496. Glenville, M. (2000). *Natural Solutions to Infertility.* London: Piatkus.
497. Hudson, T. (2008). *Women's Encyclopedia of Natural Medicine.* New York: McGraw Hill.

498. Trickey, R. (2003). *Women, Hormones & the Menstrual Cycle*. Sydney, Australia: Allen & Unwin.

499. Dalton-Brewer, N. (2016). The role of complementary and alternative medicine for the management of fibroids and associated symptomatology. *Current Obstetrics and Gynecology Reports, 5*: 110–118.

500. Curtis-Prior, P. B. (2004). *The Eicosanoids*. New York: John Wiley & Sons.

501. Benedetto, C. (1989). Eicosanoids in primary dysmenorrhea, endometriosis and menstrual migraine. *Gynecological Endocrinology, 3*(1): 71–94.

502. Lumsden, M. A., Kelly, R. W., & Baird, D. T. (2005). Primary dysmenorrhoea: the importance of both prostaglandins E_2 and $F_{2\alpha}$. *BJOG: An International Journal of Obstetrics and Gynaecology, 90*(12): 1135–1140.

503. Benedetto, C. (1989). Eicosanoids in primary dysmenorrhea, endometriosis and menstrual migraine. *Gynecological Endocrinology, 3*(1): 71–94.

504. Trickey, R. (2003). *Women, Hormones & the Menstrual Cycle*. Sydney, Australia: Allen & Unwin.

505. Toppozada, M., Khowessah, S., Shaala, S., Osman, M., & Rahman, H. A. (1977). Aberrant uterine response to prostaglandin E2 as a possible etiologic factor in functional infertility. *Fertility and Sterility, 28*(4): 434–439.

506. Curtis-Prior, P. B. (2004). *The Eicosanoids*. New York: John Wiley & Sons.

507. Puolakka, J., Mäkäräinen, L., Viinikka, L., & Ylikorkala, O. (1985). Biochemical and clinical effects of treating the premenstrual syndrome with prostaglandin synthesis precursors. *Journal of Reproductive Medicine, 30*(3): 149–153.

508. Trickey, R. (2003). *Women, Hormones & the Menstrual Cycle*. Sydney, Australia: Allen & Unwin.

509. Gonlachanvit, S., Chen, Y. H., Hasler, W. L., Sun, W. M., & Owyang, C. (2003). Ginger reduces hyperglycemia-evoked gastric dysrhythmias in healthy humans: possible role of endogenous prostaglandins. *Journal of Pharmacology and Experimental Therapeutics, 307*(3): 1098–1103.

510. Trickey, R. (2003). *Women, Hormones & the Menstrual Cycle*. Sydney, Australia: Allen & Unwin.

511. Trickey, R. (2003). *Women, Hormones & the Menstrual Cycle*. Sydney, Australia: Allen & Unwin.

512. Pitchford, P. (2002). *Healing with Whole Foods* (3rd edn). Berkeley, CA: North Atlantic.

CHAPTER FIVE

Lifestyle factors and reproductive health

Nutrition

The nutritional factors that may affect fertility have been discussed in the previous section. The main foods that may help to increase fertility, and those which are best avoided are summarised in Figure 3 below.

General nutritional advice for increasing infertility

Foods to include in the diet	Foods to avoid
• Omega-3 fatty acids from fish and flax seed oil • Whole grains, nuts, and seeds • Beans and pulses (especially soya products) • Fresh fruit and vegetables, especially leafy green, cruciferous vegetables • High fibre, low glycaemic index foods • Organic foods.	• Animal fats • Meat and dairy products • High glycaemic index carbohydrates • Non-organic foods.

Fertility increases with diets which include a lower intake of animal protein with greater vegetable protein intake; a lower intake of trans-fat with a greater intake of monounsaturated fat; and a lower intake of high glycaemic index foods with a higher intake of high-fibre, low-glycaemic index carbohydrates.[513] The latter is thought to be due to the effect of carbohydrate consumption on insulin sensitivity, which affects ovulatory function and fertility. Improved insulin sensitivity is associated with improved ovulatory function and fertility in both healthy women and women with polycystic ovary syndrome (PCOS).[514]

Nutritional deficiencies

Infertility is associated with deficiencies of various nutrients including vitamins A, C, E, B vitamins, folic acid, zinc,[515] iron, and essential fatty acids such as EPA and DHA.[516] Women who take multivitamins have a lower risk of infertility.[517,518] 400 mcg folic acid per day is also recommended for women who are trying to conceive in order to prevent spina bifida.[519]

Gluten intolerance

Consumption of foods containing gluten (wheat, rye, barley, and spelt) may contribute to infertility in patients with gluten intolerance.[520,521] It has been suggested that this may be due to resulting malabsorption of folic acid and other nutrients.[522] Nutritional deficiencies (such as iron deficiency anaemia, folate or B12 deficiency), which cannot be explained by diet or blood loss, may indicate malabsorption due to possible gluten intolerance.

Blood tests may be used to detect the presence of anti-tissue transglutaminase antibodies, which are associated with coeliac disease. However, these tests frequently show false negative results, particularly where individuals have low levels of IgA antibodies (a condition which is considerably more common in those with coeliac disease), or where patients have already reduced their gluten consumption because of the discomfort it causes.[523] Therefore an exclusion diet may be a more useful approach for women with otherwise unexplained infertility.

Caffeine

The fertility of healthy women attempting to conceive may be halved by consumption of the equivalent of one cup of coffee or more per day.[524] The mechanism of action of caffeine on fertility is unknown; however, it may be due to a combination of reduced circulatory capacity and its effects on adrenal hormones. Caffeine consumption has also been associated with increased risk of miscarriage. Therefore, women who are trying to conceive are advised to avoid consumption of coffee and other caffeine-containing substances.

Alcohol

Several studies have demonstrated that the likelihood of conception decreases with increasing alcohol intake even among women with an alcohol intake corresponding to five or fewer drinks per week.[525] As little as four units of alcohol per week has also been associated with a significantly increased risk of miscarriage.[526] Therefore women who are trying to conceive should be advised to avoid alcohol consumption.

Smoking

Cigarette smoking has been linked with reduced fertility in women.[527,528] The percentage of women experiencing conception delay for more than twelve months is over 50% higher for smokers than in non-smokers, and the impact of passive cigarette smoke exposure is almost as great as the impact of active smoking.[529] Each stage of reproductive function including folliculogenesis, hormone production, embryo transport, endometrial receptivity, and endometrial angiogenesis, is a target for cigarette smoke.[530] Uterine blood flow is also impaired, which may be due to increased levels of adrenalin and noradrenalin, with resulting vascular resistance.[531]

Cigarette smoke appears to accelerate follicular depletion and menopause occurs one to four years earlier in smoking women than in non-smokers.[532] The effects of cigarette smoke are dose-dependent, and individual sensitivity, amount, time, and type of exposure also play a role in the impact of cigarette smoke on fertility.[533] In addition to cigarette smoking, smoking cannabis causes disturbances in the endo-cannabinoid system potentially contributing to infertility.[534]

Exercise

Women who exercise tend to have lighter and less frequent periods.[535] This may be as a result of increased oestrogen clearance. Women who exercise regularly also have a reduced risk of infertility due to ovulatory disorders.[536] However, it is also important to avoid over-exercising, since vigorous exercise for more than one hour per day is associated with infertility.[537]

Drug induced infertility

The effects of various prescription drugs (such as antipsychotics, spironolactone, and chemotherapy drugs) on fertility are well documented. However, the effects of non-steroidal anti-inflammatory drugs (NSAIDs) are less widely known. NSAIDs are available over the counter, and are widely used for the treatment of pain, inflammation, and fever. The main effect of NSAIDs is inhibition of cyclooxygenase (COX), the enzyme that catalyses the synthesis of prostaglandins. Prostaglandins mediate inflammation, but they also have a wide range of other physiological functions, including essential processes in the female reproductive cycle. By interfering with the synthesis of prostaglandins, NSAIDs may interfere with maturation and egg release.[538]

Notes

513. Chavarro, J. E., Rich-Edwards, J. W., Rosner, B. A., & Willett, W. C. (2007). Diet and lifestyle in the prevention of ovulatory disorder infertility. *Obstetrics & Gynecology*, 110(5): 1050–1058.

514. Chavarro, J. E., Rich-Edwards, J. W., Rosner, B. A., & Willett, W. C. (2009). A prospective study of dietary carbohydrate quantity and quality in relation to risk of ovulatory infertility. *European Journal of Clinical Nutrition*, 63(1): 78–86.

515. Mortimore, D. (2001). *The Complete Illustrated Guide to Vitamins and Minerals*. London: Element.

516. Mehendale, S. S., Kilari Bams, A. S., Deshmukh, C. S., Dhorepatil, B. S., Nimbasrgi, V. N., & Joshi, S. R. (2009). Oxidative stress-mediated essential polyunsaturated fatty acid alterations in female infertility. *Human Fertility*, 12(1): 28–33.

517. Chavarro, J. E., Rich-Edwards, J. W., Rosner, B. A., & Willett, W. C. (2007). Diet and lifestyle in the prevention of ovulatory disorder infertility. *Obstetrics & Gynecology*, 110(5): 1050–1058.

518. Czeizel, A., Metneki, J., & Dudas, I. (1996). The effect of preconceptional multivitamin supplementation on fertility. *International Journal for Vitamin and Nutrition Research*, 66(1): 55–58.

519. NICE (2004). Fertility: assessment and treatment for people with fertility problems. National Institute for Clinical Excellence [online]. Available from www.nice.org.uk (accessed 28 January 2009).

520. Collin, P., Vilska, S., Heinonen, P. K., Hallstrom, O., & Pikkarainen, P. (1996). Infertility and coeliac disease. *Gut*, 39(3): 382–384.

521. Sher, K. S., & Mayberry, J. F. (1996). Female fertility, obstetric and gynaecological history in coeliac disease: a case control study. *Acta Paediatrica*, 85(412): 76–77.

522. Pellicano, R., Astegiano, M., Bruno, M., Fagoonee, S., & Rizzetto, M. (2007). Women and celiac disease: association with unexplained infertility. *Minerva Medica*, 98(3): 217–219.

523. Lee, D., & Marks, J. W. (2020). Could a celiac test show a false negative? *Medicinenet* [online]. Available from: https://medicinenet.com/could_a_celiac_test_show_a_false_negative/ask.htm (accessed 1 June 2020).

524. Wilcox, A., Weinburg, C., & Baird, D. (1988). Caffeinated beverages and decreased fertility. *The Lancet*, 2(8626–8627): 1453–1456.

525. Jensen, T. K., Hjollund, N. H. I., Henriksen, T. B., Scheike, T., Kolstad, H., Giwercman, A., Ernst, E., Bonde, J. P., Skakkebæk, N. E., & Olsen, J. (1998). Does moderate alcohol consumption affect fertility? Follow up study among couples planning first pregnancy. *British Medical Journal*, 317(7157): 505–510.

526. Avalos, L. A., Roberts, S. C., Kaskutas, L. A., Block, G., & Li, D.-K. (2014). Volume and type of alcohol during early pregnancy and the risk of miscarriage. *Substance Use & Misuse*, 49(11): 1437–1445.

527. Augood, C., Duckitt, K., & Templeton, A. A. (1998). Smoking and female infertility: a systematic review and meta-analysis. *Human Reproduction*, 13: 1532–1539.

528. Laurent, S. L., Thompson, S. J., Addy, C., Garrison, C. Z., & Moore, E. E. (1992). An Epidemiologic study of smoking and primary infertility in women. *Fertility and Sterility*, 57(3): 565–572.

529. Hull, M. G., North, K., Taylor, H., Farrow, A., & Ford, W. C. (2000). Delayed conception and active and passive smoking (The Avon Longitudinal Study of Pregnancy and Childhood Study Team). *Fertility and Sterility*, 74(4): 725–733.

530. Dechanet, C., Anahory, T., Mathieu Daude, J. C., Quantin, X., Reyftmann, L., Hamamah, S., Hedon, B., & Dechaud, H. (2011). Effects of cigarette smoking on reproduction. *Human Reproduction Update*, 17(1): 76–95.

531. Grassi, G., Seravalle, G., Calhoun, D. A., Bolla, G. B., Giannattasio, C., Marabini, M., Del Bo, A., & Mancia, G. (1994). Mechanisms responsible for sympathetic activation by cigarette smoking in humans. *Circulation*, 90(1): 248–253.

532. Mattison, D. R., Plowchalk, D. R., Meadows, M. J., Miller, M. M., Malek, A., & London, S. (1989). The effect of smoking on oogenesis, fertilization and implantation. *Seminars in Reproductive Endocrinology*, 7(4): 291–304.

533. Dechanet, C., Anahory, T., Mathieu Daude, J. C, Quantin, X., Reyftmann, L., Hamamah, S., Hedon, B., & Dechaud, H. (2011). Effects of cigarette smoking on reproduction. *Human Reproduction Update*, 17(1): 76–95.

534. Karasu, T., Marczylo, T. H., Maccarrone, M., & Konje, J. C. (2011). The role of sex steroid hormones, cytokines and the endocannabinoid system in female fertility. *Human Reproduction Update*, 17(3): 347–361.

535. Harlow, S. D., & Campbell, B. C. (1994). Host factors that influence the duration of menstrual bleeding. *Epidemiology, 5*(3): 352–355.

536. Chavarro, J. E., Rich-Edwards, J. W., Rosner, B. A., & Willett, W. C. (2007). Diet and lifestyle in the prevention of ovulatory disorder infertility. *Obstetrics & Gynecology, 110*(5): 1050–1058.

537. Green, B. B., Daling, J. R., Weiss, N. S., Liff, J. M., & Koepsell, T. (1986). Exercise as a risk factor for infertility with ovulatory dysfunction. *American Journal of Public Health, 76*(12): 1432–1436.

538. Mendonca, L. L. F., Khamashta, M. A., Nelson-Piercy, C., Hunt, B. J., & Hughes, G. R. (2000). Non-steroidal anti-inflammatory drugs as a possible cause for reversible infertility. *Rheumatology (Oxford), 39*(8): 880–882.

CHAPTER SIX

Energetic patterns of disharmony

Identification of the underlying cause of infertility (or other reproductive health problems) is the key to successful treatment,[539] and using scientific diagnostic techniques such as blood tests and ultrasonography can be extremely useful for choosing the correct treatment protocol.[540] However, scientific diagnostic techniques cannot always provide an explanation for the problems being encountered by the patient. This can be extremely frustrating for individuals who are suffering from reproductive health problems, or trying to conceive, since it is difficult to decide on an appropriate treatment plan without a definitive diagnosis.

Although careful case taking frequently reveals symptoms such as menstrual irregularities and abnormal menstrual flow,[541] and there may be a slight hormonal imbalance in some instances,[542] these symptoms are difficult to classify, since they do not fall into any specific disease category.[543] However, the significance of these symptoms may be better understood using a more holistic perspective; and by incorporating traditional or "energetic" approaches to diagnosis, one may find possible causal factors for infertility, or other reproductive health problems, where orthodox medicine has failed to do so.

Medical herbalists aim to use a holistic approach in treating patients, which means that the underlying cause of any problem is sought and treated rather than the symptoms alone,[544] and for many practitioners, incorporating an "energetic" system is a very important part of the holistic approach.[545]

The concept of the existence of a vitalistic principle or energy that encompasses the physical body is central to holistic medicine. Changes in this inner energy are thought to be reflected in the physical body,[546] resulting in particular patterns of health or disease. Energetics may be described as a vocabulary for describing these physiological and/or psychological patterns, which express imbalances in the energy, or vital force of the body.[547]

Traditional medicine systems, such as traditional Chinese medicine (TCM) and Ayurveda (the traditional medicine system of India), can often help to provide an explanation for difficulty in conceiving, or other reproductive health problems. Traditional diagnostic techniques may be used alongside orthodox investigations to help identify "energetic" patterns of disharmony that contribute to reproductive health problems and infertility, and help practitioners to formulate an approach to treatment, which will help to treat reproductive health problems more effectively, and improve the chances of conceiving naturally, or increase the success rates of assisted reproduction for those who wish to conceive.

Traditional medicine systems

The ancient medical systems of the world, such as traditional Chinese medicine, Ayurveda, and humoral medicine are considered to be holistic in both diagnostic and therapeutic approaches.[548] They are relatively similar systems, in that they are based on the idea of a central vital force (referred to as *Qi* in TCM, *Prana* in Ayurveda, and *Pneuma* in humoral medicine), which circulates throughout the body and is necessary for life and procreation. Health problems are thought to be caused by deficiencies or disruptions in this vital force.[549]

The ancient medical systems of the world are also based on the concept that all things are composed of the elements *Earth*, *Air*, *Fire*, and *Water*, and (in traditional Chinese medicine) *Metal* and *Wood*. These elements are considered to possess particular qualities (such as *damp*, *dry*, *hot*, and *cold*), and health problems are classified according to imbalances of the elements and their qualities.[550] The individual and the disease are treated simultaneously, using herbs that are considered to have the appropriate qualities to treat the imbalance.[551] This system can be highly effective even if the medical name of the disease is not known.[552]

To use herbs, or indeed any form of therapy effectively, it is important to know the unique constitution of the individual, as well as to establish the specific nature of the imbalance. Western medicine, and to some extent, modern Western herbal medicine, lacks this focus on the constitution of the individual and their unique presentation of disease.[553] However, there seems to be a renewed interest in traditional medicine systems in recent years; and Western herbal medicine has started to rediscover qualities of herbs and their application to contemporary herbal medicine.[554]

Integrating conventional and traditional diagnostic techniques

Modern diagnostic techniques are very useful, but they cannot define all the symptoms seen in practice, or explain the tendency of certain individuals to develop disease.[555] However, traditional diagnostic techniques can fill the gaps in the picture by providing information about the individual.[556] The best approach therefore, is one that combines scientific insights with a traditional approach.[557,558]

Traditional Chinese medicine

"Vital energy" in traditional Chinese medicine (TCM) is referred to as "Qi". It circulates in the body within numerous channels or "meridians", and the Organs are also considered to have their own Qi.[559]

Qi comprises one of the five "Fundamental Substances" in TCM, which also includes Blood, Fluids, Essence (Jing), and Spirit (Shen). The function of the Blood is to nourish and maintain the body,[560] and in pregnancy, to nourish and sustain a developing embryo.[561] The major disharmonies of Blood that are associated with infertility include: Blood Deficiency (in which the body, or a particular Organ, is insufficiently nourished by the Blood); and Blood Stasis (in which the flow of Blood is obstructed).[562]

In TCM, the Organs are understood principally in terms of their functional activity and their relationships to the Fundamental Substances, the other Organs, and other parts of the body. They are somewhat different from the organs as understood by Western medicine.[563] According to traditional Chinese medicine theory, the Kidney is the Organ responsible for reproduction.[564]

Yin/Yang

The concept of Yin and Yang is probably the most important and distinctive theory of TCM.[565] It is illustrated by the *tai ji* symbol:

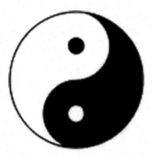

Figure 14: The *tai ji* symbol.

The term Yin means "the shady side of a slope". It is passive, cold, inward, downward, and decreasing. Yang means "the sunny side of a slope". It is active, hot, upward, outward, and increasing. Yin and Yang affect each other so that when Yin is deficient there is a relative preponderance of Yang and vice versa.[566] Yin and Yang may therefore be seen as an expression of the natural law of homeostasis.[567]

Diagnosis in TCM

A major strength of traditional Chinese medicine diagnosis is that it incorporates an incredibly detailed clinical examination of the patient. Diagnosis in Western medicine was also originally based on detailed clinical examination, before technology and modern diagnostic aids took precedence over it.[568] However, there are fundamental differences in how Western and Chinese physicians make sense of the patient's signs and symptoms.

Practitioners of traditional Chinese medicine pay close attention to the whole person in the context of the problem they present with, not just the signs and symptoms of that particular problem. All relevant information gathered from speaking to the patient, and from the clinical examination, is woven together to form what is known in Chinese medicine as a "pattern of disharmony".[569] A specific disease may be the result of one of a number of different patterns of disharmony or "syndromes", and a particular syndrome may be seen in several different diseases.[570,571]

Western medicine is primarily quantitative,[572] relying heavily on blood tests that are interpreted in terms of "reference ranges",[573] and on investigations such as ultrasound scans and laparoscopy. In contrast, TCM is more qualitative: the organs are always discussed with reference to their functions and relationships with other parts of the body,[574] expressed through signs and symptoms.

Attempts are sometimes made to impose parallels between Chinese and Western systems. However, this is largely inappropriate and often leads to misunderstanding. TCM is a coherent system, which is internally logical and consistent, and is therefore best considered in its own right.[575]

TCM diagnostic techniques

Various examinations, such as observation of the tongue and palpation of the pulse, are used to identify the manifestations and nature of a disease, enabling the practitioner to determine the syndrome in terms of TCM theory, and to decide on treatment.[576] Each sign means very little by itself: a diagnosis can only be made by considering a sign in terms of its relationship to the individual, and to the other signs present.[577]

Diagnosis by observation: tongue diagnosis

Diagnosis by observation or inspection is based on the principle that the internal organs and their disharmonies manifest themselves externally. Furthermore, each single, small part of the body such as the tongue, the face, the ear, or the hand, reflects the whole body;[578] and within each part, certain areas correspond to specific internal organs.[579]

The appearance of the tongue nearly always shows the true condition of the patient. It is particularly useful in complicated conditions where there may be contradictory signs and symptoms. The colour of the tongue body is the most important aspect of observation. It reflects the condition of the Organs, Qi, and Blood.[580] For example, a pale tongue indicates Deficient Blood or Yang, while a blue or purple hue to the tongue suggests Blood Stasis. If the tongue is pale purple and moist the obstruction is related to Cold, and if reddish purple and dry it is related to Heat.[581,582,583]

Observation of the tongue shape is also useful.[584] For example, a swollen tongue with tooth marks indicates Deficient Qi and Dampness or Phlegm.[585,586] Tongue signs may affect the whole tongue or isolated areas. Signs on isolated areas of the tongue correspond to particular Organs.

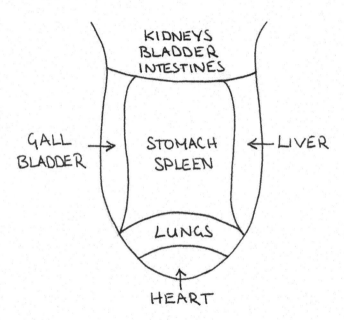

Figure 15: Areas of the tongue and their corresponding organs.

Diagnosis by palpation: pulse diagnosis

The pulse is taken at the radial artery, using the index, middle, and ring fingers, with the index finger placed closest to the wrist. The pulse is felt in three positions on each hand, and at three levels: superficial, middle, and deep, giving nine regions on each hand. The different pulse positions correspond to various Organs, and indicate disharmonies in those Organs.[587]

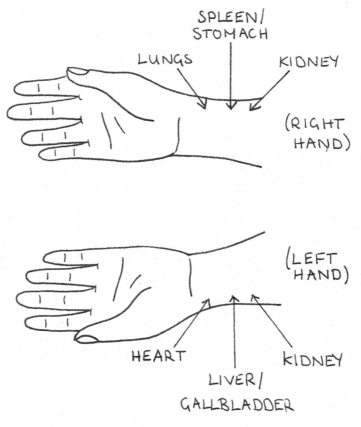

Figure 16: Pulse positions and organ correspondences.

The pulse is also assessed to establish its overall quality. For example, Dampness is indicated by a slippery pulse, while Kidney Yang Deficiency is indicated by deep pulse at the third position on the right hand.[588]

Pulse diagnosis can often be used to diagnose a pattern of disharmony, even in the absence of other symptoms. The pulse can give a picture of the body as a whole, the state of Qi and Blood, the condition of the Organs, and the presence of emotional problems.[589] Examination of the pulse also plays a crucial role in many other traditional medical systems including humoral medicine[590] and Ayurveda.[591]

Pulse and tongue diagnosis are considered to be the most important aspects of diagnosis in traditional Chinese medicine; however, the other methods of diagnosis (such as observation of the general appearance, complexion, and behaviour, listening to the quality of the voice and respiration, and enquiring about the presenting complaint and past medical history) can also provide important information.[592]

TCM approach to treatment

TCM treatments focus on rebalancing individuals and not just treating diseases.[593] They aim to correct maladjustments and restore the self-regulatory ability of the body.[594] Therefore there are no fixed measures to be followed in the treatment of reproductive health problems and infertility, and treatments vary from patient to patient based on their individual pattern of disharmony.[595]

Traditional Chinese medicine patterns of disharmony, which may contribute to infertility in women include: Blood Stasis, Qi Stagnation, Kidney Qi Deficiency, Dampness, Cold in the Uterus, and Blood Deficiency.[596,597] These patterns are discussed further in this chapter, while energetic patterns of disharmony that may contribute to infertility in men are covered in Chapter 11.

In practice, traditional Chinese medicine patterns are highly complex, and interdependent. However, they are simplified here in order to allow practitioners of Western herbal medicine (and other complementary and alternative modalities) to begin to incorporate an energetic approach into their treatment of reproductive health problems and infertility.

TCM patterns of disharmony

Blood Stasis

Blood Stasis is indicated by a blue or purple tongue-body colour, and symptoms such as poor peripheral circulation, breast tenderness, and dysmenorrhoea with dark, clotty menstrual flow.[598] This pattern is often seen in women with conditions such as pelvic inflammatory disease, uterine fibroids, and endometriosis.

Improving blood flow

Warming herbs such as *Rosmarinus officinalis*, *Cinnamonum zeylonicum*, and *Zingiber officinale* may be used to stimulate the peripheral circulation, and may also help to promote healthy circulation to the reproductive organs.[599]

Uterine spasmolytics such as *Paeonia lactiflora* and uterine tonics such as *Achillea millefolium* may also be useful to improve uterine blood flow. *Angelica sinensis* is a uterine tonic and antispasmodic herb, which is widely used to treat dysmenorrhoea,[600] and is traditionally used to treat Blood Stasis in TCM.[601] It is also thought to regulate prostaglandin synthesis,[602] and to act as a circulatory stimulant.[603]

Increasing exercise may also help to improve pelvic blood flow,[604] and other approaches such as sitz baths may be used to increase the pelvic circulation and reduce congestion.[605]

Qi Stagnation

Qi Stagnation (particularly Liver Qi Stagnation) is indicated by dys-menorrhoea and premenstrual syndrome (PMS) with irritability and mastalgia,[606] and by aches and pains.[607] Liver Qi Stagnation gives rise to a wiry pulse.

Reducing Qi Stagnation

Herbs that are used to treat Qi Stagnation in traditional Chinese medi-cine include *Angelica sinensis, Paeonia lactiflora*, and *Zingiber officinale*.[608] Western herbs that may help to reduce Qi stagnation include *Achillea millefolium, Anemone pulsatilla*, and *Leonurus cardiaca*.[609] Adequate exer-cise, and a primarily vegetarian diet, with an emphasis on fresh raw vegetables and sprouts can also help to reduce Liver Qi Stagnation.[610]

Kidney Qi Deficiency

According to traditional Chinese medicine theory, the Kidney is respon-sible for reproduction,[611] and more than half of all cases of infertility are associated with a Kidney Deficiency.[612,613] Kidney energy may be depleted by lifestyle factors such as poor diet and overwork.[614]

Kidney Yang Deficiency

Kidney Yang Deficiency is indicated by symptoms such as delayed menstruation, dizziness, tiredness, constipation, cold extremities, a tendency to excess mucus or Dampness, a wet tongue, and a deep pulse at the third position on the right hand. It is often associated with conditions such as hypothyroidism.

Since Kidney Yang is responsible for all transformations within the body, Kidney Yang Deficiency may result in insufficient production of Blood, which is required to nourish a developing embryo. Since Kidney Yang is also a source of warmth, there may be insufficient warmth to maintain the embryo. Finally Kidney Yang is responsible for pelvic blood flow, and Deficiency may therefore lead to Blood Stasis in the uterus, which as previously discussed may also contribute to infertility.[615]

Kidney Yin Deficiency

Kidney Yin Deficiency is indicated by a thin, dry, red tongue, and a fine and rapid pulse. Symptoms of Kidney Yin Deficiency include irregular periods, vaginal dryness, irritability, insomnia, hot flushes, and night sweats. Kidney Yin Deficiency is common during and after menopause, and is therefore also seen in women with premature ovarian insufficiency. Women with Yin Deficiency may have poor egg quality and thin and a poorly nourished endometrium that does not enable an embryo to thrive.

Tonifying the Kidney Qi

Warming herbs nourish the Yang and tonify the Kidneys.[616,617] Warming herbs that may be used to treat infertility due to Kidney Yang Deficiency include *Cinnamonum zeylonicum*, *Rosmarinus officinalis*, and *Zingiber officinalis*.[618] It is also important to eat plenty of warm foods, and to get adequate rest. Kidney Yin Deficiency benefits from moist, nourishing herbs such as *Asparagus racemosus*, *Dioscorea villosa*, and *Glycyrrhiza glabra*.

Dampness

Signs of Dampness include a slippery pulse, a swollen, tooth marked tongue with sticky coating, mid-cycle bleeding, and vaginal *Candida* infection. Dampness in the body may be caused by excessive consumption of greasy foods and dairy products.[619] This pattern is commonly seen in women with PCOS. Dampness may impede the flow of Qi to the Uterus and thereby contribute to infertility in some women.

Resolving Dampness

Avoiding consumption of greasy foods and dairy products, warming herbs such as *Zingiber officinale*, and astringent herbs such as *Alchemilla vulgaris*, may be used to treat Dampness in the reproductive organs. Herbs that stimulate Qi (as discussed in the section on Qi Stagnation above) are also used to remove Dampness.[620]

Cold in the Uterus

Excessive exposure to cold, or consumption of cold foods and drinks may lead to Cold in the Uterus.[621] It is indicated by symptoms such as clotty menstrual flow, feeling of cold, dysmenorrhoea that is relieved by warmth, a pale tongue, and a wiry or tight pulse.[622] Coldness causes contraction, and therefore Cold in the Uterus may impede the flow of Qi and Blood, thereby contributing to infertility. It may also dampen the Kidney Yang, which is needed for conception.[623]

Warming the Uterus

Warming herbs are recommended to treat Uterus Cold, such as *Cinnamonum zeylonicum*, *Rosmarinus officinalis*, and *Zingiber officinalis*.[624] It is also important to avoid consumption of cold foods and drinks, raw food, and exposure to cold.[625]

Blood Deficiency

Blood Deficiency is very common in women, and may be caused by loss of blood during menstruation, poor diet, overwork, or emotional stress. It is indicated by a pale, thin, moving tongue and scanty menses. Blood Deficiency results in insufficient nourishment of the reproductive organs and reduced receptivity for implantation.[626] In addition, it may cause secondary Stagnation of Qi, which could also contribute to infertility.[627]

TCM diagnoses and treatment

Diagnosis	Symptoms	Examples of herbs used	Other recommendations
Blood Stasis	Poor circulation dysmenorrhoea, mastalgia, clotty menstruation, and blue/purple tongue	*Achillea millefolium, Angelica sinensis, Cinnamomum zeylonicum, Leonurus cardiaca, Rosmarinus officinalis, Zingiber officinalis*	Increase consumption of wholegrains, nuts, seeds, and leafy green vegetables. Increase exercise
Qi Stagnation/ Liver Qi Stagnation	Dysmenorrhoea, PMS aches and pains	*Achillea millefolium Anemone pulsatilla, Angelica sinensis, Paeonia lactiflora, Zingiber officinale*	Vegetarian diet, exercise
Kidney Qi Deficiency	Delayed menstruation, constipation, tiredness, dizziness, and deep pulse at third position	*Cinnamomum zeylonicum, Glycyrrhiza glabra, Rosmarinus officinalis, Zingiber officinale*	Eat plenty of warm foods and get adequate rest
Dampness	Swollen, tooth marked tongue, slippery pulse, sticky tongue coating, mid-cycle bleeding and *Candida* infection	*Alchemilla vulgaris, Cinnamonum zeylonicum, Zingiber officinale*	Avoid greasy foods and dairy products
Uterus Cold	Clotty menses and feeling of cold, dysmenorrhoea, pale tongue	*Cinnamomum zeylonicum, Rosmarinus officinalis, Zingiber officinale*	Avoid exposure to cold, and cold foods and drinks
Blood Deficiency	Pale, thin, moving tongue and scanty menses	*Angelica sinensis, Astragalus membranaceus, Paeonia lactiflora, Rehmannia glutinosa, Withania somnifera*	Iron, vitamin B12, folic acid, and vitamin C, micro-algae, dark green leafy vegetables

Nourishing the Blood

Herbs that are traditionally used to treat Blood Deficiency in TCM include *Paeonia lactiflora* (white paeony), *Astragalus membranaceus* (Huang Qi), *Rehmannia glutinosa* (Chinese foxglove), and *Angelica sinensis* (Dang Gui).[628] *Withania somnifera* is an Ayurvedic herb that is used to treat anaemia.[629] The nutrients required to generate healthy blood include iron, vitamin B12, folic acid, and vitamin C. These are found in chlorophyll-rich foods such as micro-algae and dark green leafy vegetables.[630]

Ayurvedic dosha imbalance

Ayurveda is thought to be the oldest system of healing in existence. The term *Ayurveda* is derived from the Sanskrit words: *Ayus* meaning "life", and *Veda* meaning "knowledge" or "science".[631] It is a holistic philosophy in which body, mind, and spirit are considered to be an integrated whole.[632] Illness is viewed as a disruption in the delicate somatic, emotional, and environmental balance within the life of an individual.[633] Ayurveda is a comprehensive system, which provides many diverse approaches to healing.[634] It addresses diet, lifestyle, environmental factors, thought patterns, and behaviour, as well as using herbs to restore health.[635]

Diagnosis in Ayurveda

Diagnosis in Ayurveda is based on eight specific forms of clinical examination which are similar to those used in TCM and include observation of the general appearance, eyes, skin, tongue, urine, faeces, the sound of the voice, and the quality of the pulse.[636]

The essences of nature

The essences of nature according to Ayurveda are: *Prana* (the breath behind all vital essence), *Tejas* (the spark behind all conscious perception), and *Ojas* (the seed behind all nourishment). *Ojas*, which has an interdependent relationship with *Prana* and *Tejas*, is responsible for healthy fertility. Healthy *Ojas* is demonstrated by: strength and resistance to disease; efficient digestion; fertility; and lustre of the eyes, skin, and hair.[637]

Ojas is depleted by undernourishment, overwork, excessive exercise, stress, ejaculation, and orgasm (in both men and women).[638] Symptoms of depleted *Ojas* include weakness, anxiety, confusion, dry skin and hair, and poor complexion.[639] Clean air and good breathing habits, sufficient sleep and rest, and nourishing foods support Ojas. Herbs such as *Asparagus racemosus* (shatavari) increase *Ojas*.[640]

The three doshas

The three *doshas*: *Vata*, *Pitta*, and *Kapha*, are invisible forces, which can be perceived by their effects on the body.[641] They are derived from combinations of the five elements, ether, air, fire, water and earth.[642]

Each person is born with particular balance of *doshas*, which creates the individual nature or constitution (*prakruti*). An individual's *prakruti* remains unchanged throughout life and determines the person's nature and body type, predisposition to certain health problems, and the sort of diet and lifestyle that is appropriate. The present state of imbalance within an individual under the influence of diet, lifestyle, and environment is referred to as *vikruti*.[643] The *doshas* enable the practitioner to determine the basic nature of an individual and to establish a treatment plan that is unique to his or her needs.[644]

Vata

Vata is derived from ether and air. It is light, cold, dry, mobile, irregular, and rough. It is responsible for all movement in the body,[645] including circulation, nervous impulses, movement of the limbs, and elimination of wastes.[646]

Apana Vata is a subtype of Vata, which resides in the lower abdomen. Apana Vata is a downward moving energy, which is responsible for processes such as defecation, urination, ovulation, menstruation, and birth.[647] It is therefore not surprising that Vata aggravation is a common finding among women with reproductive health problems and infertility.

Vata disturbance may be caused by problems such as stress, anxiety, tiredness, overwork, and excessive exercise. Too many dry or cold foods, and astringent, bitter, and pungent flavours also aggravate Vata.[648] Vata disturbance is suggested by symptoms such as: fatigue, feeling anxious or stressed, feeling cold, poor peripheral circulation, palpitations, abdominal bloating, constipation, dry skin and hair, cracking joints, muscle spasm, pins and needles, absent or scanty menstruation, and infertility.[649]

Reducing Vata aggravation

Avoiding stress, worry, and excessive travelling and rushing around reduces Vata aggravation. It is important to maintain a regular daily routine, and get adequate rest and sleep. Massage with warm oil is very beneficial for balancing Vata.[650] Warm and moist foods (such as soups and stews, and oils) and sweet, sour, salty flavours (such as honey, fresh figs, sweet potatoes, yoghurt, and seaweeds), help to reduce Vata aggravation.[651]

Withania somnifera is an Ayurvedic herb that is widely used to treat Vata disturbance. *Glycyrrhiza glabra* reduces Vata aggravation, due to its sweet taste and moist nature. Warming herbs such as *Cinnamonum zeylonicum* and *Myristica fragrans* are also used in Ayurvedic medicine to reduce Vata aggravation. *Rosmarinus officinalis* is another warming herb which reduces Vata aggravation.[652]

Pitta

Pitta is derived from fire and water. It is hot, oily, fast, irritable, and intense. It is responsible for all transformations in the body,[653,654] including hormonal balance.[655] Pitta is aggravated by irritation and anger, excessive ambition, exposure to heat and humidity, and consumption of too many hot, oily foods (such as fatty meat and fried foods), and sour, salty, or pungent foods (such as yoghurt, cheese, salty meat or nuts, and spicy food).[656]

Pitta aggravation is associated with inflammation, heat, and burning sensations. It shows some similarity to the TCM pattern of Liver Qi Stagnation and Damp Heat. It is characterised by symptoms such as inflammation and irritability, hormone imbalance, liver problems, and loose bowel movements.[657,658]

Balancing Pitta

Light, bitter, sweet, and astringent foods (such as green leafy vegetables, apples, berries, and pomegranates) are useful for reducing

Pitta aggravation. It is important to avoid too many pungent, salty, sour and oily foods, red meat, caffeine, and alcohol.

Bitter herbs (such as *Andrographis paniculata*), sweet herbs (such as *Glycyrrhiza glabra*), and astringent herbs (such as *Achillea millefolium*) are useful for reducing Pitta aggravation.[659] Meditation, and avoiding aggression and competitiveness are also important to balance Pitta.[660]

Kapha

Kapha is derived from water and earth. It is heavy, cold, damp, stable, slow, and unctuous. Kapha is responsible for growth,[661] protection of the body, and maintenance of body fluids.[662]

Kapha is aggravated by possessiveness, inactivity, exposure to cold and damp, and too many sweet, sour, and salty foods. Kapha disturbance is characterised by excess phlegm, swelling and tissue growth,[663] slow digestion, constipation, and obesity.[664] It shows some similarity to the TCM pattern of Dampness. It is characterised by excess mucus, and a swollen tongue with white coating.[665]

Reducing Kapha excess

Pungent herbs (such as *Myristica fragrans* and *Zingiber officinale*), astringent herbs (such as *Cinnamonum zeylonicum* and *Alchemilla vulgaris*), and bitter herbs (such as *Andrographis paniculata* and *Taraxacum officinale*) balance Kapha. Pungent, astringent, and bitter foods (such as apples, green leafy vegetables, onions, and spicy foods) also reduce Kapha excess. It is important to avoid cold, sweet, sour, salty, and oily and damp foods such as dairy products and cold water, as they increase Kapha.[666] Exercise, activity, giving, sharing, and letting go all help to reduce excess Kapha.[667]

Ayurvedic diagnoses and treatment

Diagnosis	Symptoms	Examples of herbs used	Other recommendations
Depletion of Ojas	Weakness, anxiety, confusion, dry skin and hair, and poor complexion	Asparagus racemosus	Clean air and good breathing habits, sufficient sleep and rest, and nourishing foods
Vata disturbance/excess	Feeling of cold, poor peripheral circulation, palpitations, pins & needles, muscle spasm, cracking joints, constipation, feeling stressed, and insomnia between 2am and 6am	Withania somnifera, Glycyrrhiza glabra, Cinnamonum zeylonicum, Rosmarinus officinalis	Increase consumption of moist, warm, sweet, sour, and salty foods. Avoid dry and bitter foods, and getting tired or stressed
Pitta excess	Inflammation and irritability, heat and burning sensations	Achillea millefolium, Andrographis paniculata, Glycyrrhiza glabra	Increase bitter, sweet, astringent foods. Avoid pungent, sour, and oily foods, caffeine, alcohol, and red meat. Practise meditation
Kapha excess	Sweet cravings, constipation, excess mucous, swelling, and tissue growth.	Alchemilla vulgaris, Cinnamonum zeylonicum, Myristica fragrans, Iris versicolor, Taraxacum officinale, Zingiber officinale	Increase pungent, bitter, and astringent foods. Avoid sweet, sour, and salty, cold, damp, and oily foods. Avoid overeating and take regular exercise

Notes

539. Hoffman, D. (2009). Infertility [online]. Available from http://healthy.net/scr/Article.asp?id=1182 (accessed 28 January 2009).
540. Tillotson, A. K. (2001). *The One Earth Herbal Sourcebook*. New York: Kensington.
541. Gascoigne, S. (2001). *The Clinical Medicine Guide: A Holistic Perspective*. Clonakilty, Ireland: Jigme.
542. Hoffman, D. (2009). Infertility [online]. Available from http://healthy.net/scr/Article.asp?id=1182 (accessed 28 January 2009).
543. Gascoigne, S. (2001). *The Clinical Medicine Guide: A Holistic Perspective*. Clonakilty, Ireland: Jigme.
544. Irish Institute of Medical Herbalists (2007). About medical herbalists [online]. Available from http://iimh.org (accessed 18 February 2012).
545. Wood, M. (2004). *The Practice of Traditional Western Herbalism: Basic Doctrine, Energetics and Classification*. Berkeley, CA: North Atlantic.
546. Gascoigne, S. (2001). *The Clinical Medicine Guide: A Holistic Perspective*. Clonakilty, Ireland: Jigme.
547. Wood, M. (2004). *The Practice of Traditional Western Herbalism: Basic Doctrine, Energetics and Classification*. Berkeley, CA: North Atlantic.
548. Hoffman, D. (2003). *Medical Herbalism: The Science and Practice of Herbal Medicine*. Rochester, VT: Healing Arts.
549. Trickey, R. (2003). *Women, Hormones & the Menstrual Cycle*. Sydney, Australia: Allen & Unwin.
550. Trickey, R. (2003). *Women, Hormones & the Menstrual Cycle*. Sydney, Australia: Allen & Unwin.
551. Tillotson, A. K. (2009). Female infertility [online]. Available from http://oneearth-herbs.squarespace.com/diseases/female-infertility.html (accessed on 28 January 2009).
552. Pitchford, P. (2002). *Healing With Whole Foods* (3rd edn). Berkeley, CA: North Atlantic.
553. Frawley, D., & Lad, V. (2001). *The Yoga of Herbs: An Ayurvedic Guide to Herbal Medicine*. Twin Lakes, WI: Lotus.
554. Trickey, R. (2003). *Women, Hormones & the Menstrual Cycle*. Sydney, Australia: Allen & Unwin.
555. Gascoigne, S. (2001). *The Clinical Medicine Guide: A Holistic Perspective*. Clonakilty, Ireland: Jigme.
556. Trickey, R. (2003). *Women, Hormones & the Menstrual Cycle*. Sydney, Australia: Allen & Unwin.
557. Bone, K. (2003). *A Clinical Guide to Blending Liquid Herbs*. London: Churchill Livingstone.
558. Jiang, W. Y. (2005). Therapeutic wisdom in traditional Chinese medicine: a perspective from modern science. *Trends in Pharmacological Sciences*, 26(11): 558–563.
559. Kaptchuk, T. J. (1983). *Chinese Medicine: The Web That Has No Weaver*. London: Rider.
560. Maciocia, G. (2005). *The Foundations of Chinese Medicine: A Comprehensive Text for Acupuncturists and Herbalists*. London: Churchill Livingstone.
561. Flaws, B. (1993). *Fulfilling the Essence: The Handbook of Traditional & Contemporary Chinese Treatments for Female Infertility*. Colorado Springs, CO: Blue Poppy.

562. Kaptchuk, T. J. (1983). *Chinese Medicine: The Web That Has No Weaver*. London: Rider.
563. Kaptchuk, T. J. (1983). *Chinese Medicine: The Web That Has No Weaver*. London: Rider.
564. Liu, W., & Gong, C. (2009). Opening the blockage to reproduction: infertility. *Traditional Chinese Medicine Information Page* [online]. Available from http://tcmpage. com/hpinfertility.html (accessed 4 July 2011).
565. Maciocia, G. (2005). *The Foundations of Chinese Medicine: A Comprehensive Text for Acupuncturists and Herbalists*. London: Churchill Livingstone.
566. Kaptchuk, T. J. (1983). *Chinese Medicine: The Web That Has No Weaver*. London: Rider.
567. Tierra, M., & Tierra, L. (1998). *Chinese Traditional Herbal Medicine, Volume I: Diagnosis and Treatment*. Twin Lakes, WI: Lotus.
568. Maciocia, G. (2004). *Diagnosis in Chinese Medicine: A Comprehensive Guide*. London: Churchill Livingstone.
569. Kaptchuk, T. J. (1983). *Chinese Medicine: The Web That Has No Weaver*. London: Rider.
570. Jiang, W. Y. (2005). Therapeutic wisdom in traditional Chinese medicine: a perspective from modern science. *Trends in Pharmacological Sciences, 26*(11): 558–563.
571. Xiufen, W. (Ed.) 2003. *Traditional Chinese Diagnostics*. Beijing: People's Medical Publishing House.
572. Kaptchuk, T. J. (1983). *Chinese Medicine: The Web That Has No Weaver*. London: Rider.
573. Entwistle, I. R. (1998). *Exacta Medica* (2nd edn). Edinburgh, UK: Churchill Livingstone.
574. Kaptchuk, T. J. (1983). *Chinese Medicine: The Web That Has No Weaver*. London: Rider.
575. Kaptchuk, T. J. (1983). *Chinese Medicine: The Web That Has No Weaver*. London: Rider.
576. Xiufen, W. (Ed.) 2003. *Traditional Chinese Diagnostics*. Beijing: People's Medical Publishing House.
577. Mitchell, C., Ye, F., & Wiseman, N. (Transl.) (1999). *Shang Han Lun: On Cold Damage. Translation and Commentaries*. Brookline, MA: Paradigm.
578. Guo, B., & Powell, A. (2001). *Listen to Your Body: The Wisdom of the Dao*. Honolulu, HI: University of Hawai'i Press.
579. Maciocia, G. (2004). *Diagnosis in Chinese Medicine: A Comprehensive Guide*. London: Churchill Livingstone.
580. Maciocia, G. (2004). *Diagnosis in Chinese Medicine: A Comprehensive Guide*. London: Churchill Livingstone.
581. Kaptchuk, T. J. (1983). *Chinese Medicine: The Web That Has No Weaver*. London: Rider.
582. Maciocia, G. (2004). *Diagnosis in Chinese Medicine: A Comprehensive Guide*. London: Churchill Livingstone.
583. Xiufen, W. (Ed.) 2003. *Traditional Chinese Diagnostics*. Beijing: People's Medical Publishing House.
584. Maciocia, G. (2004). *Diagnosis in Chinese Medicine: A Comprehensive Guide*. London: Churchill Livingstone.
585. Kaptchuk, T. J. (1983). *Chinese Medicine: The Web That Has No Weaver*. London: Rider.
586. Xiufen, W. (Ed.) 2003. *Traditional Chinese Diagnostics*. Beijing: People's Medical Publishing House.
587. Kaptchuk, T. J. (1983). *Chinese Medicine: The Web That Has No Weaver*. London: Rider.
588. Kaptchuk, T. J. (1983). *Chinese Medicine: The Web That Has No Weaver*. London: Rider.
589. Maciocia, G. (2004). *Diagnosis in Chinese Medicine: A Comprehensive Guide*. London: Churchill Livingstone.
590. Kaptchuk, T. J. (1983). *Chinese Medicine: The Web That Has No Weaver*. London: Rider.

591. Lad, V. D. (2006). *Textbook of Ayurveda: A Complete Guide to Clinical Assessment. Volume 2.* Albuquerque, NM: Ayurvedic Press.

592. Dharmananda, S. (2000). *The Significance of Traditional Pulse Diagnosis in the Modern Practice of Chinese Medicine* [online]. Available from http://itmonline.org/arts/pulse.htm (accessed 4 December 2009).

593. Flaws, B. (1993). *Fulfilling the Essence: The Handbook of Traditional & Contemporary Chinese Treatments for Female Infertility.* Colorado Springs, CO: Blue Poppy.

594. Jiang, W. Y. (2005). Therapeutic wisdom in traditional Chinese medicine: a perspective from modern science. *Trends in Pharmacological Sciences,* 26(11): 558–563.

595. Flaws, B. (1993). *Fulfilling the Essence: The Handbook of Traditional & Contemporary Chinese Treatments for Female Infertility.* Colorado Springs, CO: Blue Poppy.

596. Liu, W., & Gong, C. (2009). Opening the blockage to reproduction: infertility. *Traditional Chinese Medicine Information Page* [online]. Available from http://tcmpage.com/hpinfertility.html (accessed 4 July 2011).

597. Maciocia, G. (2004). *Diagnosis in Chinese Medicine: A Comprehensive Guide.* London: Churchill Livingstone.

598. Xiufen, W. (Ed.) 2003. *Traditional Chinese Diagnostics.* Beijing: People's Medical Publishing House.

599. Holmes, P. (2007). *The Energetics of Western Herbs: A Materia Medica Integrating Western & Chinese Herbal Therapeutics, Volume 1* (4th edn). Santa Rosa, CA: Snow Lotus.

600. Bartram, T. (1995). *Encyclopedia of Herbal Medicine.* Christchurch, UK: Grace.

601. Liu, W., & Gong, C. (2009). Opening the blockage to reproduction: infertility. *Traditional Chinese Medicine Information Page* [online]. Available from http://tcmpage.com/hpinfertility.html (accessed 4 July 2011).

602. Trickey, R. (2003). *Women, Hormones & the Menstrual Cycle.* Sydney, Australia: Allen & Unwin.

603. Liu, W., & Gong, C. (2009). Opening the blockage to reproduction: infertility. *Traditional Chinese Medicine Information Page* [online]. Available from http://tcmpage.com/hpinfertility.html (accessed 4 July 2011).

604. Timonen, S., & Procopé, B. J. (1971). Premenstrual syndrome and physical exercise. *Acta Obstetricia et Gynecologica Scandinavica,* 50(4): 331–337.

605. Hassan, I. (2010). Abzan (sitz bath) a regime in unani system of medicine. *Articlesbase* [online]. Available from http://articlesbase.com/alternative-medicine-articles/abzan-sitz-bath-a-regime-in-unani-system-of-medicine-2749047.html (accessed 27 March 2012).

606. Flaws, B. (1989). *Endometriosis and Infertility and Traditional Chinese Medicine: A Laywoman's Guide.* Colorado Springs, CO: Blue Poppy.

607. Kaptchuk, T. J. (1983). *Chinese Medicine: The Web That Has No Weaver.* London: Rider.

608. Liu, W., & Gong, C. (2009). Opening the blockage to reproduction: infertility. *Traditional Chinese Medicine Information Page* [online]. Available from http://tcmpage.com/hpinfertility.html (accessed 4 July 2011).

609. Holmes, P. (2007). *The Energetics of Western Herbs: A Materia Medica Integrating Western & Chinese Herbal Therapeutics, Volume 2* (4th edn). Santa Rosa, CA: Snow Lotus.

610. Pitchford, P. (2002). *Healing With Whole Foods (3rd Edition).* Berkeley, CA: North Atlantic.

611. Liu, W., & Gong, C. (2009). Opening the blockage to reproduction: infertility. *Traditional Chinese Medicine Information Page* [online]. Available from http://tcmpage. com/hpinfertility.html (accessed 4 July 2011).

612. Maciocia, G. (2004). *Diagnosis in Chinese Medicine: A Comprehensive Guide.* London: Churchill Livingstone.

613. Coyle, M., & Smith, C. (2005). A survey comparing TCM diagnosis, health status and medical diagnosis in women undergoing assisted reproduction. *Acupuncture in Medicine, 23*: 62–69.

614. Liu, W., & Gong, C. (2009). Opening the blockage to reproduction: infertility. *Traditional Chinese Medicine Information Page* [online]. Available from http://tcmpage. com/hpinfertility.html (accessed 4 July 2011).

615. Flaws, B. (1989). *Endometriosis and Infertility and Traditional Chinese Medicine: A Laywoman's Guide.* Colorado Springs, CO: Blue Poppy.

616. Flaws, B. (1989). *Endometriosis and Infertility and Traditional Chinese Medicine: A Laywoman's Guide.* Colorado Springs, CO: Blue Poppy.

617. Pitchford, P. (2002). *Healing With Whole Foods* (3rd edn). Berkeley, CA: North Atlantic.

618. Holmes, P. (2007). *The Energetics of Western Herbs: A Materia Medica Integrating Western & Chinese Herbal Therapeutics, Volume 1* (4th edn). Santa Rosa, CA: Snow Lotus.

619. Schillemans-Eliyah, H. (2011). Stress-induced unexplained infertility—the role of acupuncture. *European Academy of Traditional Medical Science TCM Newsletter,* March [online]. Available from http://eatms.nl (accessed 20 February 2012).

620. Tillotson, A. K. (2001). *The One Earth Herbal Sourcebook.* New York: Kensington.

621. Schillemans-Eliyah, H. (2011). Stress-induced unexplained infertility—the role of acupuncture. *European Academy of Traditional Medical Science TCM Newsletter,* March [online]. Available from http://eatms.nl (accessed 20 February 2012).

622. Liu, W., & Gong, C. (2009). A natural option for endometriosis. *Traditional Chinese Medicine Information Page* [online]. Available from http://tcmpage.com/hpinfertility.html (accessed 20 February 2012).

623. Schillemans-Eliyah, H. (2011). Stress-induced unexplained infertility—the role of acupuncture. *European Academy of Traditional Medical Science TCM Newsletter,* March [online]. Available from http://www.eatms.nl (accessed 20 February 2012).

624. Holmes, P. (2007). *The Energetics of Western Herbs: A Materia Medica Integrating Western & Chinese Herbal Therapeutics, Volume 1* (4th edn). Santa Rosa, CA: Snow Lotus.

625. Pitchford, P. (2002). *Healing With Whole Foods* (3rd edn). Berkeley, CA: North Atlantic.

626. Maciocia G. (1998). *Obstetrics and Gynecology in Chinese Medicine.* London: Churchill Livingstone.

627. Schillemans-Eliyah, H. (2011). Stress-induced unexplained infertility—the role of acupuncture. *European Academy of Traditional Medical Science TCM Newsletter,* March [online]. Available from http://eatms.nl (accessed 20 February 2012).

628. Liu, W., & Gong, C. (2009). Opening the blockage to reproduction: infertility. *Traditional Chinese Medicine Information Page* [online]. Available from http://tcmpage. com/hpinfertility.html (accessed 4 July 2011).

629. Pole, S. (2006). *Ayurvedic Medicine: The Principles of Traditional Practice.* London: Churchill Livingstone.

630. Pitchford, P. (2002). *Healing With Whole Foods* (3rd edn). Berkeley, CA: North Atlantic.

631. Lad, V. D. (2002). *Textbook of Ayurveda: Fundamental Principles. Volume 1.* Albuquerque, NM: Ayurvedic Press.

632. Pole, S. (2006). *Ayurvedic Medicine: The Principles of Traditional Practice.* London: Churchill Livingstone.

633. Zimmermann, F. (1988). The jungle and the aroma of meats: an ecological theme in Hindu medicine. *Social Science and Medicine, 27*(3): 197–215.

634. Nordstrom, C. R. (1988). Exploring pluralism—the many faces of Ayurveda. *Social Science and Medicine, 27*(5): 479–489.

635. Sharma, P., Kulshreshtha, S., Mohan, G., Singh, S., & Bhagoliwal, A. (2007). Role of bromocriptine and pyridoxine in premenstrual tension syndrome. *Indian Journal of Physiology & Pharmacology, 5*(4): 368–374.

636. Lad, V. D. (2006). *Textbook of Ayurveda: A Complete Guide to Clinical Assessment. Volume 2.* Albuquerque, NM: Ayurvedic Press.

637. Sharma P. V. (Trans.) (2008). *Caraka Samhita* [text with English translation]. Varanasi, India: Chaukhambha Orientalia.

638. Pole, S. (2006). *Ayurvedic Medicine: The Principles of Traditional Practice.* London: Churchill Livingstone.

639. Sharma P. V. (Trans.) (2008). *Caraka Samhita* [text with English translation]. Varanasi, India: Chaukhambha Orientalia.

640. Pole, S. (2006). *Ayurvedic Medicine: The Principles of Traditional Practice.* London: Churchill Livingstone.

641. Svoboda, R. E. (1992). Ayurveda: Life, Health and Longevity. Penguin Books Ltd.

642. Pole, S. (2006). *Ayurvedic medicine: The Principles of Traditional Practice.* London: Churchill Livingstone.

643. Lad, V. D. (2006). *Textbook of Ayurveda: A Complete Guide to Clinical Assessment. Volume 2.* Albuquerque, NM: Ayurvedic Press.

644. Frawley, D. & Lad, V. (2001). The Yoga of Herbs: An Ayurvedic Guide to Herbal Medicine. Lotus Press, Wisconsin.

645. Svoboda, R. E. (1992). *Ayurveda: Life, Health and Longevity.* Albuquerque, NM: Ayurvedic Press.

646. Pole, S. (2006). *Ayurvedic Medicine: The Principles of Traditional Practice.* London: Churchill Livingstone.

647. Frawley, D., & Lad, V. D. (2001). The Yoga of Herbs: An Ayurvedic Guide to Herbal Medicine. Twin Lakes, WI: Lotus.

648. Pole, S. (2006). *Ayurvedic Medicine: The Principles of Traditional Practice.* London: Churchill Livingstone.

649. Lad, V. D. (2006). *Textbook of Ayurveda: A Complete Guide to Clinical Assessment. Volume 2.* Albuquerque, NM: Ayurvedic Press.

650. Pole, S. (2006). *Ayurvedic Medicine: The Principles of Traditional Practice.* London: Churchill Livingstone.

651. Lad, V. D. (2002). *Textbook of Ayurveda: Fundamental Principles. Volume 1.* Albuquerque, NM: Ayurvedic Press.

652. Frawley, D., & Lad, V. D. (2001). The Yoga of Herbs: An Ayurvedic Guide to Herbal Medicine. Twin Lakes, WI: Lotus.

653. Dick, M. (2002). Commentary on The Elements and Attributes of the Three Doshas. The Ayurvedic Institute [online]. Available from http://ayurveda.com (accessed 25 September 2009).

654. Svoboda, R. E. (1992). *Ayurveda: Life, Health and Longevity*. Albuquerque, NM: Ayurvedic Press.

655. McIntyre, A. (2005). *Herbal Treatment of Children: Western and Ayurvedic Perspectives*. London: Churchill Livingstone.

656. Pole, S. (2006). *Ayurvedic Medicine: The Principles of Traditional Practice*. London: Churchill Livingstone.

657. Lad, V. D. (2006). *Textbook of Ayurveda: A Complete Guide to Clinical Assessment. Volume 2*. Albuquerque, NM: Ayurvedic Press.

658. Stinnett, J. D. (1988). Pitta: the Dosha of transformation. *Ayurveda Today*, 1(1): 9–10.

659. Frawley, D., & Lad, V. D. (2001). *The Yoga of Herbs: An Ayurvedic Guide to Herbal Medicine*. Twin Lakes, WI: Lotus.

660. Pole, S. (2006). *Ayurvedic Medicine: The Principles of Traditional Practice*. London: Churchill Livingstone.

661. Pole, S. (2006). *Ayurvedic Medicine: The Principles of Traditional Practice*. London: Churchill Livingstone.

662. Frawley, D., & Lad, V. D. (2001). *The Yoga of Herbs: An Ayurvedic Guide to Herbal Medicine*. Twin Lakes, WI: Lotus.

663. Pole, S. (2006). *Ayurvedic Medicine: The Principles of Traditional Practice*. London: Churchill Livingstone.

664. Lad, V. D. (2006). *Textbook of Ayurveda: A Complete Guide to Clinical Assessment. Volume 2*. Albuquerque, NM: Ayurvedic Press.

665. Lad, V. D. (2006). *Textbook of Ayurveda: A Complete Guide to Clinical Assessment. Volume 2*. Albuquerque, NM: Ayurvedic Press.

666. Tillotson, A. K. (2001). *The One Earth Herbal Sourcebook*. New York: Kensington.

667. Pole, S. (2006). *Ayurvedic Medicine: The Principles of Traditional Practice*. London: Churchill Livingstone.

PART II

REPRODUCTIVE HEALTH PROBLEMS IN MEN

There is a myth that age does not affect fertility in men. However, while some men are able to conceive into their seventies, age can in fact have a significant impact on male fertility, and most men will have reduced sperm motility and less genetic integrity from their late forties.[668]

Even in younger men, fertility rates have declined dramatically over the last four decades. A meta-analysis of sperm count studies, published in the journal *Human Reproduction Update* in 2017 showed a 52.4% overall decline in sperm concentration and a 59.3% decline in total sperm count.[669] Environmental concerns such as exposure to radiation and plastics, together with lifestyle factors, are increasingly implicated in male infertility.[670]

Male factor infertility accounts for up to 50% of cases of infertility.[671,672] However, in the vast majority of cases of infertility, the woman alone is offered conventional treatment.[673] For best results, fertility treatment should include both partners, and for a minimum of three months.[674] This is in order for both partners to reach optimum health, and for fertilisation of a healthy oocyte by a healthy sperm, both of which have undergone their development, while taking herbs and supplements to protect them and improve their quality.

Spermatogenesis takes approximately three months. Similarly it takes almost three months for an ovarian follicle to develop from the preantral phase to maturation. (It takes nearly a year for a follicle to develop from the primordial phase to maturation, but it is most likely that any damage to the oocyte DNA occurs during the antral stage.)[675]

For men who do not wish to conceive, reproductive health problems such as low androgen levels, varicocele, prostatitis and sexual dysfunction cause significant distress and/or discomfort, and often respond well to natural treatment. Male reproductive health problems are divided into three categories: pre-testicular, testicular, and post-testicular.

Notes

668. Keane, D. (2016). Age & fertility [online]. Available from https://vhiblog. ie/2016/12/02/age-fertility/ (accessed 10 November 2018).
669. Levine, H., Joergensen, N., Martino-Andrade, A., Mendiola, J., Weksler-Derri, D., Mindlis, I., Pinotti, R., & Swan, S. H. (2017). Temporal trends in sperm count: a systematic review and meta-regression analysis. *Human Reproduction Update, 23*(6): 646–659.

670. FertilitySA. (2019). The top 3 reasons infertility is on the rise [online]. Available from fertilitysa.com.au (accessed 10 November 2019).

671. Ambiye, V. R., Langade, D., Dongre, S., Aptikar, P., Kulkarni, M., & Dongre, A. (2013). Clinical evaluation of the spermatogenic activity of the root extract of ashwagandha (*Withania somnifera*) in oligospermic males: a pilot study. *Evidence-Based Complementary and Alternative Medicine* [online]. Available from http://ncbi.nlm.nih.gov/pmc/articles/PMC3863556/#!po=3.84615 (accessed 15 July 2015).

672. Hirsh, A. (2003). Male subfertility. *British Medical Journal, 327*(7416): 669–672.

673. Gascoigne, S. (2001). *The Clinical Medicine Guide: A Hholistic Perspective.* Clonakilty, Ireland: Jigme.

674. Noll, A. A., & Wilms, S. (2011). *Chinese Medicine in Fertility Disorders.* New York: Thieme.

675. Erickson, G. F. (2004). Gynecology and Obstetrics Chapter 12: Follicle Growth and Development. Lippincott Williams & Wilkins [online]. Available from https://glowm.com/resources/glowm/cd/pages/v5/v5c012.html#int (accessed 15 July 2015).

CHAPTER SEVEN

Pre-testicular problems

Endocrine causes

Hypogonadotropic hypogonadism

Hypogonadotropic hypogonadism is associated with reduced production of LH and FSH from the pituitary, and resulting low levels of androgens. It may be caused by obesity, nutritional deficiency, stress, inflammatory disease, ageing, and certain medications. Symptoms of hypogonadotropic hypogonadism include reduced muscle mass, fatigue, and erectile dysfunction.[676] Hypogonadotropic hypogonadism may lead to aspermia (absence of sperm).[677]

Treatment of hypogonadotropic hypogonadism involves increasing exercise and improving nutrition, particularly ensuring adequate intake of zinc,[678] which is found in red meat, poultry, seafood, beans, nuts, dairy products, and breakfast cereals.[679] Stress levels may be improved with stress management techniques and herbal adaptogens such as *Withania somnifera*. *Withania somnifera* also improves LH and androgen production.[680] Androgen levels can also be improved with *Pinus pinaster*[681] and *Panax ginseng*.

Increased exposure to oestrogens

Increased exposure to oestrogen in utero is thought to be responsible for foetal testicular damage by inhibiting the development of Sertoli cells. It is also thought to inhibit testicular function and spermatogenesis in males after birth.[682] Excess oestrogen in men inhibits secretion of hypothalamic gonadotropin-releasing hormone (GnRH), follicle stimulating hormone (FSH), and luteinising hormone (LH),[683] resulting in low levels of androgens and impaired spermatogenesis.

Excess oestrogen in men also increases levels of sex hormone-binding globulin (SHBG), which binds to testosterone and reduces its availability, leading to symptoms of low testosterone (such as fatigue, muscle weakness, reduced libido, and erectile dysfunction).

Excessive adipose tissue and high insulin levels (both associated with obesity) are associated with increased aromatase activity,[684] which leads to aromatisation of testosterone to form oestrogen.[685] Therefore measures to reduce obesity may help to reduce oestrogen levels and improve fertility. In addition, linseed and *Serenoa serrulata* are aromatase inhibitors,[686] which help to reduce the conversion of androgens to oestrogen. Various other foods and herbs have been shown to inhibit aromatisation, including: *Camellia sinensis* (green tea); *Curcuma longa* (turmeric); *Tanacetum parthenium* (feverfew); *Taraxacum officinale* (dandelion); *Viscum album* (mistletoe); *Vitis* spp. (grape seed extract); vegetables such as asparagus, bell peppers, broccoli, celery, collard greens, endive, escarole, kale, and onions; chanterelle, portobello, shitake, and white button mushrooms; citrus fruits (such as oranges); and strawberries.[687]

Synthetic oestrogens are widely used in livestock, poultry, and dairy industries. Many commonly used pesticides, such as organochloride compounds also have oestrogenic effects within the body, and chemicals such as dioxin, DDT, and PCBs are known to interfere with spermatogenesis. It is therefore advisable to avoid hormone-containing meat and dairy products, and opt for organic foods.[688]

Hepatic cirrhosis leads to reduced oestrogen metabolism in the liver, and is therefore associated with increased endogenous oestrogens, which can suppress pituitary gonadotropin secretion and affect spermatogenesis.[689] Bitter herbs, such as *Taraxacum officinale* I which increase liver function, may help to reduce oestrogen excess. Foods high in methionine (such as beans, pulses, onions, and garlic) also assist with methylation of oestrogen in the liver.[690] In addition, cruciferous vegetables (such as cabbage, broccoli, and kale) contain indole-3-carbinol (I3 C), which has been shown to increase metabolism and elimination of oestrogen.[691]

Sex hormone-binding globulin (SHBG)

Sex hormone-binding globulin (SHBG) is a glycoprotein that binds to oestradiol, testosterone, and dihydrotestosterone. It transports these hormones in the blood as biologically inactive forms. Changes in SHBG levels can affect the amount of hormone that is available to be used by the body's tissues. Because of the higher affinity of SHBG for DHT and testosterone, compared to oestrogen, SHBG also has effects on the balance between bioavailable androgens and oestrogens.

Where blood tests show results for "total" rather than "free" levels of testosterone and other reproductive hormones, it is essential to measure SHBG. A high SHBG level means that fewer free hormones are available to the tissues. A low SHBG level means that more of the total hormone is bioavailable and not bound to SHBG.

Elevated SHBG

SHBG is increased by: high levels of oestrogen, low levels of testosterone, and nutrient deficiency. Therefore, increased SHBG levels may be seen in patients with:

- Exposure to xenoestrogens: increased SHBG may help to reduce the proliferative effects of oestrogen excess, but the effect may be negated by stress hormones (such as cortisol); growth hormones (e.g., from meat and dairy products); obesity; and insulin resistance
- Hyperthyroidism (which drives aromatisation of androgens and thereby increases production)
- Liver disease (which is associated with higher levels of oestrogen due to decreased conjugation of oestrogen in the liver), and
- Calorie restriction/anorexia nervosa (in which increased SHBG reduces bioavailability of testosterone, preventing further energy loss in reproduction).

Decreased testosterone production (due to advancing age or hypogonadism in men) also leads to increased SHBG, which further reduces the activity of testosterone. This may appear counterproductive, but it may be in order to protect against risk of prostate cancer, diabetes, and cardiovascular disease.

However, in some cases SHBG may be excessively high, due to deficiency of vitamin D; deficiency of minerals such as magnesium and zinc (which lower SHBG); a diet low in carbohydrates, protein, fat, or omega-3 oils; or reduced production of DHEA (due to stress). Increased SHBG in men may be associated with symptoms of low testosterone (such as fatigue, muscle weakness, reduced libido, and erectile dysfunction), because less testosterone is available to the body's tissue (even where total testosterone or oestrogen levels are within the normal ranges).

Low SHBG levels

SHBG is reduced by: low levels of oestrogen, high levels of testosterone, high levels of growth hormone (GH), high levels of cortisol, and high carbohydrate and high fat diets. Therefore, decreased SHBG levels may be seen in:

- Androgen (steroid) use
- Cushing's disease (which is associated with high levels of endogenous steroids)
- Insulin resistance and type 2 diabetes (insulin resistance lowers SHBG which in turn leads to increased androgen availability, and increased risk of prostate hyperplasia)
- Increased LDL cholesterol (which is associated with low testosterone and thyroxine production): this leads to increased risk of cardiovascular disease.

Low levels of SHBG in men lead to increased free testosterone, which increases the risk of prostate cancer, diabetes, and cardiovascular disease.

Thyroid abnormalities

Thyroid function is regulated by the hypothalamic-pituitary axis, and therefore changes in thyroid function can impact greatly on reproductive hormone function.[692]

Hypothyroidism

Hypothyroidism is associated with weight gain, oedema, intolerance of cold, dry skin and hair, bradycardia, depression, constipation, hoarse voice, and non-pitting pretibial oedema. Primary hypothyroidism may be congenital or autoimmune (Hashimoto's). It may be due to iodine deficiency, or may follow treatment for hyperthyroidism. It is associated with suboptimal levels of T4 and T3, and *elevated* levels of thyroid stimulating hormone (TSH). This is because low levels of thyroid hormones trigger the pituitary gland to increase TSH. Hypothyroidism is also associated with hypercholesterolaemia; low ferritin (due to the effect of thyroid hormones on ferritin synthesis); and low sex hormone-binding globulin (due the effect of hypothyroidism on oestrogen levels).

Secondary hypothyroidism is not due to a problem with the thyroid itself, but to a problem with the pituitary gland or hypothalamus. In this case, suboptimal levels of T3 and T4 are associated with *low* TSH. This is because the thyroid gland receives insufficient stimulation from pituitary thyrotropin hormones, and the hypothalamus or pituitary fails to respond to the resulting low thyroid hormone levels.

In euthyroid sick syndrome (which may be due to any severe, acute illness) free T3 is reduced, but TSH and T4 may be normal. It is therefore essential to measure TSH, T4, *and* T3 in order to accurately diagnose thyroid disease, and to differentiate between primary and secondary hypothyroidism.

In cases of primary hypothyroidism, decreased production of T3 and/or T4 by the thyroid gland also results in elevated thyroid releasing hormone (TRH) due to reduced negative feedback on the hypothalamus. The elevated TRH increases prolactin release from the pituitary.[693] Elevated prolactin in turn causes suppression of gonadotropic releasing hormone (GnRH) by the hypothalamus, resulting in low pituitary secretion of luteinising hormone (LH) and follicle stimulating hormone (FSH). The lack of LH and FSH inhibits androgen production and spermatogenesis, leading to reduced fertility.

There is also increasing evidence for the role of autoantibodies in male subfertility. This may be linked to inflammatory changes in the reproductive tissues.[694]

In cases of secondary hypothyroidism due to damage to the hypothalamus or pituitary gland, associated deficiency of GnRH and/or FSH/LH leads to decreased androgen production and spermatogenesis.

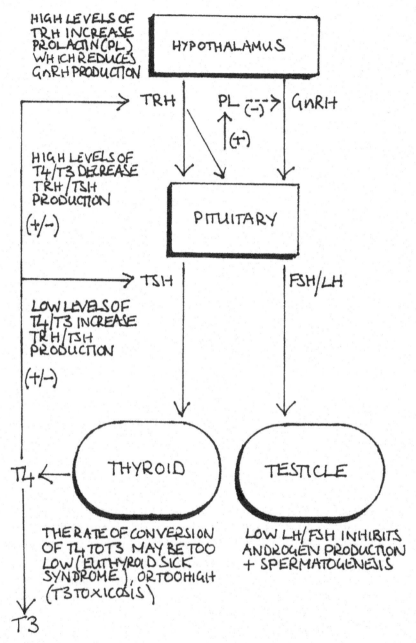

Figure 17: The thyroid and reproductive function.

Improving thyroid function

Consuming iodine rich foods including seaweeds (such as kelp), and ensuring adequate selenium intake (from nuts such as brazils), and exercising for at least 20–30 minutes a day can help to improve thyroid function in patients with hypothyroidism.[695] Other important nutrients for thyroxine synthesis include L-tyrosine, and vitamin B complex. Herbal medicines such as *Fucus vesiculosus* (bladderwrack), *Withania somnifera* (ashwagandha), and *Commiphora mukkul* (guggul) can also increase thyroid function.[696] Measures to improve oestrogen may help to improve thyroid function. *Lepidium meyenii* (maca) increases both oestrogen and thyroid hormone levels.[697] *Withania somnifera* can help to reduce autoimmunity.

Energetics

In Ayurveda, hypothyroid conditions are most commonly associated with excess Kapha, which benefits from warm, dry, and pungent foods and herbs, such as *Withania somnifera* (ashwagandha) and *Commiphora mukkul* (guggul). In TCM, hypothyroidism is most commonly associated with Yang Deficiency and accumulation of Dampness and Phlegm, which also requires warm, dry, and pungent foods and herbs.

Hyperthyroidism

Hyperthyroidism is associated with increased appetite, weight loss, heat intolerance, sweating, tachycardia, diarrhoea, restlessness, fine tremor, and exopthalmus. Primary hyperthyroidism may be autoimmune (Graves' disease), or due to subacute thyroiditis, toxic adenoma, or multinodular goitre. Amiodorone, which is used to treat cardiac arrhythmia, may also cause hyperthyroidism. In hyperthyroidism, both T4 and T3 levels are usually elevated, but in a small subset of hyperthyroid patients only T3 is elevated (T3 toxicosis).

Secondary hyperthyroidism may be due to pituitary tumours, which secrete high levels of TSH, triggering increased T4 production by the thyroid gland. TSH-secreting tumours do not respond to negative feedback from increasing T4 or T3 levels.

Hyperthyroidism is also associated with high ferritin (due to the effect of thyroid hormones on ferritin synthesis); hypocholesterolaemia;

low triglyceride; low folate (due to the increased metabolic state); high blood calcium levels (due to altered bone metabolism); and high SHBG (due to increased oestrogen levels).

An overactive thyroid increases conversion of testosterone to oestrogen.[698] Higher levels of oestrogen inhibit secretion of hypothalamic gonadotropin-releasing hormone (GnRH) and other important reproductive hormones such as follicle stimulating hormone (FSH) and luteinising hormone (LH),[699] which are responsible for sperm production, thereby contributing to infertility. Abnormalities in thyroid function can therefore have an adverse effect on reproductive health in men.

Reducing thyroid overactivity

For patients with hyperthyroidism, herbs such as *Melissa officinalis* (lemon balm) and *Lycopus virginicus* (gypsywort) reduce thyroid overactivity.[700] *Ganoderma lucidum* (reishi mushroom) and *Hemidesmus Indicus* (sariva) reduce autoimmunity.[701] *Leonurus cardiaca* is useful for reducing cardiovascular symptoms in patients with overactive thyroid.

Energetics

In Ayurveda, hyperthyroid conditions are most commonly associated with disturbances of Vata/Pitta,[702] which benefit from calming nervines such as *Melissa officinalis* (lemon balm), *Lycopus virginicus* (gypsywort), and *Leonurus cardiaca* (motherwort). In traditional Chinese medicine (TCM), hyperthyroidism is considered to be the result of Yin Deficiency.[703] For more information about energetic approaches to understanding and treating infertility, see Chapter 6.

Sperm abnormalities

Low sperm count and abnormal morphology

Spermatogenesis takes up to ninety days. The ideal temperature for sperm production is 35 degrees Celsius.[704] Total absence of sperm is termed *azoospermia*; low sperm concentration ($<10 \times 10^6$ mL) is termed *oligozoospermia*; and increased numbers of sperm with abnormal morphology is termed *teratospermia*.[705]

Azoospermia, oligozoospermia, and teratospermia may be caused by various factors including: genetic abnormalities,[706] obesity,[707] endocrine abnormalities, nutritional deficiencies, use of certain prescription medications, environmental factors, exposure to toxins, heavy metals, and radiation, recreational drug use, alcohol, excessive heat, and history of genitourinary infections. Even having a high fever can impact spermatogenesis for up to six months.[708]

Concurrent pathologies may also affect sperm production. For example, 80% of men with hemochromatosis have some degree of testicular dysfunction.[709] Over the past fifty years, sperm counts have declined significantly (by about 30%).[710]

Low sperm motility

Low sperm motility is termed *asthenozoospermia*. It may be caused by long periods of abstinence, or by the presence of anti-sperm antibodies. The presence of elevated leukocytes in semen may produce excessive reactive oxygen species (ROS) and cytotoxic cytokines.[711] This may overwhelm the antioxidant defence mechanisms and cause oxidative stress, damaging sperm and leading to infertility.[712] Studies have demonstrated a significant correlation between beta-carotene levels and antibody titres, suggesting that dietary antioxidants are involved in mediating immune function in the male reproductive system.[713]

The following table shows the normal values for semen parameters according to the World Health Organization (WHO).[714]

Normal semen parameters

Parameter	Reference value
Volume	>2.0 ml
pH	7.2–8
Concentration	$>20 \times 10^6$ ml
Total sperm per ejaculate	$>40 \times 10^6$ ml
Motility	>50% motile (grade a+b) or >25% grade a
Morphology	<15%
Viability	>75% live spermatozoa
Leukocytes	$<1 \times 10^6$ ml
Anti-sperm antibodies	<50% bound sperm
Zinc	>2.4 uM per ejaculate
Citric acid	>52 uM per ejaculate
Fructose	>13 uM per ejaculate

However, conventional semen analysis often fails to identify infertile males with "normal" samples, and conversely fails to identify fertile males with subnormal semen parameters.[715] Studies have shown that, for men whose partners were able to conceive within twelve months, the lower reference limits were: semen volume: 1.5 ml; sperm concentration: 15 million/ml; sperm count: 39 million per ejaculate; progressive motility: 32%; progressive + non-progressive motility 40%; morphology: 4.0% normal forms; viability: 58% live spermatozoa.[716]

Analysis should be performed on multiple ejaculates before diagnosing male infertility, due to the large individual variation in sperm parameters.[717] More sensitive tests are also available, including the egg penetration test; and the post-coital test, which measures the ability of sperm to penetrate cervical mucus. These tests predict fertility in an estimated 66% of cases, in comparison to 30% with conventional sperm analysis.[718]

Improving sperm count, morphology, and motility

Supplementing essential nutrients can double the sperm count, improve sperm motility by about a quarter, and increase ejaculate volume by about a third.[719] Zinc deficiency is associated with decreased testosterone levels and sperm count, and several studies have found supplemental zinc may prove helpful in treating male infertility.[720] Zinc is found in many foods, including red meat, poultry, seafood, beans, nuts, dairy products, and breakfast cereals.[721]

Carnitine is essential in sperm energy production. It contributes directly to sperm motility and may be involved in the successful maturation of sperm.[722] Arginine is also essential for sperm motility, and supplementation has been shown to increase motility in patients with asthenospermia.[723]

Fatty acids and phospholipids in the sperm cell membrane are highly susceptible to oxidative damage. Sperm produce controlled concentrations of reactive oxygen species (ROS), such as the superoxide anion, hydrogen peroxide, and nitric oxide, which are needed for penetrating the egg during fertilization. However, high concentrations of these free radicals can directly damage sperm cells.[724] Antioxidant nutrients including vitamins C and E, selenium, and glutathione have been shown to significantly improve sperm concentration and motility, and increase the chance of impregnation.[725]

Co-enzyme Q10 is involved in energy production in spermatozoa and also acts as an antioxidant.[726] Sperm concentration, motility, and morphology have all been shown to significantly improve after twelve months of co-enzyme Q10 therapy, resulting in a beneficial effect on rate of conception.[727]

Vitamin B12 is important in cellular replication, especially synthesis of RNA and DNA, and deficiency is associated with decreased sperm count and motility.[728,729]

Withania somnifera is traditionally used in Ayurvedic medicine for the treatment of male sexual dysfunction and infertility. It is particularly suited to men suffering from Vata disturbance, stress, and anxiety.[730] It reduces oxidative stress, and improves semen quality,[731] increasing semen volume, sperm count, and motility.[732] However, there have been anecdotal reports of *Withania* decreasing sperm motility in some individuals.

Lepidium meyenii (maca) also improves sperm count and motility. It does not seem to increase testosterone levels; however, it may act by increasing the bioavailability of testosterone, or augmenting testosterone receptor binding.[733] *Panax ginseng* is another useful herb for improving sperm count.[734] *Tribulus terrestris* also increases sperm count, decreases abnormal forms, and increases overall sexual health.[735]

Pygeum africanum (African prune tree bark) promotes alkaline phosphatase activity, which increases total prostatic secretions and helps to maintain the appropriate pH of seminal fluid. Sperm motility is partly determined by the pH of the prostatic fluid. Therefore *Pygeum africanum* (100–200 mg extract per day) may help to promote optimal sperm motility and improve fertility.[736] *Astragalus membranaceus* also significantly increases sperm motility.[737]

Andrographis paniculata increases testosterone levels and may improve immune response in men with anti-sperm antibodies.[738]

Ejaculation that occurs daily or more frequently (due to intercourse or masturbation) can reduce sperm counts. Conversely, abstinence for more than seven days can result in reduced sperm motility. Therefore, intercourse every thirty-six hours or so around the time of ovulation is optimal for conception.[739]

Energetics

Problems with sperm are related to Kidney Yang Deficiency.[740] Kidney energy may be depleted by lifestyle factors such as poor diet and overwork.[741]

Clinical manifestations of Kidney Yang Deficiency include: fatigue; dizziness; ringing in the ears; dull-pale complexion; lower back soreness; lack of libido; erectile dysfunction; feeling cold; loose stools; long-drawn-out urination with a thin stream or dribbling; a thick or puffy tongue body with a white tongue coating; and a thin-soft pulse.[742] Kidney Yang Deficiency may be the result of a demanding lifestyle, particularly in older men.[743] It is commonly associated with problems such as poor sperm motility.

Polygonum multiflorum nourishes the Kidney Essence and helps to improve sperm production. *Turnera diffusa, Panax ginseng, Schisandra chinesis*, and *Cinnamonu zeylonicum* are used to treat Kidney Yang Deficiency.[744]

Case study

Thirty-eight-year-old male

Presenting complaint
- Infertility: sperm analysis showed semen volume 1.5 ml; sperm concentration 12 million/ml; sperm count 30 million per ejaculate; progressive motility 20%; morphology 3% normal forms; viability 40% live spermatozoa.

Medical history
- Poor diet, smokes 10 cigarettes per day and smokes cannabis at weekends.
- Rash on arms due to allergies to chemicals used at work
- Works very long hours on farm
- Regularly takes NSAIDs for back and shoulder pain

BP: 130/80

Pulse: 70 bpm (regular)

Rx

• Panax ginseng	(1:3)	10
• Astragalus membranaceus	(1:1)	20
• Andrographis paniculata	(1:3)	20
• Polygonum multiflorum	(1:1)	15
• Harpagophytum procumbens	(1:1)	20
• Salix alba	(1:1)	15
• Zingiber officinale	(1:2)	5

105 ml per week   (Sig. 7.5 ml bid)

Recommendations
- Fertility supplement for men containing carnitine, arginine, vitamin B complex, vitamin C, vitamin E, selenium, zinc, and co-enzyme Q10
- Improve diet, reduce alcohol consumption, avoid smoking, reduce/avoid NSAID use. Use PPE to minimise exposure to chemicals
- Reduce work hours and take adequate breaks
- Aim for intercourse with partner every 36 hours around the time of ovulation

Follow-up
- Patient's partner conceived after 6 months of treatment

Undescended testes

Undescended testes (cryptorchidism) is associated with impairment of germ cell maturation and subsequent azoospermia leading to infertility, particularly if not treated before the age of one year. Normal management of infertility due to cryptorchidism consists of microsurgical sperm retrieval and intracytoplasmic sperm injection (ICSI).[745] However, herbal and nutritional approaches to improving sperm quality, as detailed in this chapter, may also be helpful.

Genetic defects

Various chromosomal abnormalities (such as Klinefelter's syndrome) can affect male sexual development, leading to low androgen production, underdeveloped testes, and subsequent infertility. It may be treated with hormone replacement therapy and assisted reproduction techniques.[746] However, herbal medicine and nutrition can also be used as an adjunct, depending on the needs of the individual.

Notes

676. Bone, K., & Mills, S. (2013). *Principles and Practice of Phytotherapy: Modern Herbal Medicine*. London: Churchill Livingstone.
677. Agarwal, A., & Said, T. M. (2011). Interpretation of basic semen analysis and advanced semen testing. In: E. S. Sabanegh, Jr. (Ed.), *Male Infertility: Problems and Solutions*. Springer [online].
678. Madding, C. I., Jacob, M., Ramsay, V. P., & Sokol, R. Z. (1986). Serum and semen zinc levels in normozoospermic and oligozoospermic men. *Annals of Nutrition and Metabolism*, 30(4): 213–218.
679. NIH (2011). Zinc. National Institutes of Health [online]. Available from https://ods.od.nih.gov/factsheets/Zinc-Consumer/ (accessed 15 July 2015).
680. Ambiye, V. R., Langade, D., Dongre, S., Aptikar, P., Kulkarni, M., & Dongre, A. (2013). Clinical Evaluation of the Spermatogenic Activity of the Root Extract of Ashwagandha (*Withania somnifera*) in Oligospermic Males: A Pilot Study. *Evidence-Based Complementary & Alternative Medicine* [online]. Available from http://ncbi.nlm.nih.gov/pmc/articles/PMC3863556/#!po=3.84615 (accessed 15 July 2015).
681. Stanislavov, R., Niklova, V., & Rohdewald, P. (2008). Improvement of erectile function with Prelox: a randomized, double-blind, placebo-controlled, crossover trial. *International Journal of Impotence Research*, 20(2): 173–178.
682. Sinclair, S. (2000). Male infertility: nutritional and environmental considerations. *Alternative Medicine Review*, 5(1): 28–38.
683. Greenstein, B., & Wood, D. F. (2006). *The Endocrine System at a Glance* (2nd edn). Oxford: Blackwell.
684. Bone, K., & Mills, S. (2013). *Principles and Practice of Phytotherapy: Modern Herbal Medicine*. London: Churchill Livingstone.
685. Tremellen, K., & Pearce, K. (2015). *Nutrition, Fertility, and Human Reproductive Function*. Boca Raton, FL: CRC Press.
686. Bone, K., & Mills, S. (2013). *Principles and Practice of Phytotherapy: Modern Herbal Medicine*. London: Churchill Livingstone.
687. Balunas, M. J., Su, B., Brueggemeier, R. W., & Kinghorn, A. D. (2011). Natural products as aromatase inhibitors. *Anti-Cancer Agents in Medicinal Chemistry*, 8(6): 646–682.
688. Sinclair, S. (2000). Male infertility: nutritional and environmental considerations. *Alternative Medicine Review*, 5(1): 28–38.
689. Sinclair, S. (2000). Male infertility: nutritional and environmental considerations. *Alternative Medicine Review*, 5(1): 28–38.
690. Trickey, R. (2003). *Women, Hormones & the Menstrual Cycle*. Sydney, Australia: Allen & Unwin.

691. Michnocicz, J. J., & Bradlow, H. L. (1991). Altered estrogen metabolism and excretion in humans following consumption of indole-3-carbinol. *Nutrition and Cancer, 16*(1): 59–66.

692. Jefferys, A., Vanderpump, M., & Yasmin, E. (2015). Thyroid dysfunction and reproductive health. *Obstetrician & Gynaecologist, 17*(1): 39–45.

693. Heffner, L. J., & Schust, D. J. (2014). *The Reproductive System at a Glance.* Oxford: John Wiley & Sons.

694. Jefferys, A., Vanderpump, M., & Yasmin, E. (2015). Thyroid dysfunction and reproductive health. *Obstetrician & Gynaecologist, 17*(1): 39–45.

695. Trickey, R. (2011). *Women, Hormones and the Menstrual Cycle.* Clifton Hill, Victoria, Australia: Melbourne Holistic Health Group.

696. Romm, A. (2016). *Botanical Medicine for Women's Health* (2nd edn). London: Churchill Livingstone.

697. Meissner, H. O., Kapczynski, W., Mscisz, A., & Lutomski, J. (2005). Use of gelatinized maca (Lepidium peruvianum) in early postmenopausal women. *International Journal of Biomedical Science, 1*(1): 33–45.

698. Trickey, R. (2011). *Women, Hormones and the Menstrual Cycle.* Clifton Hill, Victoria, Australia: Melbourne Holistic Health Group.

699. Greenstein, B., & Wood, D. F. (2006). *The Endocrine System at a Glance* (2nd edn). Oxford: Blackwell.

700. Holmes, P. (2007). *The Energetics of Western Herbs: A Materia Medica Integrating Western & Chinese Herbal Therapeutics, Volume 2* (4th edn). Santa Rosa, CA: Snow Lotus.

701. Bone, K., & Mills, S. (2013). *Principles and Practice of Phytotherapy: Modern Herbal Medicine.* London: Churchill Livingstone.

702. Aswathy Prakash, C., & Byresh, A. (2015). Understanding hypothyroidism in Ayurveda. *International Ayurvedic Medical Journal, 3*(11): 2349–2357.

703. Dharmananda, S. (1996). Treatments for thyroid diseases with Chinese herbal medicine [online]. Available from http://itmonline.org/arts/thyroid.htm (accessed 8 March 2020).

704. Noll, A. A., & Wilms, S. (2011). *Chinese Medicine in Fertility Disorders.* New York: Thieme.

705. Agarwal, A., & Said, T. M. (2011). Interpretation of basic semen analysis and advanced semen testing. In: E. S. Sabanegh, Jr. (Ed.), *Male Infertility: Problems and Solutions.* Springer [online].

706. Agarwal, A., & Said, T. M. (2011). Interpretation of basic semen analysis and advanced semen testing. In: E. S. Sabanegh, Jr. (Ed.), *Male Infertility: Problems and Solutions.* Springer [online].

707. Tremellen, K., & Pearce, K. (2015). *Nutrition, Fertility, and Human Reproductive Function.* Boca Raton, FL: CRC Press.

708. Campana, A., de Agostini, A., Bischof, P., Tawfik, E., & Mastrorilli, A. (2019). Evaluation of infertility. Graduate Foundation for Medical Education and Research (GFMER) [online]. Available from https://gfmer.ch/Books/Reproductive_health/infertility_evaluation.html (accessed 20 June 2020).

709. Sinclair, S. (2000). Male infertility: nutritional and environmental considerations. *Alternative Medicine Review, 5*(1): 28–38.

710. Carlsen, E., Giwercman, A. J., Keiding, N., & Skakkebæk, N. E. (1993). Decline in semen quality from 1930 to 1991. *Ugeskrift for Læger, 155*: 2230–2235.

711. Agarwal, A., & Said, T. M. (2011). Interpretation of basic semen analysis and advanced semen testing. In: E. S. Sabanegh, Jr. (Ed.), *Male Infertility: Problems and Solutions*. Springer [online].

712. Sharma, R. K., & Agarwal, A. (1996). Role of reactive oxygen species in male infertility. *Urology, 48*(6): 835–850.

713. Palan, P., & Naz, R. (1996). Changes in various antioxidant levels in human seminal plasma related to immunoinfertility. *Archives of Andrology, 36*(2): 139–143.

714. World Health Organization (1999). *WHO laboratory Manual for the Examination of Human Semen and Sperm-Cervical Mucus Interaction*. Cambridge: Cambridge University Press.

715. Check, J. H., Nowroozi, K., Lee, M., Adelson, H., & Katsoff, D. (1990). Evaluation and treatment of a male factor component to unexplained infertility. *Archives of Andrology, 25*(3): 199–211.

716. Cooper, T. G. Noonan, E., von Eckardstein, S., Auger, J., Gordon Baker, H. W., Behre, H. M., Haugen, T. B., Kruger, T., Wang, C., Mbizvo, M. T., & Vogelsong, K. M. (2010). World Health Organization reference values for human semen charactaristics. *Human Reproduction Update, 16*(3): 231–245.

717. Keel, B. A. (2006). Within- and between-subject variation in semen parameters in infertile men and normal semen donors. *Fertility and Sterility, 85*: 128–134.

718. Purvis, K., & Christiansen, E. (1992). Male infertility: current concepts. *Annals of Medicine, 24*: 258–272.

719. Imhof, M., Lackner, J., Lipovac, M., Chedraui, P., & Riedl, C. (2012). Improvement of sperm quality after micronutrient supplementation. *e-SPEN, the European e-Journal of Clinical Nutrition and Metabolism, 7*(1): E50–E53.

720. Madding, C. I., Jacob, M., Ramsay, V. P., & Sokol, R. Z. (1986). Serum and semen zinc levels in normozoospermic and oligozoospermic men. *Annals of Nutrition and Metabolism, 30*: 213–218.

721. NIH (2011). Zinc. National Institutes of Health [online]. Available from https://ods.od.nih.gov/factsheets/Zinc-Consumer/ (accessed 15 July 2015).

722. Sinclair, S. (2000). Male infertility: nutritional and environmental considerations. *Alternative Medicine Review, 5*(1): 28–38.

723. Scibona, M., Meschini, P., Capparelli, S., Pecori, C., Rossi, P., & Menchini Fabris, G. F. (1994). L-arginine and male fertility. *Minerva Urologica e Nefrologica, 46*(4): 251–253.

724. De Lamirande, E., Jiang, H., Zini, A., Kodama, H., & Gagnon, C. (1997). Reactive oxygen species and sperm physiology. *Reviews of Reproduction, 2*(1): 48–54.

725. Sinclair, S. (2000). Male infertility: nutritional and environmental considerations. *Alternative Medicine Review, 5*(1): 28–38.

726. Lewin, A., & Lavin, H. (1997). The effect of coenzyme Q-10 on sperm motility and function. *Molecular Aspects of Medicine, 18*: S213–S219.

727. Safarinejad, M. R. (2011). The effect of coenzyme Q10 supplementation on partner pregnancy rate in infertile men with idiopathic oligoasthenoteratozoospermia: an open-label prospective study. *International Urology and Nephrology, 44*(3): 689–700.

728. Sinclair, S. (2000). Male infertility: nutritional and environmental considerations. *Alternative Medicine Review*, 5(1): 28–38.

729. Sandler, B., & Faraher, B. (1994). Treatment of oligospermia with B12. *Infertility*, 7: 133–138.

730. Ambiye, V. R., Langade, D., Dongre, S., Aptikar, P., Kulkarni, M., & Dongre, A. (2013). Clinical evaluation of the spermatogenic activity of the root extract of ashwagandha (*Withania somnifera*) in oligospermic males: a pilot study. *Evidence-Based Complementary and Alternative Medicine* [online]. Available from http://ncbi.nlm.nih.gov/pmc/articles/PMC3863556/#!po=3.84615 (accessed 15 July 2015).

731. Ahmad, M. K., Mahdi, A. A., Shukla, K. K., Islam, N., Rajender, S., Madhukar, D., Shankhwar, S. N., & Ahmad, S. (2010). Withania somnifera improves semen quality by regulating reproductive hormone levels and oxidative stress in seminal plasma of infertile males. *Fertility and Sterility*, 94(3): 989–996.

732. Ambiye, V. R., Langade, D., Dongre, S., Aptikar, P., Kulkarni, M., & Dongre, A. (2013). Clinical evaluation of the spermatogenic activity of the root extract of ashwagandha (*Withania somnifera*) in oligospermic males: a pilot study. *Evidence-Based Complementary and Alternative Medicine* [online]. Available from http://ncbi.nlm.nih.gov/pmc/articles/PMC3863556/#!po=3.84615 (accessed 15 July 2015).

733. Gonzales, G. F., Cordova, A., Gonzales, C., & Chung, A. (2001). Lepidium meyenii (Maca) improves semen parameters in adult men. *Asian Journal of Andrology*, 3(4): 301–303.

734. Bone, K., & Mills, S. (2013). *Principles and Practice of Phytotherapy: Modern Herbal Medicine*. London: Churchill Livingstone.

735. Thirunavukkarasu, M., Sellandi, M., Thakar, A. B., & Baghel, M. S. (2012). Clinical study of *Tribulus Terrestris* Linn. in oligozoospermia: a double blind study. *Ayu*, 33(3): 356–364.

736. Lucchetta, G., Weill, A., Becker, N., & Bollack, C. (1984). Reactivation from the prostatic gland in cases of reduced fertility. *Urologia Internationalis*, 39: 222–224.

737. Hong, C. Y., Ku, J., & Wu, P. (1992). *Astragalus membranaceus* stimulates human sperm motility in vitro. *American Journal of Chinese Medicine*, 20(3): 289–294.

738. Bone, K., & Mills, S. (2013). *Principles and Practice of Phytotherapy: Modern Herbal Medicine*. London: Churchill Livingstone.

739. Campana, A., de Agostini, A., Bischof, P., Tawfik, E., & Mastrorilli, A. (2019). Evaluation of infertility. Graduate Foundation for Medical Education and Research (GFMER) [online]. Available from https://gfmer.ch/Books/Reproductive_health/infertility_evaluation.html (accessed 20 June 2020).

740. Noll, A. A., & Wilms, S. (2011). *Chinese Medicine in Fertility Disorders*. New York: Thieme.

741. Liu, W., & Gong, C. (2009). Opening the blockage to reproduction: infertility. *Traditional Chinese Medicine Information Page* [online]. Available from http://tcmpage.com/hpinfertility.html (accessed 4 July 2011).

742. Liu, W., & Gong, C. (2009). Opening the blockage to reproduction: infertility. *Traditional Chinese Medicine Information Page* [online]. Available from http://tcmpage.com/hpinfertility.html (accessed 4 July 2011).

743. Noll, A. A., & Wilms, S. (2011). *Chinese Medicine in Fertility Disorders*. New York: Thieme.

744. Holmes, P. (2007). *The Energetics of Western Herbs: A Materia Medica Integrating Western & Chinese Herbal Therapeutics, Volume 1* (4th edn). Santa Rosa, CA: Snow Lotus.

745. Chung, E., & Brock, G. B. (2011). Cryptorchidism and its impact on male fertility: a state of art review of current literature. *Canadian Urological Association Journal, 5*(3): 210–214.

746. Genetics Home Reference (2013). Klinefelter syndrome. US National Library of Medicine [online]. Available from www.ghr.nlm.nih.gov (accessed 27 July 2015).

CHAPTER EIGHT

Testicular problems

Infection

History of infections affecting the testes, such as mumps, epididymitis, or chlamydia, and chronic asymptomatic infections are significant causes of male infertility.[747,748] Undiagnosed infection may be suggested by presence of anti-sperm antibodies.[749]

Treating infection

Infections such as chlamydia require orthodox treatment to help prevent long-term complications. However, anti-inflammatories and immune stimulants (such as *Uncaria tomentosa*, *Echinacea angustifolia*, and *Andrographis paniculata*), and anti-inflammatory nutrients (such as omega-3 oils), may help to reduce inflammation. Immune enhancing and antimicrobial herbs such as *Astragalus membranaceus* and *Hydrastis canadensis* are useful for chronic infection.[750]

Energetics

From an energetic point of view, infections are often associated with Damp Heat, which may be indicated by frequent urination, poor sperm morphology, and presence of anti-sperm antibodies. Cool dry herbs such as *Hydrastis canadensis*, *Andrographis paniculata*, and *Achillea millefolium* are useful for reducing Damp Heat.

Trauma/injury

Trauma and/or injury (due to cycling, horse riding, or prior surgery, for example) may cause damage to the testes. This can negatively affect sperm production or may lead to obstruction or retrograde ejaculation, and thereby have a negative impact on fertility. Surgery (e.g., for prostate or testicular cancer, hydrocele or inguinal hernia) may also damage the sympathetic nerve plexus causing azoospermia.[751]

Because spermatozoa are haploid cells (and therefore different to normal body cells) they can trigger the formation of antibodies. In healthy males, spermatozoa are protected from the immune system by a membrane, which forms the blood-testis barrier. However, trauma or surgery may rupture this barrier, resulting in detection of sperm cells by the immune system, and production of anti-sperm antibodies.[752]

Varicocele

The presence of a varicocele (which affects around 20% of males) may reduce fertility, although this is not always the case. A varicocele may impair testicular androgen production and spermatogenesis as a result of impaired circulation, which leads to increased testicular temperature and pressure, together with hypoxia and build-up of toxic metabolites. Sperm counts and fertility may improve after surgical removal of the varicocele.[753]

Treating varicocele

Herbal medicines that are traditionally are used to treat varicose veins such as *Aesculus hippocastanum* also improve fertility in men with varicocele.[754] Nutrients which help to reduce blood stagnation such as niacin (vitamin B3), vitamin C, vitamin E, and omega-3 fatty acids, in addition to increased exercise, may also help to reduce pelvic congestion, as described in the section on female infertility.

Energetics

From an energetic point of view, varicocele, trauma, or surgery may lead to Blood Stasis.[755] This is indicated by a blue or purple tongue-body colour, and poor peripheral circulation.[756,757] Blood Stasis may be treated with herbal medicines such as *Pinus pinaster*, *Ginkgo biloba*,[758] and *Aeculus hippocastanum*.[759]

Case study

Twenty-two-year-old male jockey

Presenting complaint
- Surgery for varicocele 4 years ago. Developed post-surgical hydrocele, which was treated surgically but has reoccured

Medical history
- Poor sleep latency and low energy levels in the morning
- Stiff, painful swollen knees (especially on the right)

BP: 125/70

Pulse: 80 bpm (regular) deep, slippery pulse

Tongue: Blue tongue body with red tip

Rx

• *Aesculus hippocastanum*	(1:3)	25
• *Ginkgo biloba*	(2:1)	15
• *Achillea millefolium*	(1:3)	25
• *Apium graveolens*	(1:3)	30
• *Salix alba*	(1:1)	15
• *Scutellaria lateriflora*	(1:3)	30

140 ml per week   (Sig. 10 ml bid)

Recommendations
- Vitamin B complex, vitamin C (1,000 mg), vitamin E (200 mg), zinc (20 mg), omega-3 (3,000 mg)
- Avoid horse riding until swelling subsides

Follow-up

- Hydrocele improved over 3 months of treatment. Treatment continued for 6 months in total before discontinuing
- Sleep and energy levels much improved
- Knee pain and swelling resolved

Genetic disorders

Primary ciliary dyskinesia (PCD) is a genetic disorder, which affects the cilia lining the mucous membranes, and also the flagella of sperm (since these are related structures). It leads to poor sperm motility and infertility.[760] Patients with PCD may require intracytoplasmic sperm injection (ICSI) in order to achieve conception. However, herbal and nutritional approaches to improving sperm quality, as detailed in this chapter, may also be helpful.

DNA damage

The degree of DNA fragmentation in sperm has been shown to be a better indicator of male fertility than conventional semen parameters (such as sperm count, motility, and morphology). Men with high levels of DNA fragmentation affecting their sperm have a significantly reduced chance of achieving conception, either naturally, or through assisted reproduction procedures such as intrauterine insemination (IUI) or in vitro fertilisation (IVF).[761]

Damage to sperm DNA may be caused by various factors including age, obesity, exposure to toxins (including cigarette smoke and alcohol), and cancer treatments (such as radiotherapy and chemotherapy). Testing of DNA integrity may be appropriate for infertile patients whose partners have a history of repeated pregnancy loss and unexplained infertility.[762,763,764]

Preventing DNA damage

DNA fragmentation in spermatozoa is predominantly caused by oxidative stress, and any sources of oxidative stress (such as stress, smoking, and exposure to other toxic substances), should therefore be identified in men with high levels of DNA fragmentation, and modified where possible. Reducing oxidative stress can significantly improve a couple's chances of conception, either naturally or with assisted reproduction treatment.[765]

Antioxidants may be useful in counteracting oxidative stress in men with DNA damage to sperm. However, a balance of reduction and oxidation is necessary for essential sperm function.[766] Sperm themselves produce controlled concentrations of reactive oxygen species (ROS), such as the superoxide anion, hydrogen peroxide, and nitric oxide, which are needed for penetrating the egg during fertilisation,[767] so it is also important not to over-supplement.

Antioxidant nutrients, including vitamins C and E, selenium, and glutathione have been shown to significantly improve sperm concentration and motility, and increase the chance of impregnation.[768] Co-enzyme Q10 also acts as an antioxidant.[769] Sperm concentration, motility, and morphology have all been shown to significantly improve after twelve months of co-enzyme Q10 therapy, resulting in a beneficial effect on rate of conception.[770] *Pinus pinaster* (pine bark) is also a potent antioxidant.[771]

Exposure to heat

Scrotal temperature is highly regulated by the body, and sperm production is significantly reduced at temperatures above 35 degrees Celsius. Men attempting to improve their fertility should avoid wearing tight fitting underwear or trousers, and should avoid taking hot baths or saunas, or using hot tubs.[772]

Notes

747. Purvis, K., & Christiansen, E. (1992). Male infertility: current concepts. *Annals of Medicine*, 24: 258–272.

748. Purvis, K., & Christiansen, E. (1993). Infection in the male reproductive tract. Impact, diagnosis and treatment in relation to male fertility. *International Journal of Andrology*, 16(1): 1–13.

749. Sinclair, S. (2000). Male infertility: nutritional and environmental considerations. *Alternative Medicine Review*, 5(1): 28–38.

750. Bone, K., & Mills, S. (2013). *Principles and Practice of Phytotherapy: Modern Herbal Medicine*. London: Churchill Livingstone.

751. Agarwal, A., & Said, T. M. (2011). Interpretation of basic semen analysis and advanced semen testing. In: E. S. Sabanegh, Jr. (Eds.), *Male Infertility: Problems and Solutions*. Springer [online].

752. Campana, A., de Agostini, A., Bischof, P., Tawfik, E., & Mastrorilli, A. (2019). Evaluation of infertility. Graduate Foundation for Medical Education and Research (GFMER) [online]. Available from: https://gfmer.ch/Books/Reproductive_health/infertility_evaluation.html (accessed 20 June 2020).

753. Kantartzi, P., Goulis, C. D., Goulis, G. D., & Papadimas, I. (2007). Male infertility and varicocele: myths and reality. *Hippokratia, 11*(3): 99–104.

754. Fang, Y., Zhao, L., Yan, F., Xia, X., Xu, D., & Cui, X. (2010). Escin improves sperm quality in male patients with varicocele-associated infertility. *Phytomedicine, 17*(3–4): 192–196.

755. Liu, W., & Gong, C. (2009). Opening the blockage to reproduction: infertility. *Traditional Chinese Medicine Information Page* [online]. Available from http://tcmpage.com/hpinfertility.html (accessed 4 July 2011).

756. Xiufen, W. (Ed.) (2003). *Traditional Chinese Diagnostics.* Beijing: People's Medical Publishing House.

757. Noll, A. A., & Wilms, S. (2011). *Chinese Medicine in Fertility Disorders.* New York: Thieme.

758. Bone, K., & Mills, S. (2013). *Principles and Practice of Phytotherapy: Modern Herbal Medicine.* London: Churchill Livingstone.

759. Fang, Y., Zhao, L., Yan, F., Xia, X., Xu, D., & Cui, X. (2010). Escin improves sperm quality in male patients with varicocele-associated infertility. *Phytomedicine, 17*(3–4): 192–196.

760. National Institutes for Health (2011). What is primary ciliary dyskenesia? [online]. Available from www.nhlbi.nih.gov (accessed 27 July 2015).

761. Wright, C., Milne, S., & Leeson, H. (2014). Sperm DNA damage caused by oxidative stress: modifiable clinical, lifestyle and nutritional factors in male infertility. *Reproductive BioMedicine Online, 28*(6): 684–703.

762. Carrell, D. T., Liu, L., Peterson, C. M., Jones, K. P., Hatasaka, H. H., Erickson, L., & Campbell, B. (2003). Sperm DNA fragmentation is increased in couples with unexplained recurrent pregnancy loss. *Archives of Andrology, 49*(1): 49–55.

763. Saleh, R. A., Agarwal, A., Nada, E. A., El-Tonsy, M. H., Sharma, R. K., Meyer, A., Nelson, D. R., & Thomas, A. J. (2003). Negative effects of increased sperm DNA damage in relation to seminal oxidative stress in men with idiopathic and male factor infertility. *Fertility and Sterility, 79*(Suppl 3): 1597–1605.

764. Tremellen, K., & Pearce, K. (2015). *Nutrition, Fertility, and Human Reproductive Function.* Boca Raton, FL: CRC Press.

765. Wright, C., Milne, S., & Leeson, H. (2014). Sperm DNA damage caused by oxidative stress: modifiable clinical, lifestyle and nutritional factors in male infertility. *Reproductive BioMedicine Online, 28*(6): 684–703.

766. Wright, C., Milne, S., & Leeson, H. (2014). Sperm DNA damage caused by oxidative stress: modifiable clinical, lifestyle and nutritional factors in male infertility. *Reproductive BioMedicine Online, 28*(6): 684–703.

767. De Lamirande, E., Jiang, H., Zini, A., Kodama, H., & Gagnon, C. (1997). Reactive oxygen species and sperm physiology. *Reviews of Reproduction, 2*(1): 48–54.

768. Sinclair, S. (2000). Male infertility: nutritional and environmental considerations. *Alternative Medicine Review, 5*(1): 28–38.

769. Lewin, A., & Lavin, H. (1997). The effect of coenzyme Q-10 on sperm motility and function. *Molecular Aspects of Medicine, 18*: S213–S219.

770. Safarinejad, M. R. (2011). The effect of coenzyme Q10 supplementation on partner pregnancy rate in infertile men with idiopathic oligoasthenoteratozoospermia: an open-label prospective study. *International Urology and Nephrology, 44*(3): 689–700.

771. Hosoi, M., Belcaro, G., Saggino, A., Luzzi, R., Dugall, M., & Feragalli, B. (2018). Pycnogenol® supplementation in minimal cognitive dysfunction. *Journal of Neurosurgical Sciences, 62*(3): 279–284.

772. Sinclair, S. (2000). Male infertility: nutritional and environmental considerations. *Alternative Medicine Review, 5*(1): 28–38.

CHAPTER NINE

Post-testicular problems

Erectile dysfunction

Erectile and ejaculatory dysfunction may be associated with hypogonadism, nervous system disease (such as MS), vascular conditions (such as diabetes),[773] and various medications (such as antidepressants). It is commonly caused by emotional or psychological factors such as stress or anxiety, which trigger the release of adrenaline, restricting the blood supply to the genitals.

When assessing men suffering from erectile or ejaculatory problems, it is important to establish whether the individual still experiences morning erections, and the ability to maintain an erection and to ejaculate during masturbation, as this may suggest that erectile and ejaculatory problems may be related to stress or trauma. The loss of morning erections and inability to maintain an erection or to ejaculate during masturbation is more likely to suggest a physiological problem, such as nervous system or vascular disease, or a side effect of medication.[774]

Improving erectile function

Erectile dysfunction (ED) may be treated with herbs that improve reproductive hormone levels, and have adaptogenic and tonic effects, such as *Panax ginseng*[775] and *Lepidium meyenii* (maca).[776]

Ginkgo biloba also improves libido, erection, and orgasm in men, including those with antidepressant-induced sexual dysfunction.[777] Pine bark (*Pinus pinaster*), as 100–200 mg of pine bark extract (pycnogenol) per day, improves testosterone levels; restores erectile function; and increases levels of nitric oxide, which acts as a vasodilator.[778] Arginine (found in red meat, fish, and poultry, or 5 g a day as a supplement) also improves levels of nitric oxide, which improves symptoms of organic ED.[779]

In Ayurveda, nutmeg (*Myristica fragrans*) is considered to be rejuvenative to the reproductive tissues and is used to help restore erectile function.[780] Yohimbe bark (*Pausinystalia yohimbe*) (15–30 mg per day) has traditionally been used in Africa as an aphrodisiac and to treat sexual dysfunction, including erectile dysfunction in men.[781,782]

Emotional and psychological factors may be improved with counselling, stress management techniques, and herbal adaptogens such as *Withania somnifera*, and nervines such as *Hypericum perforatum*. *Turnera diffusa* is traditionally used to treat sexual dysfunction and as a tonic for depression and nervous exhaustion.[783,784]

Premature ejaculation

Premature ejaculation is ejaculation that occurs with minimal stimulation, often before penetration. The cause is unknown but the incidence tends to decrease with age.[785]

Treating premature ejaculation

Sour herbs (such as *Schisandra chinensis*) are traditionally used for treating premature ejaculation.[786] Relaxing nervines such as *Scutellaria lateriflora* may also help to reduce the tendency to premature ejaculation.[787] Other measures that are useful for improving premature ejaculation include pelvic floor muscle exercises to help regain control of the ejaculatory reflex.[788]

Energetics

In Ayurveda, nutmeg (*Myristica fragrans*) is considered to be rejuvenative to the reproductive tissues and is used to help prevent premature ejaculation.[789] In traditional Chinese medicine, both erectile dysfunction and premature ejaculation are often associated with Kidney Yang Deficiency. Symptoms of Kidney Yang Deficiency include: fatigue; dizziness; ringing in the ears; dull-pale complexion; lower back soreness; lack of libido; feeling cold; loose stools; long-drawn-out urination with a thin stream or dribbling; a thick or puffy tongue body with a white tongue coating; and a thin-soft pulse.[790] Kidney Yang Deficiency may be the result of a demanding lifestyle, particularly in older men.[791] Herbs such as *Turnera diffusa*, *Panax ginseng*, and *Cinnamonum zeylonicum* are useful for treating Kidney Yang Deficiency.[792]

Case study

Forty-four-year-old male

Presenting complaint
- Erectile dysfunction (no loss of morning erections)

Medical history
- Poor sleep, low energy levels, depression, and anxiety
- Often feels cold
- Poor diet (high carbohydrate, low protein)

BP: 120/70

Pulse: 68 bpm (regular, deep)

Rx
- *Ginkgo biloba*   (2:1)   15
- *Withania somnifera*   (1:1)   20
- *Hypericum perforatum*   (1:3)   30
- *Turnera diffusa*   (1:3)   30
- *Myristica fragrans*   (1:3)   10

          105 ml per week   (Sig. 7.5 ml bid)

Rx *Lepidium meyenii* (powder)   (3 g per day)

Recommendations
- Increase intake of protein (meat, poultry, fish, eggs, nuts, seeds)
- Mindfulness meditation for stress relief

Follow-up
- Erectile function much improved after 6 weeks of treatment

Retrograde ejaculation

Retrograde ejaculation occurs when the bladder neck fails to close during ejaculation, and semen travels backwards into the bladder instead of being ejaculated through the penis. Retrograde ejaculation may be caused by a spinal injury; surgery (such as prostate of bladder surgery); or neuropathy (due to diabetes or multiple sclerosis, for example).[793] Some drugs, such as those used to treat depression (e.g., SSRIs), high blood pressure (e.g., beta blockers), or enlarged prostate (e.g., alpha-adrenergic receptor antagonists), may also cause retrograde ejaculation by preventing the bladder neck from closing properly during ejaculation, and allowing semen to enter the bladder.

In cases of retrograde ejaculation, individuals can experience orgasm, but ejaculate little or no semen. The urine may be cloudy after orgasm due to the presence of sperm in the bladder. Retrograde ejaculation is not harmful in itself, but because little or no semen is ejaculated, retrograde ejaculation usually causes infertility.

Treating retrograde ejaculation

Sympathomimetic drugs (such as ephedrine) and anti-cholinergic drugs (such as ipramine) may be used to keep the bladder neck closed during ejaculation. These drugs seem to be more effective when used together, compared to either drug used alone.[794] Therefore sympathomimetic herbs such as *Ephedra sinica*, and anticholinergic herbs such as *Atropa belladonna*, may also be helpful for patients with retrograde ejaculation, particularly when used in combination.

Patients with retrograde ejaculation due to spinal cord damage or surgery are unlikely to respond to medical or herbal treatment, and may need to undergo assisted reproduction in order for their partner to conceive. Sperm can be aspirated from the testicles under local anaesthesia, or harvested from the urine, and processed before use in intrauterine insemination (IUI). In cases of retrograde ejaculation due to multiple sclerosis or diabetic neuropathy, treatment of the underlying condition may help to improve ejaculation.

Energetics

In Ayurveda, retrograde ejaculation is often related to excess Kapha, which may be reduced with pungent and astringent food, and herbs (such as *Myristica fragrans*). In traditional Chinese medicine, retrograde ejaculation is most commonly related to Qi stagnation.

Genetic diseases

Various genetic diseases may cause infertility due to their effects on the development of reproductive structures. For example, cystic fibrosis is associated with failure of the normal development of the vas deferens in men, resulting in aspermia.[795] Patients with genetic diseases may require intracytoplasmic sperm injection (ICSI) in order to conceive. However, herbal and nutritional approaches to improving sperm quality, as detailed in Chapter 7, may also be helpful.

Structural abnormalities

Structural abnormalities that lead to infertility in males include blockages of the ejaculatory duct, and may necessitate surgical correction to restore fertility. Inflammation of the prostate may also lead to infertility by causing alterations in pH or viscosity of seminal fluid, which may compromise sperm transportation.[796] Inflammation of the prostate may be treated with herbs such as *Serenoa serrulata* (saw palmetto), *Pygeum africanum* (African prune tree), *Urtica dioica* radix (nettle root), and pumpkin seeds (*Curcubita pepo*).[797]

Notes

773. Dohle, G. R., Diemer, T., Giwercman, A., Jungwirth, A., Kopa, Z., & Krausz, C. (2010). *Guidelines on Male Infertility*. Arnhem, the Netherlands: European Association of Urology.

774. Campana, A., de Agostini, A., Bischof, P., Tawfik, E., & Mastrorilli, A. (2019). Evaluation of infertility. Graduate Foundation for Medical Education and Research (GFMER) [online]. Available from https://gfmer.ch/Books/Reproductive_health/infertility_evaluation.html (accessed 20 June 2020).

775. Bone, K., & Mills, S. (2013). *Principles and Practice of Phytotherapy: Modern Herbal Medicine*. London: Churchill Livingstone.

776. Meissner, H. O., Reich-Bilinska, H., Mscisz, A., & Kedzia, B. (2006). Therapeutic effects of pre-gelatinized maca (Lepidium peruvianum chacon) used as a non-hormonal alternative to HRT in perimenopausal women—clinical pilot study. *International Journal of Biomedical Science, 2*(2): 143–159.

777. Cohen, A., & Bartlik, B. (1998). Ginkgo biloba for antidepressant-induced sexual dysfunction. *Journal of Sex and Marital Therapy, 24*(2): 139–143.

778. Stanislavov, R., Niklova, V., & Rohdewald, P. (2008). Improvement of erectile function with Prelox: a randomized, double-blind, placebo-controlled, crossover trial. *International Journal of Impotence Research, 20*(2): 173–178.

779. Chen, J., Wollman, Y., Chernichovsky, T., Iaina, A., Sofer, M., & Matzkin, H. (1999). Effect of oral administration of high-dose nitric oxide donor L-arginine in men with organic erectile dysfunction: results of a double-blind, randomized, placebo-controlled study. *BJU International, 83*(3): 269–273.

780. Pole, S. (2006). *Ayurvedic Medicine: The Principles of Traditional Practice*. London: Churchill Livingstone.

781. NCCAM (2012). Yohimbe. National Centre for Complementary and Integrative Health [online]. Available from: https://nccih.nih.gov/health/yohimbe (accessed 15 July 2015).

782. Guay, A. T., Spark, R. F., Jacobson, J. S., Murray, F. T., & Geisser, M. E. (2002). Yohimbine treatment of organic erectile dysfunction in a dose-escalation trial. *International Journal of Impotence Research, 14*(1): 25–31.

783. Chevallier, A. (1996). *The Encyclopedia of Medicinal Plants*. New York: DK.

784. Bown, D. (1995). *Encyclopedia of Herbs and Their Uses*. New York: DK.

785. Heffner, L. J., & Schust, D. J. (2014). *The Reproductive System at a Glance*. Oxford: John Wiley & Sons.

786. Bone, K., & Mills, S. (2013). *Principles and Practice of Phytotherapy: Modern Herbal Medicine*. London: Churchill Livingstone.

787. Holmes, P. (2007). *The Energetics of Western Herbs: A Materia Medica Integrating Western & Chinese Herbal Therapeutics, Volume 1* (4th edn). Santa Rosa, CA: Snow Lotus.

788. Pastore, A. L. Palleschi, G., Fuschi, A., Maggioni, C., Rago, R., Zucchi, A., Constantini, E., & Carbone, A. (2014). Pelvic floor muscle rehabilitation for patients with lifelong premature ejaculation: a novel therapeutic approach. *Therapeutic Advances in Urology, 6*(3): 83–88.

789. Pole, S. (2006). *Ayurvedic Medicine: The Principles of Traditional Practice*. London: Churchill Livingstone.

790. Liu, W., & Gong, C. (2009). Opening the blockage to reproduction: infertility. *Traditional Chinese Medicine Information Page* [online]. Available from http://tcmpage.com/hpinfertility.html (accessed 4 July 2011).

791. Noll, A. A., & Wilms, S. (2011). *Chinese Medicine in Fertility Disorders*. New York: Thieme.

792. Holmes, P. (2007). *The Energetics of Western Herbs: A Materia Medica Integrating Western & Chinese Herbal Therapeutics, Volume 1* (4th edn). Santa Rosa, CA: Snow Lotus.

793. Heffner, L. J., & Schust, D. J. (2014). *The Reproductive System at a Glance*. Oxford: John Wiley & Sons.

794. Jeffreys, A., Siassakos, D., & Wardle, P. (2012). The management of retrograde ejaculation: a systematic review and update. *Fertility and Sterility, 97*(2): 306–312.

795. Kaplan, E., Shwachman, H., Perlmutter, A. D., Rule, A., Khaw, K. T., & Holsclaw, D. S. (1968). Reproductive failure in males with cystic fibrosis. *New England Journal of Medicine, 279*(2): 65–69.

796. Agarwal, A., & Said, T. M. (2011). Interpretation of basic semen analysis and advanced semen testing. In: E. S. Sabanegh, Jr. (Eds.), *Male Infertility: Problems and Solutions*. Springer [online].

797. Institute for Quality and Efficiency in Health Care (2014). Benign enlarged prostate: medication and herbal products. PubMed Health [online]. Available from ncbi.nlm. nih.gov (accessed 27 July 2015).

CHAPTER TEN

Lifestyle factors affecting reproductive health

Stress

Psychological and physiological stress cause increased cortisol levels, which disrupts the hypothalamic-pituitary gonadal axis, reduces LH secretion, and results in a significant drop in testosterone secretion. Stress is also associated with increased generation of reactive oxygen species (ROS),[798] which cause damage to sperm.

Withania somnifera is traditionally used in Ayurvedic medicine for the treatment of male sexual dysfunction and infertility. It is a relaxing adaptogen, which makes it particularly useful for men suffering from nervous exhaustion, stress, and anxiety.[799] *Turnera diffusa* is also traditionally used to treat sexual dysfunction and as a tonic for depression and nervous exhaustion.[800,801]

Smoking, alcohol consumption, and recreational drug use

Smoking

Cigarette smoking has been associated with decreased sperm count, alterations in motility, and an overall increase in the number of abnormal sperm.[802,803] Nicotine can alter the function of the hypotha-lamic-pituitary axis, which inhibits the release of luteinising hormone (LH).[804] Smoking also reduces blood flow to the genitals, which may be due to increased levels of adrenalin and noradrenalin, with result-ing vascular resistance.[805] Finally smoking increases the level of reactive oxygen species in seminal fluid,[806] which damages the sperm plasma membrane and reduces the integrity of DNA in the sperm nucleus. This accelerates germ cell apoptosis, leading to a decline in sperm count and increased number of abnormal sperm.[807]

Alcohol and caffeine

Alcohol consumption also increases the number of abnormal sperm.[808] However, unlike female infertility, moderate caffeine consumption seems to have no significant effect on male fertility.[809] *Mentha* spp. (e.g., peppermint tea), reduces testosterone levels,[810] and therefore should not be consumed on a regular basis by men with subfertility.

Recreational drugs

Cannabinoids in *Cannabis* spp. impair spermatogenesis, decrease antioxidant capacity in the testes, and cause damage to seminiferous tubules. Reversal of these effects occurs approximately six weeks after withdrawal.[811] Sympatholytic drugs, such as amphetamines, cocaine, and ecstasy can cause aspermia (absence of semen after orgasm).[812] Anabolic steroids cause oligospermia or azoospermia (reduced or absent sperm).[813]

Drug induced infertility

Orthodox drug treatments can affect reproductive function and fertil-ity by causing damage to the leydig cells (which produce testosterone), the germ cells (which otherwise mature to become spermatozoa), or the sertoli cells (which have an important role in supporting and protecting germ cells during spermatogenesis).[814]

A number of drugs, such as immunosuppressants, anti-androgens, antibiotics, and non-steroidal anti-inflammatory drugs (NSAIDs), may cause reduced testosterone levels and/or decreased sperm count, reduced motility, and abnormal sperm morphology. Alpha blockers

Orthodox drugs which affect fertility

Immunosuppressants, anti-androgens	Reduced testosterone levels
Immunosuppressants, anti-androgens, antibiotics, non-steroidal anti-inflammatory drugs (NSAIDs), alpha blockers, chemotherapy drugs	Decreased sperm count, motility, and morphology
Alpha blockers	Decreased ejaculate volume
Antidepressant drugs (SSRIs), chemotherapy drugs	Sperm DNA fragmentation

(used to treat the symptoms of benign prostatic hyperplasia) may lead to decreased sperm count and motility, and reduced ejaculate volume, while antidepressant drugs, which are regularly used by a significant number of men, have been shown to increase sperm DNA fragmentation.[815]

Drug treatments can also impair reproductive function and fertility by affecting epididymal function or the vasculature of the testes. Anti-androgens, opioid analgesics, and some diuretics and hypertensives can cause erectile dysfunction and decreased libido. Alpha blockers used to treat the symptoms of benign prostatic hyperplasia (BPH) can cause retrograde ejaculation, while selective serotonin reuptake inhibitors (SSRIs) used to treat depression and anxiety, and antipsychotic drugs can lead to reduced libido, erectile dysfunction, retrograde ejaculation, and anorgasmia.[816]

The effect of orthodox drugs on fertility (with the exception of chemotherapy drugs and radiation) is usually reversible if the drug treatment is discontinued. However, this may take three to twelve months

Drugs which affect sexual function

Decreased libido	Anti-androgens, opioid analgesics, SSRIs, antipsychotics
Erectile dysfunction	Anti-androgens, opioid analgesics, diuretics and hypertensives, SSRIs, antipsychotics
Retrograde ejaculation	Alpha blockers, SSRIs, antipsychotics
Anorgasmia	SSRIs, antipsychotics

depending on the drug. If it is not possible to stop taking a drug, antioxidant supplements may help to minimise the effects of the drug on reproductive function.[817]

Chemotherapy drugs

Radiotherapy and chemotherapy drugs cause damage to male testicles, which can lead to absent sperm, reduced sperm count, reduced sperm motility, and/or genetic damage to sperm, which may last for months or years, or in some cases, indefinitely. In adult males, cryopreservation of sperm before cancer treatment may be offered, and sperm can then be used for IUI or IVF at a later date. Cancer treatment in young boys can also cause permanent damage to the testes, leading to infertility in adulthood. In this case, testicular tissue containing germ cells may be removed and preserved before treatment commences.[818]

For male patients with infertility due to previous cancer treatment, who do not have cryopreserved sperm or testicular tissue available, viable sperm may sometimes be retrieved by testicular sperm extraction.[819] Herbal medicine and nutrition to improve sperm count, motility, and morphology (as discussed in Chapter 7) may also help to improve fertility in men experiencing infertility due to cancer treatment.

Diet and nutrition

Obesity significantly reduces fertility in males, and decreases the success rates of assisted reproduction. It is associated with impaired secretion of GnRH, reduced levels of LH, FSH, and testosterone, and increased oestrogen production. Obesity is also associated with increased production of leptin and other adipokines, which play an essential role in reproduction, both centrally and peripherally. Obesity increases the risk of sperm DNA fragmentation, and sperm parameters are also more likely to be suboptimal in obese men. Therefore, reduction in weight through diet and exercise may help to improve fertility in men with high BMI.[820]

High dietary intakes of hydrogenated oils have been shown to have a negative impact on sperm cell function. However, adequate intake of essential fatty acids is important to ensure proper membrane fluidity in sperm cells. It is also important to avoid exogenous oestrogens, which are found in non-organic meat and dairy products, and to eat more organic foods to reduce exposure to pesticides.[821]

Nutritional supplements that have a beneficial impact on male fertility include carnitine, arginine, zinc, vitamin C, vitamin E, selenium, co-enzyme Q10, and vitamin B12.[822] Supplementing these nutrients can double the sperm count, improve sperm motility by about a quarter, and increase ejaculate volume by about a third.[823]

Notes

798. Ambiye, V. R., Langade, D., Dongre, S., Aptikar, P., Kulkarni, M., & Dongre, A. (2013). Clinical evaluation of the spermatogenic activity of the root extract of ashwagandha (*Withania somnifera*) in oligospermic males: a pilot study. *Evidence-Based Complementary and Alternative Medicine* [online]. Available from http://ncbi.nlm.nih.gov/pmc/articles/PMC3863556/#!po=3.84615 (accessed 15 July 2015).

799. Ambiye, V. R., Langade, D., Dongre, S., Aptikar, P., Kulkarni, M., & Dongre, A. (2013). Clinical evaluation of the spermatogenic activity of the root extract of ashwagandha (*Withania somnifera*) in oligospermic males: a pilot study. *Evidence-Based Complementary amd Alternative Medicine* [online]. Available from http://ncbi.nlm.nih.gov/pmc/articles/PMC3863556/#!po=3.84615 (accessed 15 July 2015).

800. Chevallier, A. (1996). *The Encyclopedia of Medicinal Plants.* New York: DK.

801. Bown, D. (1995). *Encyclopaedia of Herbs and Their Uses.* New York: DK.

802. Kulikauskas, V., Blaustein, D., & Ablin, R. J. (1985). Cigarette smoking and its possible effects on sperm. *Fertility and Sterility, 44*: 526–528.

803. Stillman, R. J. (Ed.) (1989). Seminars in reproductive endocrinology: smoking and reproductive health. New York: Thieme.

804. Weisberg, E. (1985). Smoking and reproductive health. *Clinical Reproduction and Fertility,* 3(3): 175–186.

805. Grassi, G., Seravalle, G., Calhoun, D. A., Bolla, G. B., Giannattasio, C., Marabini, M., Del Bo, A., & Mancia, G. (1994). Mechanisms responsible for sympathetic activation by cigarette smoking in humans. *Circulation, 90*: 248–253.

806. Saleh, R. A., Agarwal, A., Sharma, R. K., Nelson, D. R., & Thomas, A. J. (2002). Effect of cigarette smoking on levels of seminal oxidative stress in infertile men: a prospective study. *Fertility and Sterility, 78*(3): 491–499.

807. Agarwal, A., Saleh, R. A., & Bedaiwy, M. A. (2003). Role of reactive oxygen species in the pathophysiology of human reproduction. *Fertility and Sterility, 79*(4): 829–843.

808. Joo, K. J., Kwon, Y. W., Myung, S., & Kim, T. H. (2012). The effects of smoking and alcohol intake on sperm quality. *Journal of International Medical Research, 40*(6): 2327–2335.

809. Tremellen, K., & Pearce, K. (2015). *Nutrition, Fertility, and Human Reproductive Function.* Boca Raton, FL: CRC Press.

810. D'Cruz, S. C., Vaithinathan, S., Jubendradass, R., & Mathur, P. P. (2010). Effects of plant products on the testes. *Asian Journal of Andrology, 12*(4): 468–479.

811. D'Cruz, S. C., Vaithinathan, S., Jubendradass, R., & Mathur, P. P. (2010). Effects of plant products on the testes. *Asian Journal of Andrology, 12*(4): 468–479.

812. Agarwal, A., & Said, T. M. (2011). Interpretation of basic semen analysis and advanced semen testing. In: E. S. Sabanegh, Jr. (Eds.), *Male Infertility: Problems and Solutions.* Springer [online].

813. Semet, M., Paci, M., Saïas-Magnan, J., Metzler-Guillemain, C., Boissier, R., Lejeune, H., & Perrin, J. (2017). The impact of drugs on male fertility: a review. *Andrology, 5*(4): 640–663.

814. Semet, M., Paci, M., Saïas-Magnan, J., Metzler-Guillemain, C., Boissier, R., Lejeune, H., & Perrin, J. (2017). The impact of drugs on male fertility: a review. *Andrology, 5*(4): 640–663.

815. Semet, M., Paci, M., Saïas-Magnan, J., Metzler-Guillemain, C., Boissier, R., Lejeune, H., & Perrin, J. (2017). The impact of drugs on male fertility: a review. *Andrology, 5*(4): 640–663.

816. Semet, M., Paci, M., Saïas-Magnan, J., Metzler-Guillemain, C., Boissier, R., Lejeune, H., & Perrin, J. (2017). The impact of drugs on male fertility: a review. *Andrology, 5*(4): 640–663.

817. Semet, M., Paci, M., Saïas-Magnan, J., Metzler-Guillemain, C., Boissier, R., Lejeune, H., & Perrin, J. (2017). The impact of drugs on male fertility: a review. *Andrology, 5*(4): 640–663.

818. Okada, K., & Fujisawa, M. (2019). Recovery of spermatogenesis following cancer treatment with cytotoxic chemotherapy and radiotherapy. *World Journal of Men's Health, 37*(2): 166–174.

819. Okada, K., & Fujisawa, M. (2019). Recovery of spermatogenesis following cancer reatment with cytotoxic hemotherapy and adiotherapy. *World Journal of Men's Health, 37*(2): 166–174.

820. Tremellen, K., & Pearce, K. (2015). *Nutrition, Fertility, and Human Reproductive Function.* Boca Raton, FL: CRC Press.

821. Sinclair, S. (2000). Male infertility: nutritional and environmental considerations. *Alternative Medicine Review, 5*(1): 28–38.

822. Sinclair, S. (2000). Male infertility: nutritional and environmental considerations. *Alternative Medicine Review, 5*(1): 28–38.

823. Imhof, M., Lackner, J., Lipovac, M., Chedraui, P., & Riedl, C. (2012). Improvement of sperm quality after micronutrient supplementation. *e-SPEN, the European e-Journal of Clinical Nutrition and Metabolism, 7*(1): E50–E53.

CHAPTER ELEVEN

Energetic patterns of disharmony

TCM patterns of disharmony

Kidney Qi Deficiency

According to traditional Chinese medicine theory, the Kidney is responsible for reproduction.[824] The main pattern of disharmony associated with infertility in men is Kidney Qi Deficiency (including Deficiency of both Kidney Yin and Kidney Yang).[825] Problems with the sperm themselves are related to Yang, while problems with the seminal fluid are related to Yin or Jing.[826] Kidney energy may be depleted by lifestyle factors such as poor diet and overwork.[827]

Clinical manifestations of Kidney Yin Deficiency include: heart palpitations; fatigue; dizziness; ringing in the ears; lower back soreness; dry mouth; dry bowl movements; a feeling of heat in the palms, the soles of the feet, and the upper chest; low-grade fever in the afternoon; a red tongue body with a thin tongue coating; and a thin and rapid pulse. Kidney Yin Deficiency is commonly associated with problems such as low sperm count and low semen volume.

Clinical manifestations of Kidney Yang Deficiency include: fatigue; dizziness; ringing in the ears; dull-pale complexion; lower back soreness; lack of libido; erectile dysfunction; feeling cold; loose stools; long-drawn-out urination with a thin stream or dribbling; a thick or puffy tongue body with a white tongue coating; and a thin-soft pulse.[828] Kidney Yang Deficiency may be the result of a demanding lifestyle, particularly in older men.[829] It is commonly associated with problems such as poor sperm motility.

Treating Kidney Deficiency

Polygonum multiflorum nourishes the Kidney Essence and helps to improve sperm production. *Turnera diffusa, Panax ginseng, Schisandra chinesis,* and *Cinnamonum zeylonicum* are used to treat Kidney Yang Deficiency, while *Rehmannia glutinosa* nourishes the Kidney Yin.[830]

Blood stagnation

Kidney Yang is responsible for pelvic blood flow, and Deficiency may therefore lead to Blood Stasis,[831] which may contribute to infertility. Blood Stasis may also be caused by varicocele or surgery.[832] It is indicated by a blue or purple tongue-body colour, and poor peripheral circulation.[833,834]

Reducing Blood Stasis

Blood Stasis may be treated with herbal medicines such as *Ginkgo biloba*[835] and *Aesculus hippocastanum*.[836] Warming herbs such as *Rosmarinus officinalis, Cinnamonum zeylonicum,* and *Zingiber officinale* may be used to stimulate the peripheral circulation, and may also help to promote healthy circulation to the reproductive organs.[837]

Damp Heat

Infection, frequent urination, poor sperm morphology, and the presence of anti-sperm antibodies may all be associated with a Damp Heat pattern in traditional Chinese medicine. Cool dry herbs such as *Hydrastis Canadensis, Andrographis paniculata,* and *Achillea millefolium* are useful for reducing Damp Heat.

Ayurvedic Dosha imbalance

Nourishing Ojas

Ojas, or "essence" is responsible for healthy fertility. Healthy Ojas is demonstrated by: strength and resistance to disease; efficient digestion; fertility; and lustre of the eyes, skin, and hair.[838]

Ojas is depleted by undernourishment, overwork, excessive exercise, stress, ejaculation, and orgasm.[839] Symptoms of depleted Ojas include weakness, anxiety, confusion, dry skin and hair, and poor complexion.[840]

Clean air and good breathing habits, sufficient sleep and rest, and nourishing foods support Ojas. Nourishing herbs such as *Tribulus terrestris* and pomegranate juice improve Ojas.[841]

Vata aggravation

Vata is responsible for all movement in the body,[842] including circulation, nervous impulses, movement of the limbs, and elimination of wastes.[843] Vata disturbance may be caused by problems such as stress, anxiety, tiredness and overwork, and eating too many dry or cold foods. Astringent, bitter, and pungent flavours also aggravate Vata.[844]

Vata disturbance is suggested by symptoms such as: fatigue, feeling stressed, feeling cold, poor peripheral circulation, palpitations, abdominal bloating, constipation, dry skin and hair, cracking joints, muscle spasm, pins and needles, erectile dysfunction and infertility.[845]

Apana Vata is a subtype of Vata, which resides in the lower abdomen. Apana Vata is a downward moving energy, which is responsible for processes such as defecation, urination, and ejaculation.[846]

Reducing Vata aggravation

Avoiding stress, worry, and excessive travelling and rushing around reduces Vata aggravation. It is important to maintain a regular daily routine, and get adequate rest and sleep. Massage with warm oil is very beneficial for balancing Vata.[847] Warm and moist foods (such as soups and stews, and oils) and sweet, sour, and salty flavours (such as honey, fresh figs, sweet potatoes, yoghurt, and seaweeds), help to reduce Vata aggravation.[848]

Withania somnifera is an Ayurvedic herb, which is widely used to reduce Vata disturbance. *Glycyrrhiza glabra* also reduces Vata aggravation due to its sweet taste and moist nature. Warming herbs such as *Cinnamonum zeylonicum* and *Myristica fragrans* are also used in Ayurvedic medicine to reduce Vata aggravation. *Rosmarinus officinalis* is not an Ayurvedic herb, but it is considered to be warming and may therefore be used to reduce Vata aggravation.[849]

Pitta excess

Pitta is derived from fire and water. It is hot, oily, fast, irritable, and intense. It is responsible for all transformations in the body,[850,851] including hormonal balance.[852] Pitta is aggravated by irritation and anger, excessive ambition, exposure to heat and humidity, and consumption of too many hot, oily foods (such as fatty meat and fried foods), and sour, salty, or pungent foods (such as yoghurt, cheese, salty meat or nuts, and spicy food).[853] Pitta aggravation is associated with inflammation, heat, and burning sensations. It shows some similarity to the TCM patterns of Liver Qi Stagnation and Damp Heat. It is characterised by symptoms such as inflammation and irritability, hormone imbalance, liver problems, and loose bowel movements.[854,855]

Balancing Pitta

Bitter herbs (such as *Andrographis* paniculata), sweet herbs (such as *Tribulus terrestris*), and astringent herbs (such as *Achillea millefolium*) are useful for reducing Pitta excess. [856] Light, bitter, sweet, and astringent foods (such as green leafy vegetables, apples, berries, and pomegranates) are also useful for reducing Pitta excess. It is important to avoid too many pungent, sour, and oily foods, red meat, caffeine, and alcohol.[857]

Kapha excess

Kapha is derived from water and earth. It is heavy, cold, damp, stable, slow, and unctuous. Kapha is responsible for growth,[858] protection of the body, and maintenance of body fluids.[859]

Kapha is aggravated by possessiveness, inactivity, exposure to cold and damp, and too many sweet, sour, and salty foods. Kapha disturbance is characterised by excess phlegm, swelling, and tissue growth,[860] slow digestion, constipation, and obesity.[861] It shows some similarity to the TCM pattern of Dampness. Kapha disturbance is indicated by excessive mucus, and a swollen tongue, with white coating.[862]

Reducing Kapha excess

Pungent herbs (such as *Myristica fragrans* and *Zingiber officinale*), astringent herbs (such as *Cinnamonum zeylonicum* and *Achillea millefolium*), and bitter herbs (such as *Andrographis paniculata* and *Taraxacum officinale*) balance Kapha.

Pungent, astringent, and bitter foods (such as apples, green leafy vegetables, onions, and spicy foods) also reduce excess Kapha. It is important to avoid cold, sweet, sour, salty, and oily and damp foods such as dairy products and cold water, as they increase Kapha.[863] Exercise, activity, giving, sharing, and letting go all help to reduce excess Kapha.[864]

Summary of the causes of reproductive health problems in men

The causes of male reproductive health problems

Pre-testicular problems	**Endocrine causes** • Hypogonadotropic hypogonadism • Thyroid abnormalities • Exposure to oestrogen **Sperm abnormalities** • Low sperm count • Low motility • Abnormal morphology **Undescended testes** **Genetic defects** (e.g. Klinefelter's).
Testicular problems	• **Infection** • **Trauma/injury** • **Varicocele** • **Genetic disorders** (e.g., PCD) • **DNA damage** • **Exposure to heat**

(Continued)

Summary of the causes of reproductive health problems in men (*Continued*)

The causes of male reproductive health problems

Post-testicular problems	**Erectile dysfunction** • Emotional causes • Hypogonadism • Circulatory causes: heart disease, hypertension, cholesterol, diabetes • Nervous system causes: e.g., MS • Medication: e.g., antidepressants **Premature ejaculation** **Retrograde ejaculation** **Genetic diseases** (e.g., cystic fibrosis) **Structural abnormalities**
Lifestyle factors	• **Stress** • **Smoking, alcohol consumption, and recreational drug use** • **Diet & nutrition**
Energetic patterns of disharmony	• **Kidney Qi Deficiency (Yin or Yang)** • **Blood Stagnation** • **Damp Heat** • **Ayurvedic Dosha imbalance**

Notes

824. Liu, W., & Gong, C. (2009). Opening the blockage to reproduction: infertility. *Traditional Chinese Medicine Information Page* [online]. Available from http://tcmpage.com/hpinfertility.html (accessed 4 July 2011).

825. Liu, W., & Gong, C. (2009). Opening the blockage to reproduction: infertility. *Traditional Chinese Medicine Information Page* [online]. Available from http://tcmpage.com/hpinfertility.html (accessed 4 July 2011).

826. Noll, A. A., & Wilms, S. (2011). *Chinese Medicine in Fertility Disorders*. New York: Thieme.

827. Liu, W., & Gong, C. (2009). Opening the blockage to reproduction: infertility. *Traditional Chinese Medicine Information Page* [online]. Available from http://tcmpage.com/hpinfertility.html (accessed 4 July 2011).

828. Liu, W., & Gong, C. (2009). Opening the blockage to reproduction: infertility. *Traditional Chinese Medicine Information Page* [online]. Available from http://tcmpage.com/hpinfertility.html (accessed 4 July 2011).

829. Noll, A. A., & Wilms, S. (2011). *Chinese Medicine in Fertility Disorders*. New York: Thieme.
830. Holmes, P. (2007). *The Energetics of Western Herbs: A Materia Medica Integrating Western & Chinese Herbal Therapeutics, Volume 1* (4th edn). Santa Rosa, CA: Snow Lotus.
831. Flaws, B. (1989). *Endometriosis and Infertility and Traditional Chinese Medicine: A Laywoman's Guide*. Colorado Springs, CO: Blue Poppy.
832. Liu, W., & Gong, C. (2009). Opening the blockage to reproduction: infertility. *Traditional Chinese Medicine Information Page* [online]. Available from http://tcmpage.com/hpinfertility.html (accessed 4 July 2011).
833. Xiufen, W. (Ed.) (2003). *Traditional Chinese Diagnostics*. Beijing: People's Medical Publishing House.
834. Noll, A. A., & Wilms, S. (2011). *Chinese Medicine in Fertility Disorders*. New York: Thieme.
835. Bone, K., & Mills, S. (2013). *Principles and Practice of Phytotherapy: Modern Herbal Medicine*. London: Churchill Livingstone.
836. Fang, Y., Zhao, L., Yan, F., Xia, X., Xu, D., & Cui, X. (2010). Escin improves sperm quality in male patients with varicocele-associated infertility. *Phytomedicine, 17*(3–4): 192–196.
837. Holmes, P. (2007). *The Energetics of Western Herbs: A Materia Medica Integrating Western & Chinese Herbal Therapeutics, Volume 1* (4th edn). Santa Rosa, CA: Snow Lotus.
838. Sharma P. V. (Trans.) (2008). *Caraka Samhita* [text with English translation]. Varanasi, India: Chaukhambha Orientalia.
839. Pole, S. (2006). *Ayurvedic medicine: The Principles of Traditional Practice*. London: Churchill Livingstone.
840. Sharma P. V. (Trans.) (2008). *Caraka Samhita* [text with English translation]. Varanasi, India: Chaukhambha Orientalia.
841. Pole, S. (2006). *Ayurvedic Medicine: The Principles of Traditional Practice*. London: Churchill Livingstone.
842. Svoboda, R. E. (1992). *Ayurveda: Life, Health and Longevity*. London: Penguin.
843. Pole, S. (2006). *Ayurvedic Medicine: The Principles of Traditional Practice*. London: Churchill Livingstone.
844. Pole, S. (2006). *Ayurvedic Medicine: The Principles of Traditional Practice*. London: Churchill Livingstone.
845. Lad, V. D. (2006). *Textbook of Ayurveda: A Complete Guide to Clinical Assessment. Volume 2*. Albuquerque, NM: Ayurvedic Press.
846. Frawley, D., & Lad, V. D. (2001). *The Yoga of Herbs: An Ayurvedic Guide to Herbal Medicine*. Twin Lakes, WI: Lotus.
847. Pole, S. (2006). *Ayurvedic Medicine: The Principles of Traditional Practice*. London: Churchill Livingstone.
848. Lad, V. D. (2002). *Textbook of Ayurveda: Fundamental Principles. Volume 1*. Albuquerque, NM: Ayurvedic Press.
849. Frawley, D., & Lad, V. D. (2001). *The Yoga of Herbs: An Ayurvedic Guide to Herbal Medicine*. Twin Lakes, WI: Lotus.
850. Dick, M. (2002). Commentary on *The Elements and Attributes of the Three Doshas*. The Ayurvedic Institute [online]. Available from http://ayurveda.com (accessed 25 September 2009).
851. Svoboda, R. E. (1992). *Ayurveda: Life, Health and Longevity*. London: Penguin.

852. McIntyre, A. (2005). *Herbal Treatment of Children: Western and Ayurvedic Perspectives.* London: Churchill Livingstone.

853. Pole, S. (2006). *Ayurvedic Medicine: The Principles of Traditional Practice.* London: Churchill Livingstone.

854. Lad, V. D. (2006). *Textbook of Ayurveda: A Complete Guide to Clinical Assessment. Volume 2.* Albuquerque, NM: Ayurvedic Press.

855. Stinnett, J. D. (1988). Pitta: the Dosha of transformation. *Ayurveda Today,* 1(1): 9–10.

856. Frawley, D., & Lad, V. D. (2001). *The Yoga of Herbs: An Ayurvedic Guide to Herbal Medicine.* Twin Lakes, WI: Lotus.

857. Pole, S. (2006). *Ayurvedic Medicine: The Principles of Traditional Practice.* London: Churchill Livingstone.

858. Pole, S. (2006). *Ayurvedic Medicine: The Principles of Traditional Practice.* London: Churchill Livingstone.

859. Frawley, D., & Lad, V. D. (2001). *The Yoga of Herbs: An Ayurvedic Guide to Herbal Medicine.* Twin Lakes, WI: Lotus.

860. Pole, S. (2006). *Ayurvedic Medicine: The Principles of Traditional Practice.* London: Churchill Livingstone.

861. Lad, V. D. (2006). *Textbook of Ayurveda: A Complete Guide to Clinical Assessment. Volume 2.* Albuquerque, NM: Ayurvedic Press.

862. Lad, V. D. (2006). *Textbook of Ayurveda: A Complete Guide to Clinical Assessment. Volume 2.* Albuquerque, NM: Ayurvedic Press.

863. Tillotson, A. K. (2001). *The One Earth Herbal Sourcebook.* New York: Kensington.

864. Pole, S. (2006). *Ayurvedic Medicine: The Principles of Traditional Practice.* London: Churchill Livingstone.

PART III

TREATING REPRODUCTIVE HEALTH PROBLEMS AND IMPROVING FERTILITY IN PRACTICE

CHAPTER TWELVE

Case taking, clinical examination, and investigations

Herbalists and other healthcare practitioners are taught how to take a detailed case history, and how to carry out clinical examinations, in order to assess their patients' presenting complaint and general health. This chapter focuses on the specific areas of enquiry within the consultation, clinical examinations, and further investigations, which are important for understanding, diagnosing, and treating reproductive health problems and infertility in particular.

When assisting individuals and couples who wish to conceive, it is very important to evaluate both partners. In the vast majority of cases of infertility, it is the female partner alone who is offered treatment.[865] However, infertility is equally likely to be the result of issues affecting the male partner (or both partners). It may also be the case that there are multiple factors involved which result in difficulty in conceiving.[866]

The case history in assessing reproductive health

Assessment of reproductive health problems in women

When assessing reproductive health problems in women, it is important to make a detailed enquiry in the following areas, as part of the overall case history:

- *The menstrual cycle length and regularity*, and if there have been any recent changes. In women with amenorrhoea, note the duration of the amenorrhoea; and whether it is associated with stress, lack of nutrition, and over-exercise (suggesting hypothalamic amenorrhoea), menopausal-type symptoms (suggesting primary ovarian insufficiency), symptoms associated with excess androgens (suggesting PCOS), or any symptoms suggestive of hypopituitarism.
- *Details of the menstrual periods*, including the duration, the quantity of blood loss, the colour of the menstrual flow, and whether there is any clotting, or dysmenorrhoea. These symptoms may help with diagnosis of conditions such as abnormal blood flow, inadequate endometrium, endometriosis, and uterine fibroids. Any recent changes in the menstrual periods should also be noted.
- Any signs during *mid-cycle* which help to establish whether or not ovulation is occurring regularly (such as changes in cervical mucus, increased libido, ovulation sensation or pain, hot flushes, mid-cycle headaches, or mid-cycle bleeding).
- The presence and timing of any *premenstrual symptoms* (such as mood changes, sleep disturbance, hot flushes, mastalgia, fluid retention, abdominal bloating or pain, headaches, hyperalgesia, fatigue, or constipation), which may help to diagnose functional hormonal imbalances.
- Details of any *discharge from the breasts* which may suggest hyperprolactinaemia.
- Details of any *discharge from the vagina*, which may indicate infection.
- Any sexual difficulties (such as low libido, vaginal dryness, dyspareunia, or lack of orgasm).
- Specific questions relating to any conditions which may contribute to infertility that are suspected (such as hirsutism, androgenic alopecia, or acne in PCOS, or any symptoms suggestive of thyroid disease, for example).

Enquiry about *past medical history* and *family history* should also seek to establish whether there are any previous issues that may contribute to current reproductive health problems and infertility, such as:

- History of recurrent candida infection, bacterial vaginosis, or sexually transmitted disease (STD/STI) or other genitourinary infections.
- History of any abnormal smears, and any associated interventions (such as colposcopy, cervical biopsy, or cryotherapy).
- History of any head injuries, chest wall trauma, abdominal or pelvic surgery, or cancer treatment, which may have affected the function of the pituitary gland or ovaries, or caused any adhesions in the pelvic cavity or uterus.
- History of any significant weight gain or weight loss.
- Details of any previous pregnancies (including any problems during pregnancy, miscarriages, terminations, still births, and live births).
- Family history, including any history of infertility, recurrent miscarriage, early menopause, or conditions such as gluten enteropathy or other genetic diseases (such as cystic fibrosis).

Assessment of reproductive health problems in men

Assessment of reproductive health problems in men should include a detailed enquiry in the following areas, as part of the overall case history:

- *Energy levels*, and whether there have been any recent changes to energy levels or stamina; any problems with *low mood* or *low libido*; or any loss of muscle mass, or *muscle weakness* which may suggest androgen deficiency.
- Any *erectile or ejaculatory problems*, and if so, whether the individual still experiences morning erections, and the ability to maintain an erection and ejaculate normally during masturbation. (This helps to differentiate between erectile and ejaculatory problems that are due to stress or psychological trauma; and those that are due to a physiological cause such as neurological or vascular problems, or side effects of medication.)
- Any *urinary symptoms* (such as cloudy urine, frequent urination, irritation or pain on urination, difficulty stopping or starting the flow of

urine), which may suggest retrograde ejaculation or prostate inflammation or enlargement.
- Specific questions relating to any conditions which may contribute to infertility that are suspected (such as thyroid or adrenal disease).

Enquiry about *past medical history* and *family history* should also seek to establish whether there are any issues that may contribute to current reproductive health problems and infertility, such as:

- History of infection (such as mumps, epididymitis, prostatitis, urethritis, or STI), testicular injury, undescended testicle, surgery or cancer treatment which may have affected the function of the testes, or caused any structural abnormality of the reproductive organs.
- History of head injury, surgery, or radiation which may have affected the function of the pituitary gland.
- Details of any previous pregnancies with current or previous partners (including any miscarriages, still births, and live births).
- Family history, including any history of infertility, recurrent pregnancy loss, or conditions such as gluten enteropathy or genetic diseases (such as cystic fibrosis).

Assessment of reproductive health problems in both partners

Assessment of reproductive health problems in both partners should include questions to establish the following:

- *Age* (since fertility declines with increasing age in both men and women).
- *Duration of infertility*, and whether the individual is presenting with primary infertility (in that they have never conceived), or secondary infertility (in that they have previously conceived, but are having difficulty conceiving again).
- *Libido, frequency and timing of intercourse.* Frequent intercourse (once a day or more) may result in low sperm count, whereas infrequent intercourse (once a week or less) may cause low sperm motility. It is also important to ensure that intercourse takes place around ovulation in couples that wish to conceive.

- *Stress levels, sleep patterns, exercise, diet, smoking habits, caffeine, alcohol and recreational drug use* also need to be assessed in detail, since these factors can all have a significant impact on reproductive health and fertility.
- Details of *current medication and supplements* are needed in order to check whether patients are taking anything that may negatively impact fertility.
- Subjective feelings of heat/cold, and any problems with peripheral *circulation* may give an indication of the health of the pelvic circulation and help to establish energetic patterns of disharmony.
- Questions about *general health and any unusual symptoms*, such as fatigue, dizziness, palpitations, thirst, loose bowel movements or constipation, lower back pain or weakness, excessive sweating, etc. which may also help to diagnose energetic patterns of disharmony.
- Any changes to the skin, hair, or nails, which may point to nutritional deficiency, or other problems such as thyroid or liver disease.
- Exposure to any substances that might affect reproductive health (e.g., plastics, pesticides, or occupational exposure to toxic chemicals).

Clinical examination in assessment of reproductive health

Observation of signs

Clinical evaluation in both men and women with reproductive health problems and infertility should include careful *observation of signs* such as:

- The absence of secondary sexual characteristics, suggesting primary amenorrhoea in women.
- Scalp hair loss, and pattern of hair loss. Male pattern hair loss suggests androgen excess; while diffuse hair loss may suggest problems such as iron deficiency, or psychological or physiological stress.
- Signs such as loss of the outer corner of eyebrows, and myxoedema suggest hypothyroidism, whereas signs such as exophthalmos and tremor, suggest a hyperthyroid pathology.
- Chloasma (or melasma), which is due to oestrogen excess and appears as hyperpigmentation on sun exposed areas.

- Hirsutism (excess body hair), male pattern hair loss, and acne, which suggest androgen excess.
- Pruritus (skin itching), spider angiomas, and Terry's nails, which suggest liver stagnation.
- Vertical ridges on the nails, which suggest malabsorption.
- Signs such as epicanthus, lower implantation of ears and hairline, webbed neck, shortness of the fourth finger, and cubitus valgus, which may suggest chromosomal abnormalities.
- Hyperpigmentation, which may occur due to excess cortisol.
- Abdominal obesity, which may indicate insulin resistance.
- General obesity, which may contribute to insulin and leptin resistance, and oestrogen excess.
- Large breast size in women, or gynaecomastia in men, which may suggest oestrogen excess.

Clinical examination

Clinical evaluation of patients presenting with reproductive health problems and infertility should also include the following examinations:

- *Examination of the tongue* to check for nutritional deficiencies (such as iron deficiency which causes a pale tongue, or vitamin B12 deficiency which causes glossitis), and to help diagnose energetic patterns of disharmony.
- *Pulse diagnosis* to assess the rate and rhythm of the pulse (which may be affected by conditions such as anaemia and thyroid disease), and also to help diagnose energetic patterns of disharmony.
- Measurement of *height, weight,* and *blood pressure.*
- *Urinanalysis* in both men and women (using dipsticks to detect the presence of glucose, ketones, bilirubin, or signs of infection; and pregnancy tests to rule out pregnancy or ectopic pregnancy in female patients).
- *Bimanual examination of vagina and cervix* in women (by practitioners who have been appropriately trained).
- *Prostate examination,* and *examination of the penis and testes* in men (by practitioners who have been appropriately trained).

Medical laboratory tests

Laboratory tests are helpful tools in evaluating the health status of an individual. Disturbances in the normal relative concentration of various blood constituents can help to diagnose and monitor a wide range of health problems. In addition, practitioners need to be able to explain the purpose of the tests and the significance of the results to their patients.

However, it is not possible to diagnose or treat any disease or problem with blood tests alone. Normal ranges for any given test are set so that 95% of "healthy" patients fall within the normal range. Therefore 5% of healthy patients fall outside the normal range, even when there is no abnormality. Conversely, an individual within the large range of "normal" may well be suffering from a pathological condition, with blood tests falling outside *their own* normal range.

Other factors which may affect test results include the age and/or sex of the patient, the time or day that the sample was collected, and whether the patient is pregnant. "Abnormal" levels of hormones whose "normal" values vary according to the age and/or sex of the patient, and the time or day that the sample was collected (such as FSH, LH, oestradiol, progesterone, testosterone, and cortisol) are not usually highlighted by laboratories, which often leads GPs and other practitioners to miss abnormal results.

Varying levels of globulin binding may also make certain results less reliable, as they render more or less of a particular substance inactive. Furthermore, there may be altered receptor sensitivity (for example, oestrogen receptors may be increased following use of oestrogen antagonists).

Finally, laboratory tests are very specific, and it is often the case that the range of tests that have been performed is too narrow to make a proper diagnosis. The term "full blood count" is a common cause of confusion, and while patients will often report that their GP "tested for everything", this is impossible.

For most laboratory tests, there is no universally applicable reference value. A normal result in one lab may be abnormal in another. Therefore, it is important to use the range supplied by the laboratory that performed your test to evaluate results. However, it is also interesting to note that reference ranges tend to change over time, so that a result that was considered to be pathological a few years ago may now be considered to be within the "normal range".

For example, the upper "normal" level for oestrogen in women has increased significantly in recent years, which begs the questions "What factors are causing women to have higher levels of oestrogen?" And "What effect might this have on women's health?" It is possible that widespread use of exogenous oestrogen for contraception and hormone replacement therapy, and increasing exposure to xenoestrogens, are responsible for this phenomenon, and that it may lead to increased risk of oestrogen dependent conditions and cancer.

Likewise, the lower end of the normal reference range for T4 has reduced significantly in recent years, and the level that was once considered to represent hypothyroidism is now considered to be normal. It seems that average thyroid function is decreasing across the population, which again begs the questions "What factors are causing average thyroid function to reduce in this manner?" and "What impact does this have on the health of the population?"

In a similar vein, the lower end of the normal reference range for vitamin D in the UK and Ireland (which represents the level in 95% of "healthy" people in those countries) is considerably lower than the level which has been shown to be protective against cancer and diseases resulting from altered immune system function. Therefore medical laboratory tests should only ever be considered as a helpful tool for diagnosis, and always be interpreted in conjunction with other information gathered from careful history taking and thorough clinical examination.

Blood tests to assess reproductive health and fertility in women

The following blood tests are recommended for women with reproductive health problems, and those who are trying to conceive. Tests are best carried out during the follicular phase (ideally on day 2 or 3 of the menstrual cycle), with further tests being taken during the mid-luteal phase, approximately 6–8 days before the next expected menstrual period. This is usually on day 21, but the timing of the test should be adjusted depending on cycle length of the individual. For example, a woman with a 21-day cycle should have mid-luteal blood test on around day 15, while a woman with a 35-day cycle should have mid luteal blood test on around day 17.

Recommended blood tests for women

Early follicular phase tests (day 2–3)

- FSH, LH, oestradiol
- Prolactin

Mid-luteal phase tests (6–8 days before next expected menstrual period)

- Progesterone
- Androgens, free testosterone, SHBG
- FSH, LH, oestradiol
- Prolactin

Additional tests (may be taken either during the early luteal phase or mid-follicular phase)

- AMH
- FBC, ferritin, folate, B12
- TSH, T4, T3
- Cholesterol
- HbA1c
- CRP

Early follicular phase tests

Early follicular phase tests are best carried out on day 2 or 3 of the menstrual cycle. The reference range for follicle stimulating hormone (FSH) during the follicular phase is usually in the region of 3.5–12.5 IU/L.[867] Low follicle stimulating hormone (FSH) may suggest conditions such as hypothalamic amenorrhoea or hypopituitarism, whereas an abnormally high level, or an increased FSH/LH ratio, suggests declining oocyte quality and ovarian insufficiency or menopause.

The reference range for luteinising hormone (LH) during the follicular phase is usually in the region of 2.4–12.6 IU/L.[868] In females, cyclic LH secretion triggers ovulation, and transformation of the ovarian follicle into the corpus luteum, which in turn secretes progesterone. Low levels of luteinising hormone (LH) may suggest conditions such as hypothalamic or pituitary dysfunction, whereas an abnormally high level suggests a problem with ovulation and corpus luteum function, such as in ovarian insufficiency or menopause. An increased LH/FSH ratio is a feature of polycystic ovary syndrome (PCOS).

The reference range for oestradiol during the early follicular phase is usually in the region of 70–510 pmol/L.[869] Low levels of oestrogen suggest hypopituitarism, ovarian insufficiency, or menopause, whereas high levels may suggest oestrogen producing tumours, adrenal hyperplasia, hepatic disease, or poor hepatic metabolism of oestrogen.

The reference range for prolactin is usually in the region of 100–550 mU/L in women who are not pregnant or breastfeeding.[870] High levels in women who are not pregnant or breastfeeding may be due to physical or emotional stress, or pituitary adenoma. Women with prolactin levels within the upper part of the reference range may experience "latent hyperprolactinaemia" and infertility in spite of prolactin levels apparently within the "normal" range.

Mid-luteal phase tests

Mid-luteal phase blood tests are carried out 6–8 days before next expected menstrual period. Progesterone is predominantly secreted by the corpus luteum, with small amounts also originating from the adrenal cortex. Levels of progesterone above 28 nmol/Lin the mid-luteal phase suggest that ovulation has occurred.[871] However, higher levels (above 35 nmol/L) are desirable in terms of maintaining pregnancy and preventing early pregnancy loss.[872]

Total androgens and/or free testosterone may be raised in women with PCOS.[873] Changes in sex hormone-binding globulin (SHBG) levels can affect the amount of hormones that are available to be used by the body's tissues. A high SHBG level means that less free hormones are available to the tissues; while a low SHBG level means that more of the total hormone is bioavailable and not bound to SHBG. In women with PCOS, low levels of oestrogen and higher levels of androgens may reduce SHBG, which increases the activity of androgens.

Ideally, it is useful to retest levels of FSH, LH, oestradiol, and prolactin during the mid-luteal phase, and this may yield different results, and reveal problems that were not apparent in the early follicular tests.

Additional tests

The additional tests may be carried out at any point of the cycle, and may therefore be taken along with either the early follicular or mid-luteal blood tests.

Anti-Mullerian hormone (AMH) is secreted by the ovarian granulosa cells, and reflects the number of primary follicles present, which is an indicator of the remaining ovarian reserve.[874] Low AMH levels reflect a lower number of primary follicles, whereas abnormally high AMH suggests a higher number of primary follicles (as occurs in PCOS).[875] The approximate levels of AMH that indicate optimal, satisfactory, low, and extremely low ovarian reserve are shown below.

AMH levels as an indicator of ovarian reserve

High levels (often seen in PCOS)	Over 60 pmol/L
Optimal	40–60 pmol/L
Satisfactory	20–40 pmol/L
Low	3–20 pmol/L
Extremely low	0–3 pmol/L

Full blood count, ferritin, folate, and B12 tests help to diagnose and differentiate between different types of anaemia, including those which are due to deficiencies of iron, folate, and B12; and to assess immune system function in patients with chronic infection and immune system problems.

Thyroid function tests include tests for TSH (thyroid stimulating hormone), T4 (thyroxine), and T3 (triiodothyronine). TSH levels are used to diagnose hyper- and hypothyroidism, and to differentiate between thyroid disease and hypothalamic/pituitary dysfunction. In *hyper*thyroid conditions, high levels of T4 lead to *low* levels of TSH due to negative feedback. However if TSH is low, and T4 is also low, this suggests a problem with the hypothalamus or pituitary gland, such as a space-occupying tumour.

Similarly, in *hypo*thyroid conditions, low production of T4 by the thyroid leads to *increased* levels of TSH. However, if TSH is low, and T4 is also low, this suggests a problem with the hypothalamus or pituitary gland, such as TSH secreting pituitary adenoma. It is therefore very important to ensure that both TSH *and* thyroxine levels are tested, since pituitary causes of infertility may be missed where only levels of stimulating hormone are measured.[876]

Levels of T3 should also be tested, since levels may be low (due to inefficient conversion of T4 to T3), or high (in T3 toxicosis), despite normal levels of TSH and T4. Ideally, tests for anti-thyroperoxidase (Anti-TPO), antithyroglobulin (TgAb), and Anti-TSH receptor antibodies (TRAb) should also be carried out, since there is increasing evidence for the role of autoantibodies in subfertility and early pregnancy loss, even in euthyroid women.[877]

Cholesterol is used to synthesise bile acids and hormones (including reproductive hormones and adrenal steroids). It is therefore an important part of the assessment of liver and endocrine function. *Hyper*cholesterolaemia may be due to diabetes, hepatic or biliary cholestasis, use of oral contraceptives, or hormone deficiency (such as oestrogen deficiency or hypothyroidism). Conversely, *hypo*cholesterolaemia may indicate malnutrition or hyperthyroid conditions.

Glycated haemoglobin (HbA1c) provides a measure of the average plasma glucose concentration over the preceding three months. (The average red blood cell lifespan is 120 days. However, since red blood cells do not all undergo lysis at the same time an average of three months is used.) Elevated HbA1C is an important marker of insulin resistance.

C-reactive protein (CRP) is produced in response to inflammation. It may be elevated in any inflammatory condition, including endometriosis, uterine fibroids, and pelvic inflammatory disease. Raised CRP may also indicate low grade inflammation, which is associated with reduced fertility, decreased success rate of IVF, and increased risk of miscarriage.[878] Women with history of recurrent miscarriage should also have a blood test to check for anti-phospholipid antibodies, which can cause blood clotting and early pregnancy loss.

Tests to assess reproductive health and fertility in men

Recommended tests for men

- Full blood count, fasting glucose, cholesterol
- FSH, LH, androgens, free testosterone, oestrogen, SHBG
- TSH, T4, T3
- Semen analysis

Blood tests in men may be carried out at any time, since they are not subject to cyclical variation as is the case in women.

Full blood count and fasting glucose

The full blood count helps to diagnose and differentiate between different types of anaemia, including those that are due to deficiencies of iron, folate, and B12; and to assess immune system function in patients with chronic infection and immune system problems. Fasting glucose is used to screen for diabetes, which may lead to erectile dysfunction.

Cholesterol

Cholesterol is used to synthesise bile acids and hormones (including reproductive hormones and adrenal steroids). It is therefore an important part of the assessment of liver and endocrine function. *Hyper*cholesterolaemia may be due to diabetes, hepatic or biliary cholestasis, or hormone deficiency (such as testosterone deficiency or hypothyroidism). Conversely, *hypo*cholesterolaemia may indicate malnutrition or hyperthyroid conditions.

FSH, LH, and androgens

Decreased testosterone and total androgen production in men may be due to advancing age or hypogonadism. Reduced androgen production by the testes leads to increased levels of follicle stimulating hormone (FSH) and luteinising hormone (LH). However, low levels of FSH and LH suggest hypogonadotropic hypogonadism, in which failure of the hypothalamus or pituitary gland to stimulate the testes leads to low levels of androgens.[879]

Sex hormone-binding globulin

Changes in sex hormone-binding globulin (SHBG) levels affect the amount of hormones that are available to be used by the body's tissues. A high SHBG level means that less free hormones are available to the tissues; while a low SHBG level means that more of the total hormone is bioavailable and not bound to SHBG. In men, low testosterone levels increase SHBG, which further exacerbates the symptoms of low androgens.

Oestrogen

Excess oestrogen in men inhibits secretion of hypothalamic gonado-tropin-releasing hormone (GnRH), follicle stimulating hormone (FSH), and luteinising hormone (LH),[880] resulting in low levels of androgens and impaired spermatogenesis. Excess oestrogen in men also increases levels of sex hormone-binding globulin (SHBG), which causes less testosterone to be available.

Thyroid function tests

Thyroid function tests include tests for TSH (thyroid stimulating hormone), T4 (thyroxine), and T3 (triiodothyronine). TSH levels are used to diagnose hyper and hypothyroidism, and to differentiate between thyroid disease and hypothalamic/pituitary dysfunction. Interpretation of thyroid function tests has already been described in the previous section on blood tests to assess reproductive health and fertility in women.

Tests for anti-thyroperoxidase (Anti-TPO), antithyroglobulin (TgAb), and Anti-TSH receptor antibodies (TRAb) should also be carried out, since the presence of thyroid autoantibodies is frequently associated with sperm antibodies in infertile patients.[881]

Semen analysis

Semen analysis should be performed on multiple ejaculates before diagnosing male infertility, due to the large individual variation in sperm parameters.[882] More sensitive tests are also available, including egg penetration test; and the post-coital test, which measures the ability of sperm to penetrate cervical mucus. These tests predict fertility in an estimated 66% of cases, in comparison to 30% with conventional sperm analysis.[883] The following table shows the normal values for semen parameters according to the World Health Organization (WHO).[884]

Anti-sperm antibodies are measured as part of the semen analysis, rather than by blood testing, as there is a poor correlation between the presence of anti-sperm antibodies in semen versus serum. Furthermore, while semen anti-sperm antibodies have been shown to negatively affect fertility, serum anti-sperm antibodies do not have a significant impact on fertility prognosis.[885]

Parameter	Reference value
Volume	> 2.0 ml
pH	7.2–8
Concentration	>20 x 10^6 ml
Total sperm per ejaculate	>40 x 10^6 ml
Motility	>50% motile (grade a+b) or >25% grade a
Morphology	<15%
Viability	>75% live spermatozoa
Leukocytes	<1 x 10^6 ml
Anti-sperm antibodies	<50% bound sperm
Zinc	>2.4 uM per ejaculate
Citric acid	>52 uM per ejaculate
Fructose	>13 uM per ejaculate

Further investigations

Further investigations for women

Further investigations that may be useful for women with reproductive health problems include the following tests:

Vaginal swab

A vaginal swab is recommended for women who experience unusual vaginal discharge, abnormal vaginal bleeding, or symptoms such as pelvic pain, dyspareunia, or itching or burning affecting the vagina. A vaginal swab is used to collect a sample of vaginal secretions, which are then cultured to check for infection (such as candida, bacterial vaginosis, parasitic infection, or sexually transmitted disease).

Cervical smear

A cervical smear (or pap smear) is recommended every three years for women of childbearing age, to check for cellular changes or other cervical abnormalities. A speculum is inserted into the vagina to hold the vaginal walls open, and a spatula is used to scrape the surface of the cervix in order to obtain a sample of cells. Women who are trying to conceive, who have not had a cervical screening test within the last three years, should be encouraged to have the test carried out before getting pregnant.

If any abnormalities in the appearance of the cervix are detected while carrying out the test, or if the test results are abnormal, a colposcopy may be recommended, in which a more detailed examination of the cervix is carried out, and if necessary, cervical biopsies may be taken.

Pelvic ultrasound scan

A pelvic ultrasound scan is carried out in order to detect any abnormality in the pelvic cavity, uterus, endometrium, cervix, fallopian tubes, ovaries, or bladder. It may involve transvaginal ultrasound (during which the ultrasound probe is inserted into the vagina) and/or transabdominal ultrasound (during which the ultrasound probe is moved around on the skin of the lower abdomen). Ultrasound scans can be used to detect the presence of normal follicles on the ovaries, to look for evidence of ovulation, to diagnose ovarian cysts, to assess endometrial thickness, and to identify uterine fibroids and other uterine or pelvic abnormalities. If any abnormalities are detected, more invasive procedures such as hysteroscopy or laparoscopy may be used to investigate further.

Hysteroscopy

A hysteroscopy (which is carried out by inserting a hysteroscope into the vagina and through the cervix) may be used to diagnose endometrial hyperplasia, uterine fibroids, and other uterine abnormalities such as intrauterine adhesions. Endometrial biopsy and minor surgical procedures, such as removal of intrauterine fibroids or adhesions, may also be carried out during a hysteroscopy.

Laparoscopy

A laparoscopy may be carried out in order to investigate and treat conditions affecting the uterus, ovaries, fallopian tubes, and other pelvic structures. A laparoscope is inserted into the pelvic cavity through an incision in the abdomen in order to identify abnormalities such as endometriosis, pelvic inflammatory disease, adhesions, ovarian cysts, or growths in the pelvic cavity. During a laparoscopy, tissue samples may be taken for biopsy, endometrial lesions or scar tissue may be removed, and any damage to the uterus, fallopian tubes, or ovaries may be repaired.

Laparoscopy and dye

A laparoscopy and dye (or tubal patency test) involves injecting a dye that passes through the fallopian tubes to identify any blockages, during a laparoscopy. Where blockages are found to be present, these can often be cleared during the procedure. Laparoscopy is often only carried out where other less invasive tests have suggested the presence of an abnormality. However, up to one third of infertile women are thought to have tubal occlusion,[886] therefore it is advisable for women who are trying to conceive to undergo testing for tubal patency at an early stage of treatment.

Post-coital test

The post-coital test involves analysis of the cervical mucus, just before ovulation and six to twelve hours after intercourse. It assesses the quality of cervical mucus (including the volume, consistency, pH, and number and types of cell present), the viability of sperm,[887] and most importantly, the ability of sperm cells to function within the cervical environment.[888]A reduced number of surviving sperm may be due to inadequate cervical mucus, while abnormal penetration of cervical mucus by sperm has been associated with the presence of anti-sperm antibodies.[889]

Further investigations for men

Further investigations that may be useful for men with reproductive health problems include a urethral swab, which is recommended for men who have symptoms such as discharge from the urethra, symptoms of urinary tract infection, or swelling affecting the penis or testicles. It can be used to detect bacterial, viral, or yeast infections, including sexually transmitted disease.

A pelvic ultrasound may be recommended for men with pelvic pain, symptoms of urinary dysfunction, or to investigate masses or swellings. A transabdominal ultrasound (during which the ultrasound probe is moved around on the skin of the lower abdomen) is carried out in order to check for any abnormalities in the pelvic cavity, while a transrectal ultrasound (during which the ultrasound probe is inserted into the rectum) may be used to evaluate the prostate gland and seminal vesicles.

Predicting ovulation and the fertile window

During the follicular phase of the menstrual cycle, multiple ovarian follicles develop in response to secretion of follicle stimulating hormone (FSH) by the pituitary gland. The growing follicles secrete oestrogen, which then inhibits FSH secretion due to negative feedback. The dominant follicle is the most sensitive to FSH, and therefore continues to grow in spite of the falling levels of FSH, while the adjacent follicles undergo atresia due to lack of stimulation.

The dominant follicle continues to secrete oestrogen, eventually inducing a surge of luteinising hormone (LH) from the pituitary gland, which triggers ovulation to occur. After ovulation, the dominant follicle transforms into a corpus luteum, which secretes progesterone and if conception does not occur, it eventually collapses, leading to a drop in progesterone levels, which initiates menstruation.[890]

These hormone changes, which occur just before, during, and after ovulation (rising oestrogen in the late follicular phase, the LH surge which triggers ovulation, and subsequent secretion of progesterone), lead to specific physiological signs, such as changes in cervical mucus and body temperature. These changes can be monitored in order to identify the time during which conception is most likely to occur, often referred to as the *fertile window*.

Sperm can survive in the female body for up to five days. Therefore the fertile window begins approximately five days before ovulation. The lifespan of the oocyte is up to twenty-four hours. Therefore, the fertile window ends approximately one day after ovulation occurs.[891] Various methods can be used to help couples that wish to conceive to identify the fertile window, in order to ensure that intercourse occurs during the time that conception is possible.

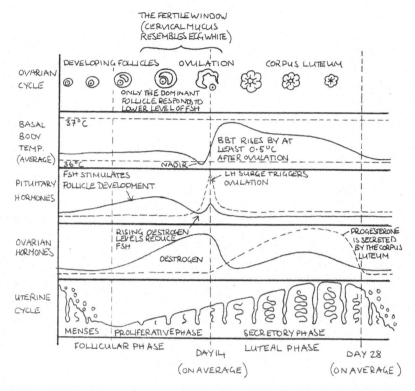

Figure 18: Hormone changes during the menstrul cycle.

Cervical mucus changes

In the days leading up to ovulation, rising serum oestrogen levels cause changes in the composition and consistency of the cervical mucus. Observation of these changes may provide a reliable indication of the fertility window.

Outside the fertile window, cervical mucus contains high levels of mucin, a glycoprotein that forms a matrix structure, providing a barrier to sperm and microorganisms. The mucus appears scanty, thick, and viscous on inspection.[892] It is usually white or cream in colour. However, during the fertile window, rising oestrogen levels cause the cervical mucus to become more abundant; and fluid, clear, and stretchy in consistency (resembling raw egg white).

Fertile mucus helps to facilitate transport of sperm during the fertile window. After ovulation, rising progesterone levels cause the cervical mucus to become thick, sticky, and opaque again. Monitoring the consistency of the cervical mucus (ideally by stretching it between thumb and forefinger) can help to identify when a woman is most likely to conceive.

Ovulation testing kits

Rising levels of oestrogen during the follicular phase eventually induce a surge of luteinising hormone (LH) from the pituitary gland, which triggers ovulation to occur.

The onset of the LH surge precedes ovulation by up to forty-eight hours, and the peak serum level of LH precedes ovulation by approximately twelve hours.[893]

Home ovulation testing kits measure LH in the urine, and can therefore help to indicate that ovulation is about to occur, in order to facilitate timing of intercourse or intrauterine insemination.[894] While the fertile window may extend up to five days before ovulation, depending on the survival time of sperm in the woman's body, the highest likelihood of conception is from two days prior to ovulation until the day of ovulation.[895] In women who are ovulating, this narrow window of peak fertility may be accurately identified using an ovulation test kit.

While ovulation testing kits that identify the LH surge can be useful for identifying the fertile window in women who are ovulating, some women may experience an LH surge without ovulation.[896] Therefore results from LH testing kits should be combined with other information to assess whether ovulation is occurring, such as cervical mucus changes, monitoring of basal body temperature, and measurement of mid-luteal serum progesterone levels.

Conversely, while detection of the luteinising hormone (LH) surge is very sensitive and specific for identifying the window of peak fertility in women who are ovulating, it is not an appropriate method for contraception, because sperm ejaculated before a woman's LH surge may survive long enough to fertilise the ovum.[897]

Basal body temperature

Progesterone is secreted by the corpus luteum only after ovulation, and therefore, detection of progesterone can confirm that ovulation has occurred.[898] A serum level of progesterone above 28 nmol/L in the mid-luteal phase suggests that ovulation has taken place;[899] however, it doesn't pinpoint exactly when it occurred. Because progesterone causes a rise in basal body temperature (BBT), measuring this temperature may be more useful for determining the timing of ovulation.[900]

The basal body temperature is the temperature of the body recorded first thing in the morning, before any activity has occurred. Charting the average basal body temperature over the course of the menstrual cycle can help to determine if and when ovulation has occurred, and when charted over several months, may be used to predict ovulation, and optimise the timing of intercourse;[901] either to increase the chances of conception, or to avoid pregnancy by only having unprotected intercourse after the fertile window has ended.

In order to measure the basal body temperature, the oral, vaginal, or rectal temperature should be measured at approximately the same time every morning (preferably within thirty minutes either side of the average time), before getting out of bed. It is very important to use the same method every day, as body temperature naturally varies between these different sites.

Each reading should be plotted on a chart. Alternatively, fertility-tracking apps are available which can be used to help calculate the fertile window when daily BBT readings are entered. After several months of tracking, a pattern may begin to emerge.[902]

During the follicular phase of the menstrual cycle, the basal body temperature remains in the lower range (usually 36.5 degrees Celsius or below). Approximately one day before ovulation, the basal body temperature reaches its lowest point (nadir).[903] After ovulation has occurred, the corpus luteum begins to secret progesterone, which causes the BBT to rise by at least 0.5 degrees Celsius. A rise in basal body temperature temperature of approximately 0.5 degrees over a forty-eight-hour period, which remains constant for at least three days, suggests that ovulation has occurred.[904]

The BBT plateaus at or around this increased temperature throughout the luteal phase. In the late luteal phase, if conception has not occurred, the corpus luteum degrades, and ceases to produce progesterone. As the serum progesterone level falls, the BBT returns to the lower range, usually a day or two before the onset of menstrual bleeding.[905]

When charted over several months, the basal body temperature may be used to predict ovulation, and optimise the timing of intercourse;[906] either to increase the chances of conception, or to avoid pregnancy. However, BBT measurements are also affected by factors such as fever, use of anti-pyretic drugs (temperature lowering medication), physical or emotional stress, lack of sleep, alcohol consumption, change in room temperature, change in waking time, and the use or discontinuation of oral contraception.[907]

Basal body temperature monitoring can indicate that ovulation has occurred, which may be helpful in establishing a pattern of fertile periods over time, but it does not predict ovulation during any one month, and therefore, using a combination of methods to predict the time that conception is most likely to occur is more effective than using any one method alone.

Notes

865. Gascoigne, S. (2001). *The Clinical Medicine Guide: A Holistic Perspective*. Clonakilty, Ireland: Jigme.

866. Campana, A., de Agostini, A., Bischof, P., Tawfik, E., & Mastrorilli, A. (2019). Evaluation of infertility. Graduate Foundation for Medical Education and Research (GFMER) [online]. Available from https://gfmer.ch/Books/Reproductive_health/infertility_evaluation.html (accessed 20 June 2020)

867. HSE (2018). *Complex Reference Ranges* [online]. Available from https://hse.ie/eng/services/list/3/acutehospitals/hospitals/waterford/laboratoryservices/complex-reference-ranges.html (accessed 21 June 2020).

868. HSE (2018). *Complex Reference Ranges* [online]. Available from https://hse.ie/eng/services/list/3/acutehospitals/hospitals/waterford/laboratoryservices/complex-reference-ranges.html (accessed 21 June 2020).

869. HSE (2018). *Complex Reference Ranges* [online]. Available from https://hse.ie/eng/services/list/3/acutehospitals/hospitals/waterford/laboratoryservices/complex-reference-ranges.html (accessed 21 June 2020).

870. O'Shea, P., Kavanagh-Wright, L., & Bell, M. (2019). Laboratory testing for hyperprolactinaemia (prolactin). *National Laboratory Handbook* [online]. Available from http://13.94.105.41/eng/about/who/cspd/ncps/pathology/resources/lab-testing-for-hyperprolactinaemia.pdf (accessed 20 June 2020).

871. NICE (2013). Fertility assessment and treatment for people with fertility problems [online]. Available from nice.org.uk (accessed 20 June 2020).

872. Lek, S. M., Ku, C. W., Allen Jr, J. C., Malhotra, R., Tan, N. S., Østbye, T., & Tan, T. C. (2017). Validation of serum progesterone <35nmol/L as a predictor of miscarriage among women with threatened miscarriage. *BMC Pregnancy and Childbirth*, 17: 78–84.

873. Legro, R. S., Arslanian, S. A., Ehrmann, D. A., Hoeger, K. M., Murad, M. H., Pasquali, R., & Welt, C. K. (2013). Diagnosis and treatment of polycystic ovary syndrome: an Endocrine Society clinical practice guideline. *Journal of Clinical Endocrinology and Metabolism*, 98(12): 4565–4592.

874. Weenen, C., Laven, J. S. E., Von Bergh, A. R. M., Cranfield, M., Groome, N. P., Visser, J. A., Kramer, P., Fauser, B. C. J. M., & Themmen, A. P. N. (2004). Anti-Müllerian hormone expression pattern in the human ovary: potential implications for initial and cyclic follicle recruitment. *Molecular Human Reproduction*, 10(2): 77–83.

875. Broer, S. L., Broekman, F. J., Laven, J. S. E., & Fauser, B. C. J. M. (2014). Anti-Mülle-rian hormone: ovarian reserve testing and its potential clinical implications. *Human Reproduction Update, 20*(5): 688–701.

876. Corenblum, B. (2018). Hypopituitarism (panhypopituitarism). Medscape [online]. Available from https://emedicine.medscape.com/article/122287-overview#a4 (accessed 14 November 2019).

877. Jefferys, A., Vanderpump, M., & Yasmin, E. (2015). Thyroid dysfunction and repro-ductive health. *Obstetrician & Gynaecologist, 17*: 39–45.

878. Gleicher, N. (2017). The importance of inflammation in human reproduction. *CHR Voice Digest*, March: 1–2.

879. Agarwal, A., & Said, T. M. (2011). Interpretation of basic semen analysis and advanced semen testing. In: E. S. Sabanegh, Jr. (Ed.), *Male Infertility: Problems and Solutions*. Springer [online].

880. Greenstein, B., & Wood, D. F. (2006). *The Endocrine System at a Glance* (2nd edn). Oxford: Blackwell.

881. Paschke, R., Schulze Bertelsbeck, D., Tsalimalma, K., & Nieschlag, E. (1994). Associa-tion of sperm antibodies with other autoantibodies in infertile men. *American Journal of Reproductive Immunology, 32*(2): 88–94.

882. Keel, B. A. (2006). Within- and between-subject variation in semen parameters in infertile men and normal semen donors. *Fertility and Sterility, 85*(1): 128–134.

883. Purvis, K., & Christiansen, E. (1992). Male infertility: current concepts. *Annals of Medicine, 24*(4): 258–272.

884. World Health Organization (1999). *WHO Laboratory Manual for the Examination of Human Semen and Sperm-Cervical Mucus Interaction*. Cambridge: Cambridge University Press.

885. Eggert-Kruse, W., Pohl, S., Näher, H., Tilgen, W., & Runnebaum, B. (1992). Microbial colonization and sperm–mucus interaction: results in 1000 infertile couples. *Human Reproduction, 7*(5): 612–620.

886. Khalaf, Y. (2003). Tubal subfertility. *British Medical Journal, 327*(7415): 610–613.

887. Campana, A., de Agostini, A., Bischof, P., Tawfik, E., & Mastrorilli, A. (2019). Eval-uation of infertility. Graduate Foundation for Medical Education and Research (GFMER) [online]. Available from https://gfmer.ch/Books/Reproductive_health/infertility_evaluation.html (accessed 20 June 2020).

888. Markham, S. (1991). Cervico-utero-tubal factors in infertility. *Current Opinion in Obstetrics and Gynecology, 3*(2): 191–196.

889. Kremer, J., & Jager, S. (1992). The significance of antisperm antibodies for sperm-cervical mucus interaction. *Human Reproduction, 7*(6): 781–784.

890. Su, H.-W., Yi, Y.-C., Wei, T.-Y., Chang, T.-C., & Cheng, C.-M. (2017). Detection of ovulation, a review of currently available methods. *Bioengineering & Translational Medicine, 2*(3): 238–246.

891. Ecochard, R., Marret, H., Rabilloud, M., Bradaï, R., Boehringer, H., Girotto, S., & Barbato, M. (2000). Sensitivity and specificity of ultrasound indices of ovulation in spontaneous cycles. *European Journal of Obstetrics & Gynecology and Reproductive Biol-ogy, 91*(1): 59–64.

892. Depares, J., Ryder, R. E., Walker, S. M., Scanlon, M. F., & Norman, C. M. (1986). Ovarian ultrasonography highlights precision of symptoms of ovulation as markers of ovulation. *British Medical Journal (Clinical Research Edition), 292*(6535): 1562.

893. Hoff, J. D., Quigley, M. E., & Yen, S. S. (1983). Hormonal dynamics at midcycle: a reevaluation. *Journal of Clinical Endocrinology and Metabolism, 57*(4): 792–796.
894. Su, H.-W., Yi, Y.-C., Wei, T.-Y., Chang, T.-C., & Cheng, C.-M. (2017). Detection of ovulation, a review of currently available methods. *Bioengineering & Translational Medicine, 2*(3): 238–246.
895. Tiplady, S., Jones, G., Campbell, M., Johnson, S., & Ledger, W. (2012). Home ovulation tests and stress in women trying to conceive: a randomized controlled trial. *Human Reproduction, 28*(1): 138–151.
896. Qublan, H., Amarin, Z., Nawasreh, M., Diab, F., Malkawi, S., Al-Ahmad, N., & Balawneh, M. (2006). Luteinized unruptured follicle syndrome: incidence and recurrence rate in infertile women with unexplained infertility undergoing intrauterine insemination. *Human Reproduction, 21*(8): 2110–2113.
897. Su, H.-W., Yi, Y.-C., Wei, T.-Y., Chang, T.-C., & Cheng, C.-M. (2017). Detection of ovulation, a review of currently available methods. *Bioengineering & Translational Medicine, 2*(3): 238–246.
898. Su, H.-W., Yi, Y.-C., Wei, T.-Y., Chang, T.-C., & Cheng, C.-M. (2017). Detection of ovulation, a review of currently available methods. *Bioengineering & Translational Medicine, 2*(3): 238–246.
899. NICE (2013). Fertility assessment and treatment for people with fertility problems [online]. Available from nice.org.uk (accessed 20 June 2020).
900. Su, H.-W., Yi, Y.-C., Wei, T.-Y., Chang, T.-C., & Cheng, C.-M. (2017). Detection of ovulation, a review of currently available methods. *Bioengineering & Translational Medicine, 2*(3): 238–246.
901. Steward, K., & Raja, A. (2019). Physiology, ovulation, basal body temperature. *StatPearls* [online]. Available from https://ncbi.nlm.nih.gov/books/NBK546686/ (accessed 22 June 2020).
902. Su, H.-W., Yi, Y.-C., Wei, T.-Y., Chang, T.-C., & Cheng, C.-M. (2017). Detection of ovulation, a review of currently available methods. *Bioengineering & Translational Medicine, 2*(3): 238–246.
903. Martinez, A. R., van Hooff, M. H., Schoute, E., van der Meer, M., Broekmans, F. J., & Hompes, P. G. (1992). The reliability, acceptability and applications of basal body temperature (BBT) records in the diagnosis and treatment of infertility. *European Journal of Obstetrics & Gynecology and Reproductive Biology, 47*(2): 121–127.
904. Su, H.-W., Yi, Y.-C., Wei, T.-Y., Chang, T.-C., & Cheng, C.-M. (2017). Detection of ovulation, a review of currently available methods. *Bioengineering & Translational Medicine, 2*(3): 238–246.
905. Su, H.-W., Yi, Y.-C., Wei, T.-Y., Chang, T.-C., & Cheng, C.-M. (2017). Detection of ovulation, a review of currently available methods. *Bioengineering & Translational Medicine, 2*(3): 238–246.
906. Steward, K., & Raja, A. (2019). Physiology, ovulation, basal body temperature *StatPearls* [online]. Available from https://ncbi.nlm.nih.gov/books/NBK546686/ (accessed 22 June 2020).
907. Su, H.-W., Yi, Y.-C., Wei, T.-Y., Chang, T.-C., & Cheng, C.-M. (2017). Detection of ovulation, a review of currently available methods. *Bioengineering & Translational Medicine, 2*(3): 238–246.

CHAPTER THIRTEEN

Supporting patients receiving orthodox fertility treatments

Assisted reproduction techniques (ART)

The success rate of assisted reproduction in individual couples is affected by the same factors that affect conception rates and pregnancy outcomes in the general fertile population.[908] Therefore addressing factors that affect fertility (as described in the earlier chapters of this book), in the months leading up to assisted reproduction techniques, can help to improve the chances of conception and pregnancy outcomes.

Assisted reproduction techniques generally either help to ensure ovulation, or in the case of IVF, help with both ovulation and fertilisation. Therefore, there is no need to use herbs to promote ovulation during assisted reproduction therapy. However, it is safe and appropriate to focus on other reproductive health issues in order to maximise the chances of conception through ART, such as improving the overall health of the couple; managing stress levels; improving the quality of oocyte and sperm; and addressing the various factors influencing implantation (such as endometrial thickness, inflammation, and endometrial blood supply); and the issues affecting pregnancy outcomes (such as uterine tone and progesterone levels).

Clomiphene citrate

Clomiphene citrate is an oestrogen antagonist. It causes an increase in FSH secretion by the pituitary gland, as a result of reduced negative feedback by oestrogen. Improved FSH levels can help to stimulate follicle development and thereby improve ovulation. However, because it antagonises oestrogen, clomiphene citrate is also associated with endometrial thinning, which can reduce the chance of conception.[909]

50 mg clomiphene citrate is given on days 2–6 of the menstrual cycle, for three consecutive cycles. (It should not be given for more than three cycles, as it is associated with an increased risk of ovarian hyper stimulation syndrome and ovarian tumours, and is associated with a very low success rate when used for more than three months).

It is only effective in cases of anovulation, and is associated with only a 5–6% pregnancy rate in couples with unexplained infertility.[910] This may be because infertility is often due to a number of factors (such as cervical factors, poor oocyte or sperm quality, fallopian tube blockage, abnormal endometrial blood flow, problems with implantation, or inadequate progesterone levels), and not just a failure to ovulate.

However, treatment with clomiphene citrate is frequently offered as a first line of treatment for women who are finding it difficult to conceive, often before carrying out any investigations to identify or rule out the other possible causes of infertility mentioned above.

Intracervical insemination (ICI) and intrauterine insemination (IUI)

Intracervical insemination (ICI) involves introducing sperm into the woman's body at the neck of the cervix, whereas intrauterine insemination (IUI) involves placing sperm directly into the uterus. These techniques may be used where it is not possible for intercourse to take place in order to conceive; for example in the case of same sex couples, men with erectile dysfunction or retrograde ejaculation, women with severe dyspareunia or structural abnormalities, individuals with disabilities, or those who have a condition that can be sexually transmitted, and/or those who need to have sperm washing before conception can take place. IUI is also useful for cervical factor infertility.

Where the female partner who wishes to conceive is ovulating normally, unstimulated IUI may be offered, in which ovulation is allowed to occur naturally, and ICI or IUI is carried out at the time of peak fertility. Unstimulated IUI is associated with a 4% pregnancy success rate in couples with unexplained infertility.[911]

If the female partner is not ovulating, she may be offered stimulated IUI in which drugs (such as clomiphene citrate or gonadotropin injections) are used to promote ovulation. Stimulated IUI is associated with a 10% pregnancy success rate in couples with unexplained infertility.[912]

ICI/IUI cannot be used where there is a very low sperm count or poor sperm quality, which does not respond to treatment, although it can be carried out using donor sperm where necessary.

In vitro fertilisation (IVF)

In vitro fertilisation (IVF) is generally recommended for couples who have been unable to conceive naturally, or as a result of other assisted reproduction techniques, and those for whom conception would otherwise be impossible for a variety of reasons. The first stage of IVF involves ovarian stimulation with gonadotropins (FSH and LH) for up to fourteen days, which results in the development of multiple follicles. Follicle development may be monitored using ultrasound scans.

When the follicles have grown sufficiently, human chorionic gonadotropin (hCG) is administered as a single subcutaneous injection, in order to trigger oocyte maturation and release. Egg collection takes place approximately thirty-six hours after the hCG injection, via ultrasound-guided, transvaginal aspiration. For women who are unable to use their own eggs (due to prior cancer treatment or critically low ovarian reserve, for example) donor eggs may be used instead.

In vitro fertilisation is carried out in a laboratory, by combining oocytes and sperm, and allowing fertilisation to occur naturally; or by intracytoplasmic sperm injection (ICSI), in which a single healthy sperm in introduced into each oocyte.

Egg transfer involves placing the fertilised embryos into the uterus (through the cervix), approximately five days after fertilisation. In some cases, embryos are frozen, and implanted during a later cycle, when the woman's body has had an opportunity to recover from the physiological and emotional stress of the IVF process. This provides an ideal opportunity for herbalists and other healthcare practitioners to help the woman to maximise her reproductive and general health in preparation for embryo transfer, particularly focusing on factors such as healthy diet, appropriate exercise, stress management, healthy blood flow, adequate endometrial lining, maintaining sufficient levels of progesterone, and reducing inflammatory prostaglandins.

If sperm count, motility, or sperm quality are low, IVF with intracytoplasmic sperm injection (ICSI) can be carried out to ensure fertilisation occurs. If the male partner's sperm cannot be used (due to azoospermia or genetic abnormalities, for example) donor sperm may be used instead.

IVF is associated with an increased risk of first trimester thromboembolism.[913] Therefore measures to prevent thromboembolism with herbal medicine and nutrition (such as *Ginkgo biloba* and fish oils) are useful during early pregnancy for women who have conceived by IVF.

Supporting patients receiving orthodox assisted reproduction

Many people who decide to use orthodox assisted reproduction techniques (ART) choose to combine orthodox interventions with natural approaches in order to improve their fertility. The success rate of assisted reproduction techniques (for each cycle) ranges from less than 10% with the drug clomiphene citrate, to just 20–25% for in vitro fertilisation (IVF),[914] and the cost of IVF treatment in Ireland ranges from about €4000–7000 per cycle.[915] Therefore many couples will turn to natural medicine to try to increase their chance of success.

In most cases, assisted reproduction techniques either help to ensure ovulation, or in the case of IVF, help with both ovulation and fertilisation. Therefore, there is no need to use herbs to promote ovulation during assisted reproduction therapy. However, these interventions pay little or no attention to other issues that may affect the outcome of the treatment, such as the overall health of the couple; their stress levels; the quality of oocyte and sperm; the various factors influencing implantation (such as endometrial thickness, inflammation, and endometrial blood supply); and the issues affecting pregnancy outcomes (such as uterine tone and progesterone levels).

Fortunately these are all issues that can be readily and safely addressed with natural approaches, such as nutrition and lifestyle changes, herbal medicine, and other modalities such as acupuncture and chiropractic, without negatively interfering with the assisted reproduction process. Therefore, there is a great deal of scope for herbalists and other natural healthcare practitioners to support patients through assisted reproduction and help to maximise their chances of conceiving.

In order to produce healthy sperm and oocytes, and to maximise the chances of conception and healthy pregnancy in people who decide to use orthodox assisted reproduction techniques, it is vital to treat any underlying condition that may contribute to infertility (as described in the earlier chapters of this book). However, it is also important to improve the nutrition and general health of both partners. For best results, it is advisable to treat both partners for at least three months before beginning any course of assisted reproduction treatment.

Improving general health and nutrition

Female fertility improves with diets that include a reduced intake of animal protein and a higher vegetable protein intake; a lower intake of trans-fat with a greater intake of monounsaturated fat; and a lower intake of high glycaemic index foods with a higher intake of high-fibre, low-glycaemic index carbohydrates.[916] It is also important to ensure the diet includes plenty of omega 3 fatty acids (from flaxseed and oily fish); whole grains; nut and seeds; beans and pulses; and plenty of fresh fruit and vegetables.

Female infertility is associated with deficiencies of various nutrients including vitamins A, C, and E, B vitamins, folic acid, zinc,[917] iron, and essential fatty acids such as EPA and DHA.[918] Women who decide to use assisted reproduction techniques should therefore be advised to take a multivitamin that is specifically designed for preconception. It is also advisable to avoid gluten, caffeine, alcohol, and smoking, which have all been associated with reduced fertility.

Regular exercise (ideally 30–50 minutes of medium intensity exercise, five days a week) is important to improve fertility and maintain a healthy body weight. However, it is important to avoid over-exercising, since high intensity exercise for more than one hour per day is associated with infertility.[919]

Women who are overweight should be advised to try to reduce their body weight with a healthy diet and adequate exercise in order to improve fertility. Conversely, women who are underweight should be encouraged to eat plenty of healthy foods, including healthy fats, in order to increase their BMI to within the optimal range if possible.

Obesity can also reduce fertility in men. It increases the risk of sperm DNA fragmentation, and sperm parameters are also more likely to be suboptimal in obese men. Therefore, reduction in weight through healthy diet and exercise may help to improve fertility in men with high BMI.[920]

High dietary intakes of hydrogenated oils have been shown to have a negative impact on sperm cell function. However, adequate intake of essential fatty acids is important to ensure proper membrane fluidity in sperm cells. It is also important to avoid exogenous oestrogens, which are found in meat and dairy products, and to eat more organic foods to reduce exposure to pesticides.[921]

Nutritional supplements that have a beneficial impact on male fertility include carnitine, arginine, zinc, vitamin C, vitamin E, selenium, co-enzyme Q10, and vitamin B12.[922] Supplementing these nutrients can double the sperm count, improve sperm motility by about a quarter, and increase ejaculate volume by about a third.[923]

Cigarette smoking has been associated with decreased sperm count, alterations in motility, and an overall increase in the number of abnormal sperm.[924,925] Cannabis, sympatholytic drugs such as amphetamines, cocaine, and ecstasy; and anabolic steroids can also cause reduced or absent sperm.

A number of orthodox drugs, such as immunosuppressants, anti-androgens, alpha blockers, antibiotics, and non-steroidal anti-inflammatory drugs (NSAIDs), may also cause reduced testosterone levels and/or decreased sperm count, motility, and morphology.[926]

For couples who are trying to conceive through assisted reproduction, it is also very helpful to address any energetic imbalances, depending on the individual patient, such as reducing Qi Stagnation, tonifying the Kidney Qi, resolving Cold or Dampness; or from an Ayurvedic perspective, nourishing Ojas, and reducing aggravation of the Doshas.

Maximising the chances of conception

Improving sperm count, morphology, and motility

Supplementing essential nutrients can double the sperm count, improve sperm motility by about a quarter, and increase ejaculate volume by about a third.[927] Zinc deficiency is associated with decreased testosterone levels and sperm count, and several studies have found supplemental zinc may prove helpful in treating male infertility.[928] Vitamin B12 is important in cellular replication, especially synthesis of RNA and DNA, and deficiency is associated with decreased sperm count and motility.[929,930]

Carnitine is essential in sperm energy production. It contributes directly to sperm motility and may be involved in the successful maturation of sperm.[931] Arginine is also essential for sperm motility, and supplementation has been shown to increase motility in patients with asthenospermia.[932]

Fatty acids and phospholipids in the sperm cell membrane and are highly susceptible to oxidative damage.[933] Antioxidant nutrients including Vitamins C and E, selenium, and glutathione have been shown to significantly improve sperm concentration and motility, and increase the chance of impregnation.[934] Co-enzyme Q10 is involved in energy production in spermatozoa and also acts as an antioxidant.[935] Sperm concentration, motility, and morphology have all been shown to significantly improve after twelve months of CoQ10 therapy, resulting in a beneficial effect on rate of conception.[936]

Withania somnifera reduces oxidative stress, and improves semen quality,[937] increasing semen volume, sperm count, and motility.[938] It is particularly suited to men suffering from stress and anxiety.[939] Other herbs that improve sperm count and motility include *Lepidium meyenii* (maca),[940] *Panax ginseng*,[941] and *Tribulus terrestris*.[942]

Ejaculation that occurs daily or more frequently (due to intercourse or masturbation) can reduce sperm counts, while abstinence for more than seven days can result in reduced sperm motility.[943] Therefore, abstinence for at least two days (but no more than five days) before collecting a sperm sample for IUI or IVF is optimal for fertilisation.

Improving oocyte quality

In order to increase the chances of conception and improve pregnancy outcomes, it is important to maximise oocyte quality, particularly in older women and those with high FSH or low AMH levels, suggesting a declining ovarian reserve. Co-enzyme Q10 is an antioxidant enzyme, which has been shown to help improve oocyte quality and embryo development.[944] Supplementation of 750 mg per day of vitamin C has also been shown to reduce the effects of oxidative stress during oocyte maturation, increase progesterone levels, and improve fertility.[945]

DHEA is essential for oestrogen production in the ovary. DHEA supplementation significantly improves levels of AMH (which reflects an increased number of developing primary follicles) and increases the quality of oocytes produced.[946] It has been shown to significantly improve outcomes in women undergoing in vitro fertilisation or intracytoplasmic sperm injection (IVF/ICSI).[947]

Withania somnifera has been shown to increase levels of DHEA[948] and may therefore have a beneficial effect on ovarian reserve, egg quality, and pregnancy outcomes, as a result of its ability to improve endogenous DHEA levels. DHEA is produced by the adrenal gland, and less is produced when cortisol is high. Therefore measures to reduce stress and improve adrenal function may help to increase DHEA and thereby improve ovarian function.[949]

Ensuring adequate endometrial blood supply

One aspect of fertility that is not addressed by assisted reproduction techniques is implantation of the fertilised embryo. Adequate endometrial blood supply is required for implantation to occur.[950] Warming herbs (such as *Rosmarinus officinalis* and *Zingiber officinale*) help to promote healthy pelvic blood flow.[951] *Ginkgo biloba* (maidenhair tree) also helps to improve uterine circulation.[952] Nutrients that help to improve blood flow include: niacin (vitamin B3), vitamin C, vitamin E, and omega-3 fatty acids.[953] Increasing exercise may also help to improve uterine circulation.[954]

In women with pelvic blood congestion, uterine tonics such as *Rubus idaeus* may be more useful.[955] *Achillea millefolium* also reduces pelvic congestion, possibly due to an anti-thrombotic effect,[956] as well as relaxation of the veins, which allows congestion to move out of the capillaries.[957]

Reducing inflammation

Reducing inflammation may help to increase the chances of implantation and reduce the risk of early pregnancy loss. Reducing series 2 (inflammatory) prostaglandins can help to reduce inflammation, and alleviate uterine muscle spasm and ischaemia. Reducing consumption of animal fats, and increasing essential fatty acids, selectively decreases dietary precursors of series 2 (inflammatory) prostaglandins, and increases series 1 prostaglandins, which have anti-inflammatory, anti-thrombotic, and antispasmodic effects.[958]

Omega-3 fatty acids (found in oily fish) reduce the production of inflammatory cytokines.[959] A fish oil supplement containing a total of 400–600 mg EPA and 200–300 mg DHA per day is recommended for women who are trying to conceive, either naturally or through assisted reproduction. Increasing intake of oily fish and supplementing with evening primrose oil can also help to reduce inflammatory markers.[960]

Vitamin E can also positively influence prostaglandin ratios; and Vitamin B6 and zinc are necessary co-factors in the production of series 1 prostaglandins.[961] *Zingiber officinale* has also been shown to reduce the production of series 2 prostaglandins.[962]

Reducing uterine spasm

Reducing uterine spasm may also help to increase implantation and reduce the risk of early pregnancy loss. *Paeonia lactiflora*, *Viburnum opulus*, and *Viburnum prunifolium* are useful uterine spasmolytics. Magnesium may also help to decrease uterine cramping.[963]

Uterine tonics

Uterine tonics are useful for increasing the chances of conception, and improving pregnancy outcomes in women who are trying to conceive through assisted reproduction. Uterine tonic herbs include *Achillea millefolium*, *Angelica sinensis*, *Leonurus cardiaca*, *Rubus idaeus*, and *Viburnum prunifolium*.

Nourishing the endometrium

Consumption of moist, sweet, heavy, and nourishing foods such as root vegetables, soaked nuts, and oils (such as flaxseed oil); and herbs such as *Asparagus racemosus* (shatavari) and *Trigonella foenum graecum* (fenugreek), help to support a healthy endometrium. In traditional Chinese medicine (TCM), an inadequate endometrium is often associated with Blood Deficiency, which similarly requires moist, warming, and nourishing foods and herbs such as *Angelica sinensis* (Dang Gui) and *Rehmannia glutinosa*.

Ensuring adequate progesterone

Adequate progesterone levels are vital for maintaining pregnancy during the early stages. Herbs that are thought to improve progesterone function include *Achillea millefolium, Alchemilla vulgaris,*[964] and *Paeonia lactiflora.*

Magnesium helps to decrease conversion of progesterone to aldosterone. It is found in soya products, whole-grain cereals, seeds, and leafy green vegetables. Adaptogens and adrenal tonics improve adrenal function,[965] and may thereby help to increase adrenal production of progesterone and its metabolites. They include herbs such as *Eleutherococcus senticosus, Withania somnifera,* and *Glycyrrhiza glabra.*

Improving hepatic metabolism of fertility drugs

The liver metabolises fertility drugs and the hormones they stimulate. Poor hepatic metabolism can result in hormone imbalances, which contribute to the physiological and psychological side effects of fertility treatment. Gently assisting healthy liver function can help to improve these symptoms.

Inducers of liver metabolism include resveratrol (from berries, grapes, and red wine), cruciferous (brassica) vegetables, green tea, and *Rosmarinus officinalis.* Flaxseed also improves liver metabolism. In addition, it contains soluble fibre, which benefits bowel flora and reduces constipation.[966] This is important to reduce enterohepatic recirculation of hormones in women during fertility treatment.

Reducing the effects of stress

For individuals and couples with infertility, trying to conceive can be unbelievably stressful, and assisted reproduction techniques can add an extra layer of stress that can actually reduce the chances of conceiving. The herbal and dietary management of stress involves reducing the adverse effects of stress with nervine tonics and sedatives, as well as improving the body's capacity to adapt to stress with herbal adaptogens.[967] *Hypericum perforatum* is a nervine tonic, which is thought to inhibit monoamine oxidase (MAO).[968] Nervine sedatives include *Anemone pulsatilla, Leonurus cardiaca, Matricaria recutita,* and *Melissa officinalis,* while herbal adaptogens include *Eleutherococcus senticosus* and *Withania somnifera*. B vitamins and magnesium also help to reduce tension and to improve sleep patterns.[969]

Relaxation or stress management techniques may also be useful for reducing the effects of stress.[970] Other types of stress management could include meditation or yoga.[971] Social activities, such as dancing and relaxing with friends may be useful if the idea of meditating is unappealing.[972] Acupuncture also significantly alleviates depression, anxiety, and stress, by modulating both specific and non-specific neurological signalling and affecting stress hormones such as cortisol, prolactin, epinephrine, and beta-endorphin.[973]

Notes

908. Petrozza, J. C. (2020). Assisted reproduction technology. *Medscape* [online]. Available from https://emedicine.medscape.com/article/263907-overview#a4 (accessed 28 June 2020).

909. Petrozza, J. C. (2020). Assisted reproduction technology. *Medscape* [online]. Available from https://emedicine.medscape.com/article/263907-overview#a4 (accessed 28 June 2020).

910. Petrozza, J. C. (2020). Assisted reproduction technology. *Medscape* [online]. Available from https://emedicine.medscape.com/article/263907-overview#a4 (accessed 28 June 2020).

911. Petrozza, J. C. (2020). Assisted reproduction technology. *Medscape* [online]. Available from https://emedicine.medscape.com/article/263907-overview#a4 (accessed 28 June 2020).

912. Petrozza, J. C. (2020). Assisted reproduction technology. *Medscape* [online]. Available from https://emedicine.medscape.com/article/263907-overview#a4 (accessed 28 June 2020).

913. Petrozza, J. C. (2020). Assisted reproduction technology. *Medscape* [online]. Available from https://emedicine.medscape.com/article/263907-overview#a4 (accessed 28 June 2020).

914. Beers, M. H., & Berkow, R. (1999). *The Merck Manual of Diagnosis and Therapy*. Kenilworth, NJ: Merck.

915. Clane General Hospital (2008). IVF fee schedule [online]. Available from http://clanehospital.ie/ivfprices (accessed 13 February 2009).

916. Chavarro, J. E., Rich-Edwards, J. W., Rosner, B. A., & Willett, W. C. (2007). Diet and lifestyle in the prevention of ovulatory disorder infertility. *Obstetrics & Gynecology*, *110*(5): 1050–1058.

917. Mortimore, D. (2001). *The Complete Illustrated Guide to Vitamins and Minerals*. London: Element.

918. Mehendale, S. S., Kilari Bams, A. S., Deshmukh, C. S., Dhorepatil, B. S., Nimbargi, V. N., & Joshi, S. R. (2009). Oxidative stress-mediated essential polyunsaturated fatty acid alterations in female infertility. *Human Fertility*, *12*(1): 28–33.

919. Green, B. B., Daling, J. R., Weiss, N. S., Liff, J. M., & Koepsell, T. (1986). Exercise as a risk factor for infertility with ovulatory dysfunction. *American Journal of Public Health*, 76(12): 1432–1436.

920. Tremellen, K., & Pearce, K. (2015). *Nutrition, Fertility, and Human Reproductive Function*. Boca Raton, FL: CRC Press.

921. Sinclair, S. (2000). Male infertility: nutritional and environmental considerations. *Alternative Medicine Review*, 5(1): 28–38.

922. Sinclair, S. (2000). Male infertility: nutritional and environmental considerations. *Alternative Medicine Review*, 5(1): 28–38.

923. Imhof, M., Lackner, J., Lipovac, M., Chedraui, P., & Riedl, C. (2012). Improvement of sperm quality after micronutrient supplementation. *e-SPEN, the European e-Journal of Clinical Nutrition and Metabolism*, 7(1): E50–E53.

924. Kulikauskas, V., Blaustein, D., & Ablin, R. J. (1985). Cigarette smoking and its possible effects on sperm. *Fertility and Sterility*, 44(4): 526–528.

925. R. J. Stillman (Ed.) (1989). *Seminars in Reproductive Endocrinology: Smoking and Reproductive Health*. New York: Thieme.

926. Semet, M., Paci, M., Saïas-Magnan, J., Metzler-Guillemain, C., Boissier, R., Lejeune, H., & Perrin, J. (2017). The impact of drugs on male fertility: a review. *Andrology*, 5(4): 640–663.

927. Imhof, M., Lackner, J., Lipovac, M., Chedraui, P., & Riedl, C. (2012). Improvement of sperm quality after micronutrient supplementation. *e-SPEN, the European e-Journal of Clinical Nutrition and Metabolism*, 7(1): E50–E53.

928. Madding, C. I., Jacob, M., Ramsay, V. P., & Sokol, R. Z. (1986). Serum and semen zinc levels in normozoospermic and oligozoospermic men. *Annals of Nutrition and Metabolism*, 30(4): 213–218.

929. Sinclair, S. (2000). Male infertility: nutritional and environmental considerations. *Alternative Medicine Review*, 5(1): 28–38.

930. Sandler, B., & Faraher, B. (1994). Treatment of oligospermia with B12. *Infertility*, 7: 133–138.

931. Sinclair, S. (2000). Male infertility: nutritional and environmental considerations. *Alternative Medicine Review*, 5(1): 28–38.

932. Scibona, M., Meschini, P., Caparelli, S., Pecori, C., Rossi, P., & Menchini Fabris, G. F. (1994). L-arginine and male fertility. *Minerva Urologica e Nefrologica*, 46(4): 251–253.

933. De Lamirande, E., Jiang, H., Zini, A., Kodama, H., & Gagnon, C. (1997). Reactive oxygen species and sperm physiology. *Reviews of Reproduction*, 2(1): 48–54.

934. Sinclair, S. (2000). Male infertility: nutritional and environmental considerations. *Alternative Medicine Review*, 5(1): 28–38.

935. Lewin, A., & Lavin, H. (1997). The effect of coenzyme Q-10 on sperm motility and function. *Molecular Aspects of Medicine*, 18: S213–S219.

936. Safarinejad, M. R. (2011). The effect of coenzyme Q10 supplementation on partner pregnancy rate in infertile men with idiopathic oligoasthenoteratozoospermia: an open-label prospective study. *International Urology and Nephrology*, 44(3): 689–700.

937. Ahmad, M. K., Mahdi, A. A., Shukla, K. K., Islam, N., Rajender, S., Madhukar, D., Shankhwar, S. N., & Ahmad, S. (2010). Withania somnifera improves semen quality by regulating reproductive hormone levels and oxidative stress in seminal plasma of infertile males. *Fertility and Sterility*, 94(3): 989–996.

938. Ambiye, V. R., Langade, D., Dongre, S., Aptikar, P., Kulkarni, M., & Dongre, A. (2013). Clinical evaluation of the spermatogenic activity of the root extract of ashwagandha (*Withania somnifera*) in oligospermic males: a pilot study. *Evidence-Based Complementary and Alternative Medicine* [online]. Available from http://ncbi.nlm.nih.gov/pmc/articles/PMC3863556/#!po=3.84615 (accessed 15 July 2015).

939. Ambiye, V. R., Langade, D., Dongre, S., Aptikar, P., Kulkarni, M., & Dongre, A. (2013). Clinical evaluation of the spermatogenic activity of the root extract of ashwagandha (*Withania somnifera*) in oligospermic males: a pilot study. *Evidence-Based Complementary and Alternative Medicine* [online]. Available from http://ncbi.nlm.nih.gov/pmc/articles/PMC3863556/#!po=3.84615 (accessed 15 July 2015).

940. Gonzales, G. F., Cordova, A., Gonzales, C., Chung, A., Vega, K., & Villena, A. (2001) Lepidium meyenii (maca) improved semen parameters in adult men. *Asian Journal of Andrology*, 3(4): 301–303.

941. Bone, K., & Mills, S. (2013). *Principles and Practice of Phytotherapy: Modern Herbal Medicine*. London: Churchill Livingstone.

942. Thirunavukkarasu, M., Sellandi, M., Thakar, A. N., & Baghel, M. S. (2012). Clinical study of *Tribulus terrestris* Linn. in oligozoospermia: a double blind study. *Ayu*, 33(3): 356–364.

943. Campana, A., de Agostini, A., Bischof, P., Tawfik, E., & Mastrorilli, A. (2019). Evaluation of infertility. Graduate Foundation for Medical Education and Research (GFMER) [online]. Available from https://gfmer.ch/Books/Reproductive_health/infertility_evaluation.html (accessed 20 June 2020).

944. Xu, Y., Nisenblat, V., Lu, C., Li, R., Qiao, J., Zhen, X., & Wang, S. (2018). Pretreatment with coenzyme Q10 improves ovarian response and embryo quality in low-prognosis young women with decreased ovarian reserve: a randomized controlled trial. *Reproductive Biology and Endocrinology*, 16: 29.

945. Dennehy, C. E. (2006). The use of herbs and dietary supplements in gynecology: an evidence-based review. *Journal of Midwifery & Women's Health*, 51(6): 402–409.

946. Gleicher, N., Weghofer, A., & Barad, D. H. (2010). Improvement in diminished ovarian reserve after dehydroepiandrosterone supplementation. *Reproductive BioMedicine Online*, 21(3): 360–365.

947. Xu, L., Hu., C., Liu, Q., & Li, Y. (2019). The effect of dehydroepiandrosterone (DHEA) supplementation on IVF or ICSI: a meta-analysis of randomized controlled trials. *Geburtshilfe und Frauenheilkunde*, 79(7): 705–712.

948. Lopresti, A. L., Smith, S. J., Malvi, H., & Kodgule, R. (2019). An investigation into the stress-relieving and pharmacological actions of an ashwagandha (*Withania somnifera*) extract. A randomized, double-blind, placebo-controlled study. *Medicine (Baltimore)*, 98(37): e17186.

949. Trickey, R. (2011). *Women, Hormones and the Menstrual Cycle*. Clifton Hill, Victoria, Australia: Melbourne Holistic Health Group.

950. Raine-Fenning, N. J., Campbell, B. K., Kendall, N. R., Clewes, J. S., & Johnson, I. R. (2004). Endometrial and subendometrial perfusion are impaired in women with unexplained infertility. *Human Reproduction*, 19(11): 2605–2614.

951. Holmes, P. (2007). *The Energetics of Western Herbs: A Materia Medica Integrating Western & Chinese Herbal Therapeutics, Volume 1* (4th edn). Santa Rosa, CA: Snow Lotus.

952. Bone, K., & Mills, S. (2013). *Principles and Practice of Phytotherapy: Modern Herbal Medicine*. London: Churchill Livingstone.
953. Weiss, R. (1988). *Herbal Medicine*. Gothenburg, Sweden: Arcanum.
954. Timonen, S., & Procopé, B. J. (1971). Premenstrual syndrome and physical exercise. *Acta Obstetricia et Gynecologica Scandinavica, 50*(4): 331–337.
955. Trickey, R. (2003). *Women, Hormones & the Menstrual Cycle*. Sydney, Australia: Allen & Unwin.
956. Weiss, R. (1988). *Herbal Medicine*. Gothenburg, Sweden: Arcanum.
957. Wood, M. (2004). *The Practice of Traditional Western Herbalism: Basic Doctrine, Energetics and Classification*. Berkeley, CA: North Atlantic.
958. Puolakka, J., Mäkäräinen, L., Viinikka, L., & Ylikorkala, O. (1985). Biochemical and clinical effects of treating the premenstrual syndrome with prostaglandin synthesis precursors. *Journal of Reproductive Medicine, 30*(3): 149–153.
959. Trickey, R. (2011). *Women, Hormones and the Menstrual Cycle*. Clifton Hill, Victoria, Australia: Melbourne Holistic Health Group.
960. Romm, A. (2016). *Botanical Medicine for Women's Health* (2nd edn). London: Churchill Livingstone.
961. Trickey, R. (2003). *Women, Hormones & the Menstrual Cycle*. Sydney, Australia: Allen & Unwin.
962. Gonlachanvit, S., Chen, Y. H., Hasler, W. L., Sun, W. M., & Owyang, C. (2003). Ginger reduces hyperglycemia-evoked gastric dysrhythmias in healthy humans: possible role of endogenous prostaglandins, *Journal of Pharmacology and Experminental Therapeutics, 307*(3): 1098–1103.
963. Trickey, R. (2003). *Women, Hormones & the Menstrual Cycle*. Sydney, Australia: Allen & Unwin.
964. Lapraz, J. C. (2008). *Clinical Phytotherapy and Osteoporosis*. London: British Endobiogenic Medicine Society.
965. Tillotson, A. K. (2009). Female infertility [online]. Available from http://oneearthherbs.squarespace.com/diseases/female-infertility.html (accessed 28 January 2009).
966. Brice-Ytsma, H., & McDermott, A. (2020). *Herbal Medicine in Treating Gynaecological Conditions*. London: Aeon.
967. Trickey, R. (2003). *Women, Hormones & the Menstrual Cycle*. Sydney, Australia: Allen & Unwin.
968. Linde, K., Ramirez, G., Mulrow, C. D., Pauls, A., Weidenhammer, W., & Melchart, D. (1996). St John's wort for depression: an overview and meta-analysis of randomised clinical trials. *British Medical Journal, 313*(7052): 253–258.
969. Trickey, R. (2003). *Women, Hormones & the Menstrual Cycle*. Sydney, Australia: Allen & Unwin.
970. Glenville, M. (2000). *Natural Solutions to Infertility*. London: Piatkus.
971. Hudson, T. (2008). *Women's Encyclopedia of Natural Medicine*. New York: McGraw Hill.
972. Trickey, R. (2003). *Women, Hormones & the Menstrual Cycle*. Sydney, Australia: Allen & Unwin.
973. Dalton-Brewer, N. (2016). The role of complementary and alternative medicine for the management of fibroids and associated symptomatology. *Current Obstetrics and Gynecology Reports, 5*: 110–118.

CHAPTER FOURTEEN

Preventing recurrent pregnancy loss

For individuals and couples who are able to conceive, either naturally or with the help of orthodox fertility treatments, recurrent miscarriage can prevent successful pregnancy outcomes. Recurrent pregnancy loss affects approximately 1% of women of reproductive age, and is usually defined as the loss of three or more pregnancies before twenty weeks gestation. It may be caused by many factors, including DNA damage to sperm; poor oocyte quality; smoking; alcohol or caffeine consumption; luteal insufficiency; uterine or cervical problems; PCOS; thyroid disease; immune system abnormalities; inflammatory disease; infection; or thrombophilia.[974]

DNA damage to sperm

Chromosomal abnormalities are among the most common causes of early pregnancy loss. They may be due to DNA damage, either to the sperm, oocyte, or both. Supplementing essential nutrients for at least three months prior to conception may help to improve the quality of sperm. Vitamin B12 is important in cellular replication, especially synthesis of RNA and DNA.[975,976] Carnitine and arginine are also essential for healthy sperm development.[977,978] Antioxidant nutrients, including vitamins C and E, selenium, and co-enzyme Q10 help to prevent DNA damage to sperm.[979,980] *Pinus pinaster* (pine bark) is also a potent antioxidant.[981]

Although antioxidants may be useful in counteracting oxidative stress in men with DNA damage to sperm, a balance of reduction and oxidation is necessary for essential sperm function.[982] Sperm themselves produce controlled concentrations of reactive oxygen species (ROS), which are needed for penetrating the egg during fertilisation,[983] so it is also important not to over-supplement. For more information about improving sperm quality, see Chapter 7.

Oocyte quality

The risk of pregnancy loss increases with the age of the mother, and may be due to declining oocyte quality. Co-enzyme Q10 is an antioxidant enzyme that has been shown to help increase oocyte quality and improve embryo development.[984] Supplementation of 750 mg per day of vitamin C has also been shown to reduce the effects of oxidative stress during oocyte maturation, and to increase progesterone levels.[985]

Withania somnifera increases levels of DHEA[986] and may therefore have a beneficial effect on egg quality and pregnancy outcomes. DHEA is produced by the adrenal gland, and less is produced when cortisol is high. Therefore measures to reduce stress and improve adrenal function may help to increase DHEA and thereby improve ovarian function and egg quality.[987] For more information about improving oocyte quality, see Chapter 1.

Tobacco, alcohol, caffeine consumption

Each stage of female reproductive function, including hormone production, folliculogenesis, embryo transport, endometrial receptivity, and endometrial angiogenesis, is a target for cigarette smoke.[988] Cigarette smoke also appears to increase ovarian cellular damage,[989] resulting in an accelerated decline in egg quality, which increases the risk of miscarriage. Uterine blood flow, which is essential for maintenance of pregnancy, is also impaired in women who smoke.[990]

In men, smoking increases the level of reactive oxygen species in seminal fluid,[991] which reduces the integrity of DNA in the sperm nucleus, and thereby increases the risk of early pregnancy loss.

Therefore both men and women who are trying to conceive should be advised to avoid smoking.

Alcohol consumption also increases the number of abnormal sperm in men,[992] increasing the risk of pregnancy loss. In women, consuming as little as four units of alcohol per week has been associated with a significantly increased risk of miscarriage.[993] Therefore both men and women who are trying to conceive should be advised to avoid alcohol consumption.

Finally, consuming more than 200 mg caffeine a day (equivalent to one to two cups of coffee, or two to four cups of black tea) is associated with an increased risk of pregnancy loss in women.[994] However, moderate caffeine consumption seems to have no significant impact on male fertility.[995]

Luteal insufficiency

Adequate progesterone levels are vital for maintaining pregnancy during the early stages. Women with poor luteal function may therefore have an increased risk of early pregnancy loss. Herbs that are thought to improve progesterone function include *Achillea millefolium* (yarrow), *Alchemilla vulgaris* (lady's mantle), and *Paeonia lactiflora* (paeony).

Magnesium helps to decrease conversion of progesterone to aldosterone, thereby helping to maintain healthy progesterone levels. Adaptogens and adrenal tonics improve adrenal function,[996] and may therefore help to increase adrenal production of progesterone. They include herbs such as *Eleutherococcus senticosus* (Siberian ginseng), *Withania somnifera* (ashwagandha), and *Glycyrrhiza glabra* (liquorice). For more information about promoting healthy luteal function and maintaining adequate progesterone levels, see Chapter 4.

Uterine or cervical problems

Problems affecting the uterus or cervix, such as cervical incompetence, may cause early pregnancy loss. Depending on the nature of the problem, surgical treatment may be necessary in order to prevent miscarriage. However, herbal therapies may be used alongside orthodox interventions to help improve pregnancy outcomes.

Uterine tonics may be useful for preventing recurrent miscarriage in women with uterine or cervical problems. Uterine tonic herbs include

Achillea millefolium (yarrow), *Angelica sinensis* (dong quai), *Leonurus cardiaca* (motherwort), and *Rubus idaeus* (raspberry leaf). Reducing uterine spasm may also help to reduce the risk of miscarriage. *Paeonia lactiflora* (paeony), *Viburnum opulus* (cramp bark), and *Viburnum prunifolium* (black haw), are useful uterine spasmolytics. *Asparagus racemosus* (shatavari) reduces uterine contractions, which is useful for preventing early pregnancy loss.[997] Magnesium may also help to decrease uterine cramping.[998] For more information about treating uterine or cervical problems, see Chapter 3.

Polycystic ovary syndrome

Polycystic ovary syndrome (PCOS) is a complex endocrine and metabolic disorder, which causes abnormal ovarian function. It accounts for about 75% of cases of anovulatory infertility. Additionally, if pregnancy does occur, the first trimester miscarriage rate is as high as 30% to 50%.[999]

Dietary modification and increased exercise are essential for women with PCOS, in order to reduce insulin resistance. Insulin resistance may also be improved by using herbs such as *Cinnamonum zeylonicum* (cinnamon), *Eleutherococcus senticosus* (Siberian ginseng), *Trigonella foenum-graecum* (fenugreek), and/or *Galega officinalis* (goat's rue);[1000] and supplements such as inositol, omega-3 essential fatty acids, biotin, magnesium, and chromium.[1001]

Excess androgen production in PCOS can be reduced with herbs such as *Paeonia lactiflora* (white paeony), *Glycyrrhiza glabra* (liquorice),[1002] *Serenoa repens* (saw palmetto), *Ganoderma lucidum* (reishi mushroom), *Camellia sinensis* (green tea), and *Mentha spicata* (spearmint).[1003] *Humulus lupulus* (hops) and *Cimicifuga racemosa* (black cohosh) also reduce both LH and androgens.[1004] For more information about treating PCOS, see Chapter 2.

Thyroid disease

Abnormalities in thyroid function can have an adverse effect on reproductive health and may result in reduced rates of conception, increased early pregnancy loss, and adverse neonatal outcomes.

Keeping thyroid-stimulating hormone (TSH) levels at the lower end of normal (<2.5 mU/l) in euthyroid women may reduce the risk of miscarriage.[1005] There is also increasing evidence for the role of autoantibodies in early pregnancy loss, even in euthyroid women. This may be linked to inflammatory changes in the reproductive tissues.[1006]

In women with low levels of T3 or T4, and/or elevated TSH, consuming iodine rich foods such as seaweeds, ensuring adequate selenium intake, and exercising for at least twenty to thirty minutes a day can help to improve thyroid function.[1007] Other important nutrients for thyroxine synthesis include L-tyrosine, and vitamin B complex. Herbal medicines such as *Fucus vesiculosus* (bladderwrack)—*Withania somnifera* (ashwagandha), and *Commiphora mukkul* (guggul) can also increase thyroid function.[1008] Measures to improve oestrogen may help to improve thyroid function. *Lepidium meyenii* (maca) increases both oestrogen and thyroid hormone levels.[1009]

In women with hyperthyroidism, herbs such as *Melissa officinalis* (lemon balm) and *Lycopus virginicus* (gypsywort) reduce thyroid over–activity.[1010] *Ganoderma lucidum* (reishi mushroom) and *Hemidesmus indicus* (sariva) are useful for reducing autoimmunity.[1011] Measures to reduce oestrogen and prolactin can also help to reduce autoimmune thyroid problems. For more information about treating thyroid problems, see Chapter 1.

Immune system problems and inflammatory diseases

Immune system problems and inflammatory diseases, such as systemic lupus erythematosus (SLE) and pelvic inflammatory disease, are associated with an increased risk of miscarriage. In women with immune system problems and inflammatory disease, reducing series 2 (inflammatory) prostaglandins, can help to reduce inflammation, and lower the risk of early pregnancy loss.

Reducing consumption of animal fats, and increasing essential fatty acids, selectively decreases dietary precursors of series 2 (inflammatory) prostaglandins, and increases series 1 prostaglandins, which have anti-inflammatory, anti-thrombotic, and antispasmodic effects.[1012] Omega-3 fatty acids (found in oily fish and flaxseed) reduce the production of inflammatory cytokines.[1013] Vitamin E can also positively influence prostaglandin ratios; and vitamin B6 and zinc are necessary co-factors in the production of series 1 prostaglandins.[1014] *Zingiber officinale* has also been shown to reduce the production of series 2 prostaglandins.[1015]

Infection

A large number of different bacterial, viral, and parasitic infections have been associated with an increased risk of miscarriage, and adverse effects in the foetus. These include a number of food borne infections (such as listeria and salmonella); infections transmitted by animals (such as brucellosis and toxoplasmosis); infections transmitted by mosquito bites (such as Zika virus and malaria); sexually transmitted infections (such as gonorrhoea and chlamydia); and bacterial vaginosis.

Specific antimicrobial treatment depends on the nature of the infection, and orthodox interventions may be necessary. However, immune enhancing herbs such as *Echinacea angustifolia* (purple coneflower) and *Astragalus membranaceus* (Huang Qi), and herbal anti-inflammatories (as shown in the previous section), may be used alongside orthodox treatment where necessary to help treat infections and prevent complications. Topical treatment to the vagina using antimicrobial and anti-inflammatory herbs also provides a route for treating vaginal infections and PID.[1016]

Thrombophilia

Thrombophilia may be caused by an inherited gene mutation or by anti-phospholipid syndrome. Abnormal clotting leads to placental insufficiency, which results in early pregnancy loss.

In women with inherited gene mutations, mutation of the genes that code for anticoagulant proteins in the blood leads to hyper-coagulation, placental insufficiency, and recurrent miscarriage. In women with anti-phospholipid syndrome, pregnancy specific antigens trigger an autoimmune response, which causes production of anti-phospholipid antibodies. These antibodies inhibit the release of anticoagulant factors, which leads to platelet aggregation and thrombosis.[1017]

Women with thrombophilia may be treated with low dose aspirin or heparin for the duration of pregnancy. However, there is limited evidence to support these treatments, and women with thrombophilia remain at high risk for preterm labour, foetal growth restriction, and pre-eclampsia.[1018]

High levels of homocysteine are linked to vascular damage and thrombogenesis, which leads to recurrent pregnancy. Vitamins B6 and B12 and folate are important in homocysteine metabolism.[1019]

Other nutrients that help to improve blood flow include niacin (vitamin B3), vitamin C, vitamin E, and omega-3 fatty acids.[1020] Herbs that have an anti-thrombotic effect, and may help to improve uterine circulation, include *Ginkgo biloba* (maidenhair tree),[1021] *Zingiber officinale* (ginger root),[1022] and *Achillea millefolium* (yarrow).[1023]

Notes

974. Oner, G. (2011). Thrombophilia and recurrent pregnancy loss. *Intechopen* [online]. Available from https://ntechopen.com/books/thrombophilia/thrombophilia-and-recurrent-pregnancy-loss (accessed 1 July 2020).

975. Sinclair, S. (2000). Male infertility: nutritional and environmental considerations. *Alternative Medicine Review*, 5(1): 28–38.

976. Sandler, B., & Faraher, B. (1994). Treatment of oligospermia with B12. *Infertility*, 7: 133–138.

977. Sinclair, S. (2000). Male infertility: nutritional and environmental considerations. *Alternative Medicine Review*, 5(1): 28–38.

978. Scibona, M., Meschini, P., Caparelli, S., Pecori, C., Rossi, P., & Menchini Fabris, G. F. (1994). L-arginine and male fertility. *Minerva Urologica e Nefrologica*, 46(4): 251–253.

979. Sinclair, S. (2000). Male infertility: nutritional and environmental considerations. *Alternative Medicine Review*, 5(1): 28–38.

980. Safarinejad, M. R. (2011). The effect of coenzyme Q_{10} supplementation on partner pregnancy rate in infertile men with idiopathic oligoasthenoteratozoospermia: an open-label prospective study. *International Urology and Nephrology*, 44(3): 689–700.

981. Hosoi, M., Belcaro, G., Saggino, A., Luzzi, R., Dugall, M., & Feragalli, B. (2018). Pycnogenol® supplementation in minimal cognitive dysfunction. *Journal of Neurosurgical Sciences*, 62(3): 279–284.

982. Wright, C., Milne, S., & Leeson, H. (2014). Sperm DNA damage caused by oxidative stress: modifiable clinical, lifestyle and nutritional factors in male infertility. *Reproductive BioMedicine Online*, 28(6): 684–703.

983. De Lamirande, E., Jiang, H., Zini, A., Kodama, H., & Gagnon, C. (1997). Reactive oxygen species and sperm physiology. *Reviews of Reproduction*, 2(1): 48–54.

984. Xu, Y., Nisenblat, V., Lu, C., Li, R., Qiao, J., Zhen, X., & Wang, S. (2018). Pretreatment with coenzyme Q10 improves ovarian response and embryo quality in low-prognosis young women with decreased ovarian reserve: a randomized controlled trial. *Reproductive Biology and Endocrinology*, 16: 29.

985. Dennehy, C. E. (2006). The use of herbs and dietary supplements in gynecology: an evidence-based review. *Journal of Midwifery & Women's Health*, 51(6): 402–409.

986. Lopresti, A. L., Smith, S. J., Malvi, H., & Kodgule, R. (2019). An investigation into the stress-relieving and pharmacological actions of an ashwagandha (*Withania somnifera*) extract. A randomized, double-blind, placebo-controlled study. *Medicine (Baltimore)*, 98(37): e17186.

987. Trickey, R. (2011). *Women, Hormones and the Menstrual Cycle*. Clifton Hill, Victoria, Australia: Melbourne Holistic Health Group.

988. Dechanet, C., Anahory, T., Mathieu Daude, J. C., Quantin, X., Reyftmann, L., Hamamah, S., Hedon, B., & Dechaud, H. (2011). Effects of cigarette smoking on reproduction. *Human Reprodtion Update*, *17*(1): 76–95.

989. Mattison, D. R., Plowchalk, D. R., Meadows, M. J., Miller, M. M., Malek, A., & London, S. (1989). The effect of smoking on oogenesis, fertilization and implantation. *Seminars in Reproductive Endocrinology*, *7*(4): 291–304.

990. Grassi, G., Seravalle, G., Calhoun, D. A., Bolla, G. B., Giannattasio, C., Marabini, M., Del Bo, A., & Manci, G. (1994). Mechanisms responsible for sympathetic activation by cigarette smoking in humans. *Circulation*, *90*(1): 248–253.

991. Saleh, R. A., Agarwal, A., Sharma, R. K., Nelson, D. R., & Thomas, A. J. (2002). Effect of cigarette smoking on levels of seminal oxidative stress in infertile men: a prospective study. *Fertility and Sterility*, *78*(3): 491–499.

992. Joo, K. J., Kwon, Y. W., Myung, S., & Kim, T. H. (2012). The effects of smoking and alcohol intake on sperm quality. *Journal of International Medical Research*, *40*(6): 2327–2335.

993. Avalos, L. A., Roberts, S. C., Kaskutas, L. A., Block, G., & De-Kun, L. (2014). Volume and type of alcohol during early pregnancy and the risk of miscarriage. *Substance Use & Misuse*, *49*(11): 1437–1445.

994. NICHD (2016). Couples' pre-pregnancy caffeine consumption linked to miscarriage risk [online]. Available from https://nichd.nih.gov/news/releases/Pages/032416-miscarriage-caffeine.aspx (accessed 1 July 2019).

995. Tremellen, K., & Pearce, K. (2015). *Nutrition, Fertility, and Human Reproductive Function*. Boca Raton, FL: CRC Press.

996. Tillotson, A. K. (2009). Female infertility [online]. Available from http://oneearth-herbs.squarespace.com/diseases/female-infertility.html (accessed on 28 January 2009).

997. Pole, S. (2006). *Ayurvedic Medicine: The Principles of Traditional Practice*. London: Churchill Livingstone.

998. Trickey, R. (2003). *Women, Hormones & the Menstrual Cycle*. Sydney, Australia: Allen & Unwin.

999. Homburg, R., Armar, N. A., Eshel, A., Adams, J., & Jacobs, H. S. (1988). Influence of serum luteinising hormone concentrations on ovulation, conception, and early pregnancy loss in polycystic ovary syndrome. *British Medical Journal*, *297*(6655): 1024–1026.

1000. Trickey, R. (2011). *Women, Hormones and the Menstrual Cycle*. Clifton Hill, Victoria, Australia: Melbourne Holistic Health Group.

1001. Trickey, R. (2011). *Women, Hormones and the Menstrual Cycle*. Clifton Hill, Victoria, Australia: Melbourne Holistic Health Group.

1002. Trickey, R. (2011). *Women, Hormones and the Menstrual Cycle*. Clifton Hill, Victoria, Australia: Melbourne Holistic Health Group.

1003. Grant, P., & Ramasamy, S. (2012). An update on plant derived anti-androgens. *International Journal of Endocrinology and Metabolism*, *10*(2): 497–502.

1004. Trickey, R. (2011). *Women, Hormones and the Menstrual Cycle*. Clifton Hill, Victoria, Australia: Melbourne Holistic Health Group.

1005. Jefferys, A., Vanderpump, M., & Yasmin, E. (2015). Thyroid dysfunction and reproductive health. *Obstetrician & Gynaecologist*, *17*: 39–45.

1006. Jefferys, A., Vanderpump, M., & Yasmin, E. (2015). Thyroid dysfunction and reproductive health. *Obstetrician & Gynaecologist, 17*: 39–45.

1007. Trickey, R. (2011). *Women, Hormones and the Menstrual Cycle*. Clifton Hill, Victoria, Australia: Melbourne Holistic Health Group.

1008. Romm, A. (2016). *Botanical Medicine for Women's Health* (2nd edn). London: Churchill Livingstone.

1009. Meissner, H. O., Kapczynski, W., Mscisz, A., & Lutomski, J. (2005). Use of gelatinized maca (Lepidium peruvianum) in early postmenopausal women. *International Journal of Biomedical Science, 1*(1): 33–45.

1010. Holmes, P. (2007). *The Energetics of Western Herbs: A Materia Medica Integrating Western & Chinese Herbal Therapeutics, Volume 2* (4th edn). Santa Rosa, CA: Snow Lotus.

1011. Bone, K., & Mills, S. (2013). *Principles and Practice of Phytotherapy: Modern Herbal Medicine*. London: Churchill Livingstone.

1012. Puolakka, J., Mäkäräinen, L., Viinikka, L., & Ylikorkala, O. (1985). Biochemical and clinical effects of treating the premenstrual syndrome with prostaglandin synthesis precursors. *Journal of Reproductive Medicine, 30*(3): 149–153.

1013. Trickey, R. (2011). *Women, Hormones and the Menstrual Cycle*. Clifton Hill, Victoria, Australia: Melbourne Holistic Health Group.

1014. Trickey, R. (2003). *Women, Hormones & the Menstrual Cycle*. Sydney, Australia: Allen & Unwin.

1015. Gonlachanvit, S., Chen, Y. H., Hasler, W. L., Sun, W. M., & Owyang, C. (2003). Ginger reduces hyperglycemia-evoked gastric dysrhythmias in healthy humans: possible role of endogenous prostaglandins, *Journal of Pharmacology and Experimental Therapeutics, 307*(3): 1098–1103.

1016. Bone, K., & Mills, S. (2013). *Principles and Practice of Phytotherapy: Modern Herbal Medicine*. London: Churchill Livingstone.

1017. Oner, G. (2011). Thrombophilia and recurrent pregnancy loss. *Intechopen* [online]. Available from https://intechopen.com/books/thrombophilia/thrombophilia-and-recurrent-pregnancy-loss (accessed 1 July 2020).

1018. Di Nisio, M., Peters, L. W., & Middeldorp, S. (2005). Anticoagulants for the treatment of recurrent pregnancy loss in women without antiphospholipid syndrome. *Cochrane Database of Systemic Reviews, 2*(2): CD004734.

1019. de la Calle, M., Usandizaga, R., Sancha, M., Magdaleno, F., Herranz, A., & Cabrillo, E. (2003). Homocysteine, folic acid and B-group vitamins in obstetrics and gynaecology. *European Journal of Obstetrics & Gynecology and Reproductive Biology, 107*(2): 125–134.

1020. Weiss, R. (1988). *Herbal Medicine*. Gothenburg, Sweden: Arcanum.

1021. Bone, K., & Mills, S. (2013). *Principles and Practice of Phytotherapy: Modern Herbal Medicine*. London: Churchill Livingstone.

1022. Beers, M. H., & Berkow, R. (1999). *The Merck Manual of Diagnosis and Therapy*. Kenilworth, NJ: Merck.

1023. Weiss, R. (1988). *Herbal Medicine*. Gothenburg, Sweden: Arcanum.

CHAPTER FIFTEEN

Herbal medicines and reproductive health

The practice of herbal medicine is based on the recognition of powerful self-correcting forces in the body. The emphasis is on influencing the body's innate capability for healing, rather than simply treating the symptoms or pathologies.[1024] This is particularly true in the case of infertility, since healthy reproductive function is fundamental to the survival of the human species. In many cases, supporting the body to heal and regain its natural state of balance, with herbal medicines, nutrition, and lifestyle changes, is enough to restore reproductive health and optimum fertility.

Herbal medicines are particularly well suited to the treatment of broad physiological patterns in the body (such as those which contribute to infertility), by virtue of their complexity,[1025] and herbal medicine has an excellent reputation for enhancing fertility.[1026] However, herbalists and other alternative healthcare practitioners often advise that couples should avoid trying to conceive for the first three months of treatment, to ensure that both partners reach peak physical health, and that healthy sperm and ovum (which have been protected throughout their final maturation phase, and nourished with a healthy diet and suitable herbs to improve their quality) are available for conception, rather than those which began maturing before treatment began.

Ovarian follicular development begins while the female foetus is in utero. Girls are born with one to two million primordial follicles. By the time they reach puberty, approximately 400,000 to 500,000 primordial follicles remain. After menarche, around 1000 follicles are lost each month due to natural degeneration of follicles (atresia), and this rate increases after thirty-five years of age.

It takes approximately one year for a primordial follicle to mature before ovulation. The first phase of development is the gonadotropin-independent (pre-antral growth) phase, which takes up to 300 days. The second phase (the antral growth phase) takes approximately fifty days, and is dependent on gonadotropins (FSH and LH). Eventually the dominant follicle is released in response to the LH surge, which triggers ovulation.[1027] Atresia (degeneration of the follicle) can occur at any stage of folliculogenesis (preantral or antral); however, the highest incidence is seen in the antral follicles, during the final fifty days of folliculogenesis.[1028]

Spermatogenesis is also dependent on gonadotropins (FSH and LH), and takes approximately three months. During this time, many factors can interfere with spermatogenesis and cause damage to sperm. Therefore for optimum fertility, it is advisable to wait for around three months before trying to conceive, so that a healthy sperm and ovum (which have been protected throughout their final maturation phase, and nourished with a healthy diet and suitable herbs to improve their quality) are available for conception, rather than those that began maturing before treatment began.

Some herbal medicine practitioners advise that all herbal remedies should be stopped at once if conception occurs.[1029] However, healthy luteal function and adequate progesterone levels are essential for maintaining pregnancy in the early stages,[1030,1031,1032] and where herbal medicines are supporting healthy progesterone levels, sudden withdrawal is not a good idea.

Some herbalists use herbs that are contraindicated in pregnancy for treatment of infertility, which would indeed make it necessary for the patient to discontinue herbal treatment upon conception. However, the potential problem here is that the patient may not know that she has conceived for at least two weeks after conception, and a miscarriage could occur before this time.[1033]

Herbs that should be avoided in pregnancy, and therefore also in women who are actively trying to conceive, include those containing alkaloids which have harmful effects in pregnancy (such as *Hydrastis canadensis* which contains berberine) and emmenagogues which stimulate uterine contraction (such as *Angelica sinensis*).

Herbs containing high levels of essential oils that are harmful in pregnancy (such as *Thuja occidentalis* which contains high levels of thujone) should be avoided in women who are actively trying to conceive. However, many essential oil-containing herbs (such as *Matricaria recutita*) may be safely used as the whole herb, or whole plant extract, within the recommended dosage range. High doses of herbs that contain high levels of anthraquinones (such as *Senna* spp.) should also be avoided as they may overstimulate the bowel, which can cause reflex irritation of the uterus and lead to miscarriage.[1034]

It is generally safer to treat infertility using herbs that are considered to be safe in early pregnancy wherever possible. If herbs are chosen which are contraindicated in pregnancy, the patient must be advised to use barrier methods of contraception while taking those herbs, and the prescription should be revised before the patient resumes trying to conceive.

When a woman discovers she is pregnant, the prescription should be reviewed in any case, and any herbs which are considered to be supporting healthy hormone balance, maintaining adequate pelvic blood flow, or helping to manage stress levels, should be maintained for the whole of the first trimester, provided they are safe in pregnancy (or substituted with safer herbs if they are not). Any herbs that are no longer necessary should be discontinued, and if required, herbs that help with any new problems (such as morning sickness, constipation, or threatened miscarriage) may be introduced.

Unfortunately there is actually very little consensus regarding the safety of herbal medicines in pregnancy. Sources vary widely in terms of which herbs are safe in pregnancy, and which are not. Many consider any herb that does not have clear evidence of safety from controlled clinical trials to be contraindicated in pregnancy; and in some cases, even herbs that do have an established safety record in clinical trials when used within recommended dosage ranges (such as *Senna* spp. and *Glycyrrhiza glabra*), are considered by some to be unsuitable for use during pregnancy.[1035] There are also instances of herbs that have been widely used by pregnant women, with no reports of adverse effects (such as *Matricaria recutita*, *Urtica dioica*, and *Zingiber officinale*), being said to be unsuitable for use during pregnancy.[1036]

For the purposes of this chapter, herbs which are considered to be safe in pregnancy, and therefore safe to use in women who are actively trying to conceive, are either those which have shown no risk to the foetus in controlled studies, or those which have been widely used by pregnant women, with no reports of causing harmful effects. Herbs which are considered to be unsafe during pregnancy (and therefore also unsuitable for women who are actively trying to conceive) are those which have demonstrated adverse effects on the foetus in humans, and those which have shown adverse effects in animal studies, but there have been no studies on women to see whether or not the adverse effect is reproduced in humans.

The recommended dosage ranges are a general guide only. Some practitioners may use higher or lower doses, depending on the level of sensitivity and the needs of the individual patient. In general, the lower end of the dosage range is sufficient for regular use, especially when combined with other herbs that support its action, and address the overall health needs of the patient. Slightly higher doses may be needed to achieve an effect in some patients, but the higher dosage ranges are generally only used short term, in more acute situations.

Some herbs may interact with orthodox medicines, and therefore it is important to check for potential interactions before recommending herbs to an individual who is taking any prescribed or over the counter medication.

Herbal medicines for improving reproductive health

The plants discussed here are just a small selection of those that are useful for improving reproductive health. Like most herbs, they have a wide range of actions, which affect many body processes, and they are therefore useful for the treatment of a great variety of different health problems. However, for the purposes of this book, which is aimed at understanding and overcoming reproductive health problems, this section focuses more specifically on how these plants help to improve reproductive health and fertility.

Achillea millefolium

Achillea millefolium (yarrow herb) is considered to be cool and dry.[1037] It has a strong tradition for use in a variety of gynaecological conditions, particularly spasmodic dysmenorrhoea.[1038] It is a uterine tonic, which has both stimulating and spasmolytic effects on uterine muscle,[1039] resulting in increased uterine tone without excessive spasm.[1040] It is also an astringent herb, which is traditionally used to treat menorrhagia. It is thought to improve progesterone function,[1041,1042] which also helps to reduce excessive menstruation, as well as improving fertility.

Achillea millefolium is a circulatory stimulant, which improves peripheral circulation,[1043] and reduces pelvic congestion.[1044] This may be due to an anti-thrombotic effect,[1045] as well as relaxation of the veins, which allows congestion to move out of the capillaries.[1046]

It is a bitter herb with a choleretic action,[1047] which helps to reduce congestion of the liver. Bitter herbs are useful for reducing Pitta.[1048] *Achillea millefolium* is recommended for PMS, which is due to Liver Qi Stagnation; and for congestive dysmenorrhoea and menorrhagia, which are the result of Uterus Qi Stagnation.[1049]

Thujone-containing varieties of *Achillea millefolium* should be avoided in pregnancy, and are therefore also best avoided in women who are currently trying to conceive. Otherwise, limited use of yarrow in women is not associated with harmful effects in pregnancy, and therefore it may be used by women who are trying to conceive. Very high doses have been associated with harmful effects in animal studies, but the relevance to humans is unknown.[1050] However, it may be prudent to discontinue its use on conception, as a precaution.

The usual dosage range for yarrow is around 20–60 ml per week of a 1:3 tincture, or 1–3 g a day of the dried herb. Some practitioners may use higher or lower doses, depending on the needs of the individual patient. There are no known interactions between yarrow and other herbs or medicines. It should not be used in those with sensitivity to plants of the Compositae family.[1051]

Aesculus hippocastanum

Aesculus hippocastanum (horse chestnut seed) is considered to be cool and dry.[1052] It is traditionally used for the treatment of venous stasis, congestion, and engorgement, and is particularly effective for haemorrhoids.[1053] This demonstrates its usefulness for addressing blood stasis due to venous congestion in the pelvic region.

Herbal medicines that are traditionally used to treat varicose veins and haemorrhoids also help to improve fertility in men with varicocele.[1054]

In women, *Aesculus hippocastanum* helps to reduce oedema associated with premenstrual fluid retention, and reduces the risk of thrombosis.[1055]

Horse chestnut has been successfully used to treat venous conditions in pregnant women for a duration of up to four weeks. However, evidence of safety for longer periods of use during pregnancy is lacking.[1056] It may therefore be safely used by women who are trying to conceive; but, it may be prudent to discontinue its use on conception, as a precaution.

The usual dosage range for horse chestnut is around 20–50 ml per week of a 1:3 tincture. The lower end of the dosage range (20–30 ml per week) is generally sufficient for most patients, and some practitioners may use higher or lower doses, depending on the needs of the individual patient.

Alchemilla vulgaris

Alchemilla vulgaris (lady's mantle herb) has a strong reputation among modern Western herbalists for the treatment of menstrual disorders.[1057,1058] It is considered to be cold and dry, and to tonify reproductive Qi.[1059] Very little modern research has been conducted on the actions of *Alchemilla vulgaris*, and its use appears to be predominantly based on traditional knowledge.

Lady's mantle is astringent and styptic, due at least in part to its tannin content.[1060] It is therefore useful for reducing heavy menstrual bleeding.[1061] It also tones the muscles and tissues of the uterus, improving prolapse and removing excessive dampness and stagnation.[1062]

Alchemilla vulgaris is thought to increase progesterone function,[1063] and it is widely used to help promote conception.[1064] It is safe during pregnancy,[1065] and therefore women who have been taking it to support progesterone levels and improve fertility prior to conception should continue taking it until around twelve weeks' gestation.

The usual dosage range for *Alchemilla vulgaris* is around 35–75 ml per week of a 1:3 tincture, or 1.5–3.5 g a day of the dried herb. The lower end of the dosage range (35–45 ml per week) is generally sufficient for most patients, though higher doses may be needed to control heavy menstrual bleeding in some cases. Some practitioners may use higher or lower doses, depending on the needs of the individual patient.

Andrographis paniculata

Andrographis paniculata (kalamegha) is an Ayurvedic herb, which is also known as the "king of bitters". It is considered to be a very cooling herb, which is useful for relieving conditions in which Pitta is aggravated, leading to symptoms such as fever, inflammation, and burning sensations. It is also useful for reducing Kapha, and relieving symptoms such as vaginal infections with thick discharge.[1066]

Andrographis paniculata is an immune stimulant, which may be used to treat acute and chronic infections.[1067] It also increases testosterone levels and may improve immune response in men with anti-sperm antibodies.[1068]

The usual dosage range for *Andrographis* is around 20–60 ml per week of a 1:3 tincture, or 1–3 g a day of the dried herb. The lower end of the dosage range (20–30 ml per week) is generally sufficient for most patients, particularly given its exceptionally bitter taste, though higher doses and frequent dosing may be needed for acute infections. Some practitioners may use higher or lower doses, depending on the needs of the individual patient. *Andrographis paniculata* is best avoided in early pregnancy due to insufficient evidence regarding safety. Women who are taking *Andrographis* should be advised to discontinue use before trying to conceive.[1069]

Anemone pulsatilla

Anemone pulsatilla (pasque flower dried herb) is considered to be dry and neutral (with both cooling and warming potential). It is useful for Liver Qi Stagnation, and Dampness in the reproductive organs.[1070]

Anemone pulsatilla is traditionally considered to be an antispasmodic herb,[1071,1072] which is useful for dysmenorrhoea, and indeed any painful or spasmodic condition affecting the reproductive organs,[1073,1074] in both men and women.

It is also considered to be a sedative nervine,[1075,1076] which is useful for the treatment of conditions such as: nervous tension, anxiety, PMS, headache, and exhaustion.[1077]

Anemone pulsatilla is contraindicated in pregnancy.[1078] It may cause uterine contraction and miscarriage, and can also lead to harmful effects on the foetus.[1079] It should therefore be discontinued in women who are actively trying to conceive. The usual dosage range for *Anemone pulsatilla* is 5–15 ml per week of a 1:3 tincture, made from the dried aerial parts. The fresh plant is not used because it is high in protoanemonin, which has irritant side effects. The dose should not be exceeded, as large doses can cause severe gastritis.[1080]

Angelica sinensis

Angelica sinensis (Dong Quai root) is considered to be warm and moist.[1081] It is traditionally used as a nourishing tonic for women in particular,[1082,1083] as it seems to help regulate the menstrual cycle.[1084] It is widely recommended by herbalists for the treatment of infertility.[1085,1086,1087]

Angelica sinensis is a uterine tonic and antispasmodic herb, which is used to treat dysmenorrhoea.[1088] The water-soluble and non-volatile elements of the root increase the contraction of the uterus, while the volatile elements have an antispasmodic effect on the uterine muscles.[1089] It therefore restores normal uterine function by relaxing the uterus, but encouraging more orderly and effective uterine contractions when required. It is also thought to regulate prostaglandin synthesis, and to act as a circulatory stimulant, which reduces pelvic congestion by regulating the activity of thromboxane A2. *Angelica sinensis* is also helpful for treating constipation, which may be both a contributing factor and consequence of pelvic congestion.[1090]

Angelica sinensis is used to treat Qi Stagnation in traditional Chinese medicine (TCM).[1091] It is particularly useful for Liver Qi Stagnation, which may contribute to infertility.[1092] It is also considered to be a Blood tonic,[1093] which is used to treat Blood Deficiency.[1094]

Angelica sinensis is contraindicated in pregnancy, and in women with heavy bleeding.[1095] The usual dosage range is around 45–90 ml per week of a 1:3 tincture (15–30 ml per week of 1:1 fluid extract), or 2–4 g a day of the dried herb. The lower end of the dosage range (45–60 ml per week) is generally sufficient for most patients. Some practitioners may use higher or lower doses, depending on the needs of the individual patient.

Aparagus racemosus

Aparagus racemosus (shatavari) is a cool, moist, nourishing herb. According to Ayurveda, it reduces Vata and Pitta excess, and increases Ojas, which is responsible for healthy fertility.[1096] In men, *Aparagus racemosus* may be used to increase Ojas and promote sperm production.[1097] In women, it is useful for amenorrhoea, which is often associated with Vata disturbance, and therefore benefits from consumption of moist, sweet, heavy, and nourishing herbs.[1098]

Aparagus racemosus reduces uterine contractions, which is useful for treating dysmenorrhoea and menorrhagia, and preventing early pregnancy loss.[1099] *Aparagus racemosus* is also an effective aphrodisiac for women with low libido.[1100]

Steroidal saponins in *Aparagus racemosus* weakly stimulate hypothalamic oestrogen receptors, increasing FSH secretion from the pituitary, which improves ovulation and oestrogen production. Oestrogen promoting herbs are also useful for vaginitis and cervical atrophy due to low oestrogen levels.[1101]

Aparagus racemosus is safe in pregnancy, and may therefore be used by women who are trying to conceive.[1102] The usual dosage range for *Aparagus racemosus* is around 45–100 ml per week of a 1:3 tincture (15–30 ml per week of fluid extract), or 3–5 g a day of the dried herb. It is a very nourishing herb that is safe even at higher doses.

Astragalus membranaceus

Astragalus membranaceus (Huang Qi root) is a sweet and nourishing herb, which is considered to be warm and somewhat dry.[1103] Traditional indications for *Astragalus membranaceus* in traditional Chinese medicine include fatigue, poor appetite, diarrhoea, uterine prolapse, abnormal uterine bleeding, and spontaneous sweating. It tonifies the Qi and Blood in men and women with Qi or Blood Deficiency,[1104] and significantly increases sperm motility in men.[1105]

Astragalus membranaceus also significantly improves immune function and is therefore a useful adjunct in cases of chronic infection.[1106] It is safe in pregnancy, and may therefore be used by women who are trying to conceive.[1107] The usual dosage range is around 45–90 ml per week of a 1:3 tincture (15–30 ml per week of fluid extract), or 3–4 g a day of the dried herb.

Camellia sinensis

Camellia sinensis (green tea) acts as an aromatase inhibitor (the enzyme which catalyses the conversion of androgens to form oestrogen).[1108]

It can therefore help to reduce oestrogen in conditions involving oestrogen excess, such as endometriosis, fibroids, and infertility.

Camellia sinensis also reduces 5-alpha reductase (which converts testosterone to the more potent dihydrotestosterone), and can therefore also be helpful in reducing symptoms of hyperandrogenism in women with PCOS.[1109]

Camellia sinensis is best taken as tea (2–3 cups per day). Concentrated green tea extracts should be avoided as they have been associated with hepatotoxicity.[1110] Average levels of tea consumption during early pregnancy are not associated with any adverse effects.[1111]

Capsella bursa-pastoris

Capsella bursa-pastoris (shepherd's purse herb) is a plant of the Brassicaceae family, which induces phase 1 liver metabolism of oestrogen, tending to favour formation of the more protective *2-hydroxyoestrone*, rather than more harmful *16-α-hydroxyoestrone*.[1112,1113]

It is a useful anti-haemorrhagic herb, which has a long history of use for reducing bleeding.[1114,1115] It is very effective for menorrhagia and dysfunctional uterine bleeding associated with fibroids.[1116] It also helps to reduce venous blood stagnation, and is therefore useful in cases of uterine congestion and congestive dysmenorrhoea. It is considered to be cool and dry.[1117]

The usual dosage range of shepherd's purse is 30–60 ml per week of 1:3 tincture. It is considered to be an emmenagogue and has been used to stimulate uterine contractions during birth,[1118] and to assist delivery of the placenta. Therefore women should be advised to stop taking medicines containing *Capsella bursa-pastoris* if they conceive.

Cimicifuga racemosa

Cimicifuga racemosa (black cohosh root) is helpful in alleviating symptoms of ovarian insufficiency. It reduces luteinising hormone (LH) levels, which have been linked to hot flushes. In addition, its oestrogenic effects promote proliferation of vaginal epithelium, reducing vaginal dryness and atrophy,[1119] and improving associated discomfort and dyspareunia.[1120]

Apart from its effect on the vaginal mucosa, *Cimicifuga racemosa* can also help to reduce pelvic pain directly, which is useful in cases of pelvic inflammatory disease, and other painful, spasmodic, or inflammatory conditions of the reproductive organs and tissues, such as endometriosis and vaginismus.[1121,1122]

Cimicifuga racemosa reduces both LH and androgens in women with polycystic ovary syndrome (PCOS).[1123] It also acts as an agonist at serotonin and dopamine receptors, helping to improve mood disturbances such as depression, anxiety, and irritability.[1124] Its dopaminergic action inhibits prolactin release,[1125] which is useful for women with premenstrual syndrome (PMS) or infertility due to hyperprolactinaemia.

The recommended dose of *Cimicifuga racemosa* is 15–30 ml per week of a 1:3 tincture (up to 1.5 g per day of dried root). It can cause headaches in some patients, particularly at higher doses.[1126] *Cimicifuga racemosa* is not recommended during pregnancy, except to assist with birth. However, limited use in pregnant women has not been associated with any harmful effects,[1127] and therefore it may be used by women who are actively trying to conceive, and discontinued once conception occurs.

Cinnamonum zeylonicum

Cinnamonum zeylonicum (cinnamon bark) is a warming herb, which may be used in cases of poor circulation. It is considered to be specific for the pelvic region, which is useful for treating dysmenorrhoea related to "stagnant blood".[1128] It has a powerful astringent action and is traditionally used to reduce excessive bleeding in women with menorrhagia and uterine haemorrhage.[1129,1130]

Cinnamonum zeylonicum also improves fasting blood sugar and reduces insulin resistance,[1131,1132] which may in turn help to improve ovulatory function and fertility,[1133] particularly in women with insulin resistance and polycystic ovary syndrome (PCOS).

Cinnamonum zeylonicum is considered to be hot and dry.[1134] It may be used to treat Kidney Yang Deficiency, which manifests with symptoms such as cold extremities, palpitations, and fatigue.[1135] It is also used in Ayurvedic medicine to reduce Vata and Kapha.[1136,1137]

The recommended dose of *Cinnamonum zeylonicum* is 20–60 ml of 1:3 tincture per week, or 3–8 g a day of dried herb. 1–2 teaspoons per day of ground cinnamon may be taken in divided doses, as tea, or added to suitable food. *Cinnamonum zeylonicum* is safe during pregnancy at normal therapeutic doses,[1138] and is therefore suitable for women who are trying to conceive. It is known to cause allergy in rare cases.[1139]

Dioscorea villosa

Dioscorea villosa (wild yam root) is considered to be cool and dry.[1140] It is traditionally used as an antispasmodic, to relieve pain in spasmodic dysmenorrhoea.[1141] The antispasmodic action may help to relieve vaginismus and dyspareunia. *Dioscorea villosa* is also useful as an anti-inflammatory for inflammatory conditions affecting the reproductive system, such as endometriosis and PID.[1142]

Dioscorea villosa contains steroidal saponins such as diosgenin, which are structurally and functionally similar to human oestrogens. They have an affinity for oestrogen receptors, exerting a weak oestrogenic affect in comparison to oestradiol.[1143] They act as selective oestrogen receptor modulators (SERMS), which both reduce the symptoms of oestrogen deficiency, and compete with endogenous oestrogen to help reduce its proliferative effects in women with oestrogen excess.[1144]

In women with low oestrogen levels, phytoestrogens can help to reduce associated symptoms, with limited side effects.[1145] This has a beneficial effect on symptoms of ovarian insufficiency, such as hot flushes, night sweats, depression, insomnia, and reduced libido.[1146] Oestrogen promoting herbs such as *Dioscorea villosa* (wild yam) are also useful for cervical atrophy due to low oestrogen levels,[1147] and they help to stabilise vaginal flora.[1148]

The weaker effect on hypothalamic oestrogen receptors compared to endogenous oestrogen causes the body to continue to respond to the low oestrogen levels, stimulating the pituitary to increase FSH secretion, which in turn increases oestrogen production.[1149] Improved levels of FSH also lead to improved ovulation, especially when given on days 5–14.[1150]

Conversely, in women with conditions related to oestrogen excess, phytoestrogens compete with endogenous oestrogens for hypothalamic oestrogen receptors, and thereby exert a protective effect.[1151,1152] They may also reduce aromatisation of androstenedione to oestrone in fat cells, and stimulate liver production of sex hormone-binding globulin (SHBG), which binds to excess oestrogen, reducing its ability to bind to hormone-sensitive tissues.[1153]

Dioscorea villosa is considered to be safe for pregnant women, and is traditionally used for treating nausea and vomiting in pregnancy.[1154] It is therefore suitable for use in women who are actively trying to conceive. The usual dosage range for wild yam is 1.5–3 g per day of dried root, or 30–60 ml per week of a 1:3 tincture. Saponin-containing herbs may occasionally cause gastric irritation and reflux in susceptible individuals.[1155]

Echinacea spp.

Echinacea angustifolia/Echinacea purpurea (purple coneflower root) is an immune enhancing herb, which is useful in cases of genitourinary infection and PID.[1156]

In the case of inflammatory conditions such as endometriosis, the cell-mediated immune response is responsible for clearing menstrual debris from the peritoneal cavity and preventing implantation of endometrial cells.[1157] Therefore immune modulating herbs and lymphatics such as *Echinacea* spp. may also help to prevent and resolve endometrial cysts.[1158,1159]

Echinacea spp. is traditionally used to control benign growths, including uterine fibroids.[1160] As an immune modulating herb, it may also be useful for reducing anti-sperm antibodies.[1161] It is considered to be cool and dry.[1162]

Echinacea spp. is considered to be safe for use during pregnancy.[1163] The usual dosage range for *Echinacea* spp. is 1.5–3 g per day of dried herb, or 30–60 ml per week of a 1:3 strength tincture. Some practitioners may use higher or lower doses, depending on the needs of the individual patient, and frequent dosing (every 2 hours or so) is necessary for treating acute infections. *Echinacea* spp. (particularly the aerial parts) may very occasionally cause allergy in susceptible individuals. Caution is advised for transplant patients taking immunosuppressive drugs.[1164]

Eleutherococcus senticosus

Eleutherococcus senticosus (Siberian ginseng root) is an adaptogenic herb, which increases the individual's ability to adapt to various environmental factors, and to avoid the damage they may cause.[1165] It is therefore widely used as a tonic in times of stress and pressure,[1166,1167] and can reduce symptoms of overwork and exhaustion, such as low mood, fatigue, and sweet cravings.[1168]

The beneficial effects of adaptogens such as *Eleutherococcus senticosus* are often considered to be mainly associated with their effects on the hypothalamic-pituitary-adrenal (HPA) axis.[1169] They are thought to improve adrenal function and to increase levels of cortisol.[1170]

However, *Eleutherococcus senticosus* also appears to regulate the other hypothalamic-pituitary-endocrine axes, and can be used for chronic pituitary, adrenocortical, thyroid, or pancreatic insufficiency.[1171] It reduces blood glucose levels and HbA1c, indicating an improvement in insulin sensitivity.[1172] It is therefore useful for treatment infertility.[1173]

Eleutherococcus senticosus is considered to be safe for use during pregnancy,[1174] and is safe for use by women who wish to conceive. The usual dosage range for *Eleutherococcus senticosus* is 1–3 g of dried herb per day, or 20–60 ml per week of a 1:3 strength tincture. Some practitioners may use higher or lower doses, depending on the needs of the individual patient. *Eleutherococcus senticosus* is traditionally contraindicated during the acute phase of infections. Due to the stimulating nature of the herb, it is advisable to take a break of at least two weeks after six weeks of continuous use.[1175]

Gelsemium sempervirens

Gelsemium sempervirens (yellow jasmine root) is considered to be cold and dry.[1176] It is principally used as an anodyne to treat conditions characterised by acute pain, spasm, and inflammation. It is very effective for pelvic pain,[1177] and can therefore be used for women with dysmenorrhoea, dyspareunia, and pelvic inflammatory disease.

Gelsemium sempervirens is contraindicated in pregnancy,[1178] and should therefore not be given to women who are actively trying to conceive, except for relief of pain during menses. In the UK, *Gelsemium sempervirens* is included in Schedule 20 of the Human Medicines Regulations 2012, and is subject to a maximum daily dose of 75 mg (equivalent to 5 ml per week of a 1:10 tincture). However, some practitioners consider this to be a low dose, and practitioners in other countries may use higher doses.

Ginkgo biloba

Ginkgo biloba (maidenhair tree leaf) is considered to be dry and neutral. It is useful for problems caused by Blood Stagnation, and treating Kkidney Essence Deficiency.[1179]

Ginkgo biloba may help to improve uterine circulation,[1180] and it is therefore useful for relieving pain in conditions associated with Blood Stasis, such as congestive dysmenorrhoea and fibroids. *Ginkgo biloba* also reduces oedema,[1181] and is useful for women with cyclical breast tenderness and fluid retention, and for men with varicocele.

Its circulatory stimulant action and beneficial effects on Kidney Essence make it useful in the treatment of erectile dysfunction.[1182] *Ginkgo biloba* has also been shown to improve libido and orgasm in both men and women with antidepressant induced sexual dysfunction.[1183]

The recommended dose of *Ginkgo biloba* is 1.5–4 ml per day (10–28 ml per week) of a 2:1 standardised extract. It considered to be safe during pregnancy and can therefore be used by women who are trying to conceive. However, it should be avoided in patients on anticoagulant or antiplatelet medication.[1184]

Glycine max

Glycine max (soy beans) are an especially rich source of phytoestrogens, particularly isoflavones (such as genistein and daidzein), which are structurally and functionally similar to human oestrogens, exerting a weak oestrogenic affect in comparison to oestradiol.[1185] They act as selective oestrogen receptor modulators (SERMs), which both reduce the symptoms of oestrogen deficiency, and compete with endogenous oestrogen to help reduce its proliferative effects in women with oestrogen excess.[1186]

In women with low oestrogen levels, phytoestrogens can help to reduce associated symptoms, with limited side effects.[1187] This has a beneficial effect on the manifestations of ovarian insufficiency, such as hot flushes, night sweats, depression, insomnia, and reduced libido.[1188] Phytoestrogens are also useful for cervical atrophy due to low oestrogen levels,[1189] and they help to stabilise vaginal flora.[1190] Consumption of phytoestrogens is also associated with lower fracture risk.[1191]

In women with low oestrogen levels, the weaker effect on hypothalamic oestrogen receptors of phytoestrogens compared to endogenous oestrogen causes the body to continue to respond to the low oestrogen levels, stimulating the pituitary to increase FSH secretion, which in turn increases oestrogen production.[1192] Improved levels of FSH also lead to improved ovulation.[1193]

In women with conditions related to oestrogen excess on the other hand, phytoestrogens bind weakly to oestrogen receptors, competing with endogenous oestrogens and preventing them from exerting stronger oestrogenic effects.[1194,1195] They may also reduce aromatisation of androstenedione to oestrone in fat cells, and stimulate liver production of sex hormone-binding globulin (SHBG), which binds to excess oestrogen, reducing its ability to bind to hormone-sensitive tissues.[1196]

In other words, phytoestrogens improve oestrogen production and ameliorate symptoms in women with low oestrogen levels; but they compete with endogenous oestrogen, help to reduce its production and availability, and thereby help to reduce its proliferative effects in women with oestrogen excess.[1197]

In order to be absorbed from the digestive system, isoflavones must first undergo hydrolysis of the sugar moiety by ß-glucosidase enzymes,[1198] which are produced by bifidobacteria in the intestine. Therefore, the efficacy of dietary phytoestrogens varies between different individuals depending on their gut flora.[1199] Consuming fermented soya products or taking a probiotic supplement may help to enhance the bioavailability of isoflavones.[1200]

Soya products, together with whole-grain cereals, seeds, and leafy green vegetables are also a good source of magnesium,[1201] which can help to reduce uterine cramping.[1202]

Glycyrrhiza glabra

Glycyrrhiza glabra (liquorice root) is a demulcent and nutritive herb,[1203] which can act as a mild laxative in cases of constipation due to dryness.[1204] In traditional Chinese medicine it is considered to be moist and neutral. In Ayurvedic terms, it reduces Vata and Pitta, but increases Kapha.[1205]

In more recent times, *Glycyrrhiza glabra* is widely used for its effects on adrenal function. It is thought to increase production of steroid hormones by the adrenal gland, and mimic the activity of cortisol.[1206] It also reduces activity of 11ß-hydroxysteroid dehydrogenase (11ß-OHSD), the enzyme responsible for deactivating cortisol, thereby prolonging the activity of cortisol by reducing its breakdown.[1207] It is therefore useful for patients with symptoms of low cortisol function such as low blood pressure, hypoglycaemia, depression, fatigue, allergies, loss of body hair, and hyperpigmentation.

Reduction of 11ß-OHSD and reduced cortisol clearance lead to improved cortisol levels. This inhibits ACTH release from the pituitary due to negative feedback. Reduced ACTH levels in turn lead to a decrease in the production of adrenal androgens.[1208] *Glycyrrhiza glabra* is therefore useful for patients with androgen excess. It also reduces levels of 5-alpha reductase (the enzyme which converts testosterone to the more potent dihydrotestosterone), which helps to reduce the symptoms of androgen excess in conditions such as PCOS.[1209]

The recommended dose of liquorice is 2–6 g per day, or 15–40 ml per week of a 1:1 fluid extract. In patients taking corticosteroid drugs, it increases plasma concentration of the drug by inhibiting its metabolism, and may thereby potentiate the effects of corticosteroids. It should not be used in patients taking potassium-depleting drugs (such as thiazide diuretics or laxatives) as it can lead to severe potassium loss. Due to its mineralcorticoid effect, it is contraindicated in hypertension, congestive heart failure, hypokalaemia, oedema, and severe kidney insufficiency and liver disease.[1210]

Liquorice is listed as being contraindicated in pregnancy in the Commission E monographs.[1211] There are some reports of very high doses being associated with increased risk of preterm labour; and theoretical concerns about liquorice lowering androgen levels, which are necessary for normal development of the testes in a male foetus (which occurs from about six weeks' gestation). However, doses of up to 3 g per day (20 ml per week of 1:1 fluid extract) are generally considered to be safe.[1212] It is therefore advisable for women who are taking liquorice while trying to conceive, to take low doses (15–20 ml per week of 1:1 fluid extract), and ideally, to discontinue its use once conception occurs (before six weeks' gestation).

Humulus lupulus

Humulus lupulus (hops flower) is traditionally used as a sedative nervine, for relieving restlessness, pain, and insomnia. It is also an aromatic bitter which acts as a stomachic and tonic.[1213] It is therefore particularly useful for people with agitation or anxiety that manifests as gastrointestinal problems and sleeplessness. It is considered to be cold and dry.[1214]

Hop strobiles have a significant oestrogenic action,[1215] and are effective for reducing vasomotor symptoms (flushing) associated with ovarian insufficiency.[1216] Topically, vaginal applications containing hops can reduce vaginal dryness and associated inflammation, discomfort, and dyspareunia.[1217] Due to the oestrogenic effects, there is also a potential role for hops in the long-term prevention of bone loss in postmenopausal women,[1218] or those at increased risk of osteoporosis due to hypothalamic amenorrhoea or primary ovarian insufficiency.

Humulus lupulus is effective for reducing anxiety and sleeplessness, which are also common symptoms associated with primary ovarian insufficiency. Hop strobiles improve both sleep latency and sleep quality.[1219] The sedative action of the plant is due in part to its effect on GABA receptors.[1220]

While *Humulus lupulus* is very useful for patients with anxiety and sleeplessness, it is traditionally contraindicated in depression, and appears to worsen low mood and lethargy in some patients.[1221]

Humulus lupulus is considered to be safe during pregnancy at normal therapeutic doses,[1222] and may be recommended for women who are trying to conceive. However, marked oestrogenic effects have been observed, and therefore it is best to discontinue its use once pregnancy has been confirmed, as a precaution. The oestrogenic effect may also cause gynaecomastia in men.[1223] The usual dose of hops is 750 mg–1.5 g of dried hop strobiles per day, or 15–30 ml per week of a 1:3 tincture.

Hydrastis canadensis

Hydrastis canadensis root is considered to be cold and dry.[1224] It has a restorative effect on the mucous membranes, relieving conditions involving excessive mucus secretions and bleeding, reducing inflammation, and healing ulceration.[1225] It is traditionally used for the relief of excessive vaginal bleeding and congestive dysmenorrhoea, and to heal cervical erosion.[1226]

Hydrastis canadensis has demonstrated antimicrobial activity against a wide range of pathogens, including bacteria, fungi, and parasites.[1227] It is therefore a useful adjunct in cases of chronic infection.[1228] It was traditionally used to treat infections such as *Neisseria gonorrhoeae* (gonorrhoea),[1229] and may still be a useful adjunct to orthodox interventions in the treatment of sexually transmitted disease. It is a beneficial component of vaginal pessaries for women with infections such as candida, *Trichomonas*, or bacterial vaginosis.[1230]

From an energetic perspective, it is useful for resolving conditions characterised by Damp Heat, such as yellow vaginal discharge, and spermatorrhoea. It also helps with conditions involving Blood Stagnation. *Hydrastis canadensis* is a very bitter herb, which can be useful for treating Liver Qi Stagnation.[1231]

The recommended dose of *Hydrastis canadensis* is 15–30 ml per week of a 1:3 tincture. It is indicated for the treatment of chronic problems, and is traditionally not recommended for use in acute inflammation.[1232] *Hydrastis canadensis* is contraindicated in pregnancy (except for short-term use to help induce labour at full term), and should therefore not be used by women who are actively trying to conceive. It is endangered, and therefore only cultivated sources should be used.[1233]

Hypericum perforatum

Hypericum perforatum (St John's wort herb) is considered to be cool and dry.[1234] It is a nervous system restorative,[1235] which was traditionally used in the treatment of nervous depression.[1236] It is thought to inhibit monoamine oxidase (MAO),[1237] the enzyme which catalyses the breakdown of neurotransmitters such as serotonin, dopamine, and epinephrine. The available evidence suggests that it is similar to orthodox antidepressants in terms of efficacy, but with fewer side effects.[1238,1239]

Hypericum perforatum is beneficial in relieving the mood disturbances that are often associated with premature ovarian insufficiency.[1240] It may also have some hormonal effects, since it seems to improve both psychological and psychosomatic symptoms of ovarian insufficiency, reducing vasomotor symptoms, and improving sexual well-being.[1241]

Hypericum perforatum may help to reduce oestrogen excess (which can contribute to conditions such as endometriosis, uterine fibroids, PMS, and subfertility), since monoamine oxidase activity is correlated with the progesterone to oestradiol ratio.[1242] A combination of *Hypericum perforatum* and *Vitex agnus-castus* has been shown to improve PMS symptoms such as depression and anxiety.[1243] *Hypericum perforatum* has also been traditionally used for dysmenorrhoea,[1244] due to its sedative and anodyne actions.[1245]

Hypericum perforatum is traditionally used to treat liver problems.[1246] It induces phase 1 liver metabolism (hydroxylation), the process by which oestrogen is metabolised, and tends to favour formation of the more protective *2-hydroxyoestrone*, rather than the more harmful *16-α-hydroxyoestrone*.[1247,1248]

The usual recommended dose of *Hypericum perforatum* is 1–3 g per day of dried herb, or 20–60 ml per week of 1:3 tincture. However, higher doses (equivalent to 6–12 g a day of dried herb) have been safely used in some cases. Normal therapeutic doses may cause photosensitivity, and therefore avoiding excessive sun exposure and appropriate use of sunscreens should be recommended.[1249]

Hypericum perforatum may increase mania in susceptible individuals, and should be avoided in patients with bipolar disorder. Due to its effect on hepatic metabolism, it may interact with a number of drugs. It should therefore be avoided in patients taking anticoagulants (such as warfarin), immune suppressants (such as cyclosporine), cardiac glycosides (such as digoxin), chemotherapy drugs (such as irinotecan), and antivirals for HIV (such as nevirapine and indinivir). It may also cause breakthrough bleeding in women taking low dose oral contraceptives, and may affect serotonin levels in people taking selective serotonin reuptake inhibitors (SSRIs), increasing the risk of serotonin syndrome. It should be discontinued at least three days before general anaesthesia. It is considered to be safe in pregnancy, and may therefore be recommended to women who are trying to conceive.[1250]

Leonurus cardiaca

Leonurus cardiaca (motherwort herb) is a nervine tonic[1251] which reduces tension and irritability.[1252] The term *"cardiaca"* refers to its usefulness for heart and circulatory problems.[1253] It is a cardio tonic,[1254] with a diffusive action, which maintains healthy circulation.[1255] It can help to normalise blood pressure, and has been recommended to treat both hypertension[1256] (possibly by reducing tension, and thereby relaxing blood vessels) and hypotension[1257] (probably by improving cardiac output).

The common name, "motherwort", indicates its relevance in the treatment of uterine conditions.[1258] It is widely used to treat various gynaecological disorders, such as spasmodic dysmenorrhoea.[1259] It seems to possess the apparently contradictory effects of both stimulating uterine activity and relieving spasm. This combination of actions helps to regulate uterine function by encouraging more orderly and effective contractions, which are then followed by an adequate rest period so that blood can circulate through the uterine muscle again.[1260] It is also traditionally used to tone and strengthen the uterus,[1261] and it is recommended for the treatment of infertility.[1262] In energetic terms, *Leonurus cardiaca* reduces stagnation in the uterus. It is considered to be cool and dry.[1263]

The recommended dose of *Leonurus cardiaca* is 1–2 g per day of dried herb, or 20–40 ml per week of a 1:3 tincture. Due to its stimulating effect on uterine muscle, *Leonurus cardiaca* is contraindicated in pregnancy.[1264]

Therefore, women should ideally be advised to discontinue its use before actively trying to conceive.

Lepidium meyenii

Lepidium meyenii (maca) is a Peruvian plant of the Brassicaceae family. It is a highly nutritive herb, which can help to improve ovarian function in women with premature ovarian insufficiency.[1265] It reduces elevated FSH, improves the LH:FSH ratio, increases oestrogen and progesterone levels, and increases production of ACTH and thyroid hormones.[1266]

Short-term use of maca initially increases secretion of both FSH and LH by the pituitary. This improves ovarian function in women, and thereby increases production of both oestrogen and progesterone, reducing symptoms associated with low ovarian hormone levels, such as hot flushes, sweating, sleep disturbance, mood changes, reduced libido, joint pains, and heart palpitations.[1267] Improved oestrogen levels also lead to improved bone density.[1268] After several months of treatment, improved ovarian hormone levels allow FSH levels to fall due to negative feedback, and the FSH:LH ratio improves.[1269]

In men, improved FSH and LH levels due to maca consumption increase production of androgens, improving libido, reducing erectile dysfunction,[1270] and improving sperm count and sperm motility in men with subfertility.[1271]

Dried maca contains gamma-aminobutyric acid (GABA), and constituents that inhibit monoamine oxidase (MAO), the enzyme that breaks down neurotransmitters such as serotonin and dopamine. This leads to a reduction in symptoms of both anxiety and depression.[1272] Maca also improves libido and sexual function in both men and women with sexual dysfunction due to antidepressant medication.[1273]

Constituents of maca include various alkaloids, sterols, glucosinolates, amino acids, fatty acids, vitamins, and minerals.[1274] It is thought to act as an adaptogen, positively affecting pituitary function, and thereby improving ovarian, adrenal, and thyroid activity.[1275]

The usual therapeutic dose of maca is around 3 g per day of dried maca powder.[1276] However, in the Peruvian Andes, much higher quantities are regularly consumed by indigenous people without causing any adverse effects.[1277] Since there is very little research on the safety of maca during pregnancy, it is best to advise women to discontinue its use after conception occurs.

Linum usitatissimum

Linum usitatissimum (flaxseed) is rich in lignans, which inhibit 5-α reductase (the enzyme that catalyses the conversion of testosterone into the more biologically active dihydrotestosterone). It is therefore beneficial for helping to reduce the effects of androgens in patients with PCOS or prostate problems.

Lignans also act as selective oestrogen receptor modulators (SERMS), which both reduce the symptoms of oestrogen deficiency, and compete with endogenous oestrogen to help reduce its proliferative effects in women with oestrogen excess.[1278] Lignans also help to reduce excess oestrogen by inhibiting aromatase (the enzyme which catalyses the conversion of androgens to oestrogen)[1279] and reduce oestrogen activity by increasing the production of sex hormone-binding globulin (SHBG).[1280]

Furthermore, consumption of flaxseed increases production of 2-hydroxyestrone (an oestrogen metabolite with protective properties), compared to the more potent 16α-hydroxyestrone, during hepatic metabolism of oestrogen.[1281] Flaxseed also contains soluble fibre, which benefits bowel flora and reduces constipation by drawing water into the bowel and softening the stool.[1282] For women with oestrogen excess, healthy bowel flora and regular bowel movements are important to reduce enterohepatic recirculation of oestrogen.

Flaxseed is a good source of essential fatty acids, including α-linolenic acid (ALA), linoleic acid, and oleic acid, providing 3:10 ratio of omega-6 to omega-3, which helps to reduce series 2 prostaglandins and inflammatory markers.[1283] Omega-3 fatty acids also help to reduce blood stagnation. This action, in combination with its anti-inflammatory and oestrogen modulating effects, makes flaxseed a useful adjunct for the treatment of conditions such as endometriosis and pelvic inflammatory disease.[1284]

Small amounts of flaxseed (up to 1 tablespoon per day) are safe during pregnancy. However, large doses of flaxseed or flax oil should be avoided in pregnant women.

Matricaria recutita

Matricaria recutita (German chamomile flower) is considered to be cool and neutral.[1285] It is traditionally used for problems affecting the nervous system and the gastro-intestinal tract.[1286] It is widely used by modern

Western herbalists for treating irritability, tension headaches, and various digestive disorders.[1287,1288] Studies also support its usefulness in reducing anxiety.[1289] These actions make it very useful for reducing the effects of stress, and for women with premenstrual mood changes and other symptoms. The name *"Matricaria"*, being derived from the term meaning "mother", points to its usefulness in problems of the female reproductive system, such as spasmodic dysmenorrhoea.[1290]

The usual dose of chamomile is 1.5–3 g per day of dried flowers by infusion, or 30–60 ml per week of a 1:3 tincture. Chamomile rarely causes allergic reactions in susceptible individuals. It is safe for use in pregnancy and by women who are trying to conceive.[1291]

Melissa officinalis

Melissa officinalis (lemon balm leaf) is considered to be a relaxing nervine,[1292] and was traditionally used to treat painful menstruation.[1293] It is still widely used by herbalists as a nervous system relaxant,[1294] which helps to reduce the effects of stress. It is useful for treating anxiety and tension headache, and has been shown to reduce PMS symptoms.[1295] It seems to possess both relaxing and uplifting qualities, not only relieving tension and stress, but also lifting depression and increasing alertness.[1296]

Melissa officinalis reduces thyroid overactivity.[1297] It appears to inhibit TSH receptor binding in cases of hyperthyroidism, which causes decreased production of T3 and T4 in the thyroid gland. It is also thought to block antibodies associated with Graves' disease.[1298] Topically, it has been shown to be effective for recurrent herpes labialis.[1299]

Melissa officinalis is considered to be cool and dry. It tonifies the reproductive Qi and may therefore be useful in treating patients with infertility.[1300] The usual dose of lemon balm is 1.5–3 g per day of dried aerial parts by infusion, or 30–60 ml per week of a 1:3 tincture. It is safe for use in pregnancy and by women who are trying to conceive.[1301]

Mentha spicata

Mentha spicata (spearmint leaf) is traditionally considered to have a similar, albeit less powerful action to peppermint, and is principally used as a carminative.[1302] It is a relaxing herb, which is regarded as being gentler and more soothing than peppermint, and therefore useful for nausea, vomiting, and colic in infants.[1303] *Mentha spicata* is considered to be cool and neutral,[1304] and is traditionally used as a febrifuge.[1305]

Mentha spicata has been shown to reduce free testosterone, and to reduce symptoms of hyperandrogenism in women with PCOS, without reducing DHEA.[1306] Two cups of spearmint tea per day is sufficient to have significant anti-androgenic effects.[1307]

Spearmint tea is safe in pregnancy, when taken in moderate doses.[1308] However, due to its significant anti-androgenic effect, spearmint, and other mints, should not be consumed on a regular basis by men with subfertility.

Myristica fragrans

In Ayurveda, *Myristica fragrans* (nutmeg) is a profoundly relaxing and warming herb, which is used to reduce heavy menstrual bleeding and relieve spasmodic pain.[1309] It reduces excess Kapha, and calms Vata aggravation.[1310]

Myristica fragrans is considered to be rejuvinative to the reproductive tissues and is used to help improve libido in both men and women, and to restore erectile function. It is also considered to have an astringent action and is used to help prevent premature ejaculation.[1311]

The usual dose of nutmeg is 10–40 ml per week of a 1:3 tincture, or a quarter-teaspoon of nutmeg powder, one to three times a day. It is often given at night in warm milk to aid restful sleep.[1312]

Paeonia lactiflora

Paeonia lactiflora (paeony root) is traditionally used as an antispasmodic.[1313,1314] It is regarded as a uterine antispasmodic in particular, and is also recommended for "obstructions of the liver".[1315]

Modern Western herbalists also consider *Paeonia lactiflora* to be a uterine antispasmodic, which is useful for dysmenorrhoea and uterine overactivity during pregnancy. In addition, it is thought to have a regulating effect on a variety of hormones including oestrogen, androgens, progesterone, and prolactin.[1316] It is therefore widely used to treat a variety of conditions such as premenstrual headaches and irritability,[1317] mastalgia, and infertility.[1318]

Paeonia lactiflora appears to increase aromatisation of androgens,[1319] and reduce levels of 5-alpha reductase (which converts testosterone to the more potent dihydrotestosterone).[1320] It is therefore useful in the treatment of hyperandrogenism and PCOS.

Paeonia lactiflora is considered to be cool and dry.[1321] It is included in traditional Chinese medicine formulas to treat both Kidney Yang Deficiency and Qi Stagnation.[1322] It is recommended for the treatment of infertility due to Liver Stagnation in particular.[1323]

Paeonia lactiflora is considered to be safe in pregnancy, and is therefore suitable for women who are actively trying to conceive. The usual dose is 45–90 ml per week of a 1:3 tincture.

Panax ginseng

Panax ginseng (Korean ginseng root) is considered to be warm and dry. It is used in traditional Chinese medicine to treat Kidney Yang Deficiency,[1324] which is associated with symptoms such as fatigue, lack of libido, erectile dysfunction, and infertility.[1325]

It is an adaptogen, which helps to improve physical performance, memory, and well-being when under stress—including increasing alertness, reducing fatigue, enhancing relaxation and sleep quality, and improving recovery from infections.[1326] *Panax ginseng* improves androgen levels,[1327] increases sperm count, and reduces symptoms if erectile dysfunction in men.[1328]

The recommended dose of *Panax ginseng* is 10–60 ml per week of a 1:3 tincture.[1329] It is safe to take during pregnancy, although overstimulation can occur in susceptible people, especially at higher doses. It is contraindicated in individuals with hypertension, and is traditionally considered to be inappropriate for use during acute infections, or in people with signs of excess heat.[1330]

Pinus pinaster

Pinus pinaster (pine bark) is a potent antioxidant and anti-inflammatory. It also helps to significantly increase blood flow. These actions lead to improved cognitive function,[1331] and a significant reduction of symptoms in patients with chronic venous insufficiency.[1332] *Pinus pinaster* has also been shown to decrease cardiovascular risk factors in perimenopausal women.[1333]

Pinus pinaster significantly reduces pain in women with dysmenorrhoea when continued for at least two cycles,[1334] and helps reduce symptoms in women with endometriosis.[1335] There also seems to be a hormonal action, which decreases symptoms of ovarian insufficiency, including tiredness, headache, depression, and anxiety, and hot flashes;[1336] and can help improve sexual function in women.[1337]

In patients with metabolic syndrome, which has a negative impact on fertility and is a significant feature of PCOS, *Pinus pinaster* lowers triglycerides, blood sugar levels, and blood pressure, decreases waist circumference, and increases high-density lipoprotein (HDL) or "good" cholesterol.[1338]

In men, improved venous blood flow may help to reduce symptoms of varicocele. *Pinus pinaster* also increases levels of nitric oxide (which acts as a vasodilator), restores erectile function, and improves testosterone levels.[1339] Treatment with *Pinus pinaster* can also significantly increase semen volume and sperm count, and improve sperm motility and morphology.[1340]

The recommended dose of *Pinus pinaster* is 50–350 mg per day of standardised pine bark extract, usually in tablet form. It is considered to be safe to take during pregnancy.[1341]

Rehmannia glutinosa

Rehmannia glutinosa (Chinese foxglove root) is traditionally considered to be warm and moist,[1342] and is used as a nourishing tonic for Blood and Yin in traditional Chinese medicine.[1343] Conditions which are associated with scanty or absent menstruation, such as hypothalamic amenorrhoea and ovarian insufficiency are often associated with Kidney Yin Deficiency and Blood Deficiency,[1344,1345] and require moist, warming, and nourishing herbs such as *Rehmannia glutinosa*.[1346]

Rehmannia glutinosa also inhibits cortisol metabolism and improves cortisol levels in patients with low cortisol function. This is a similar action to liquorice, but unlike liquorice, *Rehmannia glutinosa* is not contraindicated in patients with hypertension.[1347]

The recommended dose of *Rehmannia glutinosa* is 2–4 g per day of prepared rehmannia root, or 45–90 ml per week of a 1:3 tincture made from prepared rehmannia root. (Prepared rehmannia root consists of fresh root that has been stewed in wine.) It is considered to be safe during pregnancy, and is therefore appropriate for use by those who are actively trying to conceive. However, in Chinese medicine, Rehmannia is traditionally contraindicated in pregnant women with Blood

Deficiency,[1348] and it may therefore be preferable to discontinue its use once conception occurs, as a precaution.

Rosmarinus officinalis

Rosmarinus officinalis, now officially named *Salvia rosmarinus* (rosemary), is an exceptionally useful herb for infertility due to its wide range of actions, particularly on the circulatory system and the liver.

Rosmarinus officinalis was traditionally considered to be diffusively stimulating.[1349] It is still considered by modern Western herbalists to be a circulatory stimulant, which is useful for circulatory weakness with low blood pressure and cold extremities. These are all symptoms that may accompany Kidney Yang Deficiency syndromes, and indeed, *Rosmarinus officinalis* is recommended to treat infertility due to Kidney Yang Deficiency or Uterus Cold.[1350] *Rosmarinus officinalis* is also used to treat symptoms such as headache and muscular pain,[1351] which may be due to its effect on the circulation. Rosemary essential oil may also have some antifungal activity against *Candida albicans*, the microorganism that causes thrush.[1352]

Rosmarinus officinalis was traditionally used as an antispasmodic for painful menstruation,[1353] and is also useful for a variety of other menstrual disorders.[1354] It enhances the detoxifying capacity of the liver,[1355] and improves phase 2 metabolism and elimination of oestrogen in particular,[1356] which is helpful for conditions associated with excess oestrogen, such as endometriosis, fibroids, premenstrual syndrome, and infertility. Energetically, *Rosmarinus officinalis* is considered to be warm and dry.[1357] It reduces Vata and Kapha,[1358] and helps to remove Blood Stagnation.[1359]

The recommended dose of rosemary is 1–2 g of dried herb per day, or 20–45 ml per week of a 1:3 tincture. Rosemary has a reputation of being contraindicated in pregnancy due to its essential oil content. However, normal culinary use of rosemary, and aqueous extracts of rosemary (which contain low levels of essential oil), consumed within the recommended dosage range, are not associated with any harmful effects in pregnancy.

Rubus idaeus

Rubus idaeus (raspberry leaf) is considered to be cool and dry.[1360] It is traditionally used in Western herbal medicine for excessive menstrual bleeding and for uterine prolapse.[1361] It is a uterine tonic, which has a restorative and harmonising effect.[1362] In common with other uterine tonics, it regulates uterine function by relaxing the uterus, but encouraging more effective uterine contractions when required.[1363]

Rubus idaeus is considered to be a nourishing herb,[1364] which is most commonly used during pregnancy as a partus preparator to strengthen and tone the uterus.[1365,1366,1367] However, it has also been used for nausea in pregnancy that extends beyond the first trimester, and to relax the uterus in cases of threatened miscarriage.[1368]

The recommended dose of raspberry leaf is 2–7 g per day of dried leaf by infusion, or 45–150 ml per week of a 1:3 tincture.[1369] Herbs such as raspberry leaf, which contain high levels of tannins, are not recommended for patients with iron deficiency anaemia, malnutrition, or constipation.[1370]

Salvia officinalis

Salvia officinalis (sage) has been traditionally used to decrease production of breast milk.[1371] It binds to GABA receptors,[1372] which reduces prolactin synthesis and release, and also increases dopamine, which in turn further inhibits prolactin.[1373]

Salvia officinalis is very useful for reducing excessive sweating, including hot flushes and night sweating associated with ovarian insufficiency.[1374] It also improves cognitive function, memory, mood, and energy levels, which can deteriorate with declining oestrogen levels in women with ovarian insufficiency.[1375]

Salvia officinalis (sage) is warm, dry, and pungent, and is therefore suitable for treating both Yang Deficiency and Damp patterns, as well as Kapha excess.

The recommended dose of *Salvia officinalis* is 1–2 g per day of dried herb (as capsules or infusion), or 20–45 ml per week of a 1:3 tincture.[1376] Where sage tea is recommended for treatment of hot flushes and night sweats due to ovarian insufficiency, it is best taken cold rather than hot.

Salvia officinalis is contraindicated in pregnancy.[1377] If it is being used for the treatment of reproductive problems in patients who wish to become pregnant, it is preferable to discontinue before actively trying to conceive, in order to avoid any risk in early pregnancy.

Schisandra chinensis

Schisandra chinensis (schisandra berry) is used as an adaptogen and nervine tonic, which improves energy and relieves fatigue.[1378] It is a sour, astringent herb, which is traditionally used for treating damp conditions such as premature ejaculation,[1379] vaginal discharge, and excessive sweating.[1380]

Schisandra chinensis is considered to be warm and dry. It nourishes the Kidney Yang, and may be used to treat conditions associated with Kidney Yang Deficiency,[1381] such as low libido and erectile dysfunction.[1382]

Schisandra chinensis also improves both phase 1 and phase 2 detoxification in the liver.[1383] It is therefore useful for the treatment of conditions associated with oestrogen excess. During phase 1 liver metabolism of oestrogen (hydroxylation), *Schisandra chinensis* tends to favour metabolism of oestradiol to form the more protective *2-hydroxyoestrone*, rather than the more harmful *16-α-hydroxyoestrone*.[1384,1385]

The recommended dose of *Schisandra chinesis* is 1.5–4 g per day, or 35–90 ml per week of a 1:3 tincture. *Schisandra chinesis* is oxytocic and helps to assist labour and reduce complications. It is therefore contraindicated in pregnancy, except to aid childbirth.[1386]

Scutellaria lateriflora

Scutellaria lateriflora (skullcap herb) is traditionally used as a nervine tonic, and antispasmodic herb.[1387] It is considered to be cool and dry.[1388]

Relaxing nervines, such as *Scutellaria lateriflora* can help to reduce stress levels, and help to prevent stress-induced hormonal changes and other stress-related reproductive health problems. For example, hypothalamic amenorrhoea is associated with elevated cortisol levels.[1389] Therefore herbs that relieve stress may help to reverse hypothalamic amenorrhoea. Relaxing nervines such as *Scutellaria lateriflora* may also help with problems such as insomnia,[1390] premenstrual or perimenopausal anxiety and mood changes,[1391] and premature ejaculation.[1392]

The recommended dose of skullcap is 2–4 g per day of dried herb, or 20–45 ml per week of a 1:3 tincture.[1393] It is considered to be safe during pregnancy,[1394] and is therefore suitable for use by women who are trying to conceive.

Serenoa repens

Serenoa repens (saw palmetto fruit) is a warming, astringent herb, which is traditionally considered to be a tonic for the genitourinary system. It is used to improve fertility,[1395] and is thought to remedy any atony of the ovaries or breasts in women, and the testes in men.[1396] It is also recommended for improving libido in women,[1397] and treating erectile dysfunction in men, particularly where this is the result of nervous exhaustion.[1398]

Serenoa repens is an anti-inflammatory and antispasmodic herb,[1399] which is useful for reducing pelvic congestion, ovarian pain,[1400] and dysmenorrhoea.[1401] It inhibits aromatase,[1402] (the enzyme which reduces conversion of androgens to oestrogen). It may therefore also be useful for conditions involving oestrogen excess.

As well as reducing oestrogen excess, *Serenoa repens* may also be useful for reducing the effects of excess androgens. It reduces 5-alpha reductase (the enzyme which converts testosterone to the more potent dihydrotestosterone);[1403] reduces 11ß-hydroxysteroid dehydrogenase (11ß-OHSD), which leads to reduced adrenal androgen production (via reduced cortisol clearance); and is also thought to inhibit androgen receptor binding.[1404]

It may therefore help to reduce symptoms of hyperandrogenism, such as inflammation or benign enlargement of the prostate in men;[1405] and androgenic alopecia or hirsutism in women with PCOS, or other causes of androgen excess.[1406]

The recommended dose of saw palmetto is 1–2 g per day of dried berries; or 20–45 ml per week of a 1:3 tincture.[1407] Saw palmetto is considered to be safe during pregnancy,[1408] and is therefore suitable for use by women who are trying to conceive.

Taraxacum officinale

Taraxacum officinale (dandelion root) is considered to be cold and dry.[1409] It is traditionally used for liver disorders such as chronic hepatic obstruction, and as a mild laxative.[1410,1411] It is also traditionally considered to remove "uterine obstructions".[1412] This is interesting given that constipation is often considered to be part of a picture of "pelvic congestion", and we now understand that hepatic congestion and constipation can significantly contribute to oestrogen excess.

Modern Western herbalists still consider *Taraxacum officinale* to reduce liver congestion,[1413] and to have a restorative effect on hepatic function.[1414,1415,1416] It has a choleretic effect,[1417] and may help to remove excess oestrogen from the body.[1418,1419] It is also thought to act as an aromatase inhibitor, which reduces conversion of androgens to oestrogen.[1420] It is therefore useful for conditions such as endometriosis, fibroids, premenstrual syndrome, and infertility, especially where accompanied by constipation and signs of liver congestion.

The recommended dose of dandelion root is 1.5–3 g per day of dried root; or 30–60 ml per week of a 1:3 tincture.[1421] Dandelion root is considered to be safe during pregnancy,[1422] and is therefore suitable for use by women who are trying to conceive.

Tribulus terrestris

Tribulus terrestris (puncture vine) is sweet and cooling. It is an Ayurvedic herb, which reduces all three Dosha, but it is particularly useful for Vata excess. It is considered to be a nourishing tonic for the reproductive system in both men and women, and it is traditionally used for the treatment of infertility.

Tribulus terrestris contains steroidal saponins such as diosgenin, which compete with endogenous oestrogens for hypothalamic oestrogen receptors. They have a weaker effect on hypothalamic oestrogen receptors than endogenous oestrogen, causing the body to respond as if oestrogen levels are lower than they really are, stimulating the pituitary to increase FSH secretion, which in turn increases oestrogen production.[1423]

This has a beneficial effect on symptoms of ovarian insufficiency, such as hot flushes, night sweats, depression, insomnia, and reduced libido. Improved levels of FSH also lead to improved ovulation, especially when given on days 5–14.[1424]

Tribulus terrestris is also considered to be a rejuvenating tonic for the male reproductive system, and is traditionally used for the treatment of impotence and infertility in men.[1425] It increases sperm count, decreases abnormal forms, and increases libido and overall sexual health.[1426]

The recommended dose of *Tribulus terrestris* is 1–5 g per day of dried aerial parts; or 20–100 ml per week of a 1:3 tincture.[1427] *Tribulus terrestris* is traditionally only used with caution during pregnancy.[1428]

Trigonella foenum graecum

Trigonella foenum graecum (fenugreek seed) is a very warming, demulcent, and nourishing herb. It is traditionally used in Ayurveda for reducing Vata and Kapha excess.[1429] It reduces pelvic congestion, which helps to relieve congestive conditions such as constipation and dysmenorrhoea.[1430]

Trigonella foenum graecum is nourishing to the reproductive system,[1431] improving libido and sexual function in women.[1432] It contains phytoestrogens such as diosgenin,[1433] which compete with endogenous oestrogens for hypothalamic oestrogen receptors.

As previously described, phytoestrogens weakly stimulate hypothalamic oestrogen receptors, causing the body to respond as if oestrogen levels are lower than they really are, stimulating the pituitary to increase FSH, which in turn increases oestrogen production.[1434] This has a beneficial effect on symptoms of low oestrogen, such as hot flushes, night sweats, depression, insomnia, and reduced libido. Improved levels of FSH also lead to improved ovulation when given during the follicular phase.[1435]

Trigonella foenum graecum also reduces elevated blood sugar levels,[1436] which is useful for women with insulin resistance and PCOS. The recommended dose of fenugreek seed is 1–4 g per day, or 20–75 ml per week of a 1:3 tincture. Fenugreek seed is considered to be safe during pregnancy,[1437] and is therefore suitable for use by women who are trying to conceive.

Trillium erectum

Trillium erectum (beth root or "birth root") is an astringent and tonic to the mucous membranes,[1438] which was traditionally used to assist with birth.[1439] It controls uterine bleeding in cases of menorrhagia and metrorrhagia, and helps to reduce excessive vaginal discharge.[1440]

Trillium erectum contains steroidal saponins, which are structurally and functionally similar to human oestrogens.[1441] They have an affinity for oestrogen receptors, exerting a weak oestrogenic affect in comparison to oestradiol.[1442] They act as selective oestrogen receptor modulators (SERMS), which both reduce the symptoms of oestrogen deficiency, and compete with endogenous oestrogen to help reduce its proliferative effects in women with oestrogen excess.[1443]

Trillium erectum is a uterine stimulant,[1444] and is therefore contraindicated in pregnancy, except to assist birth. The recommended dose is 0.5–1 g dried root per day, or 10–20 ml per week of a 1:3 tincture. However it is an endangered plant, and therefore only cultivated sources should be used.[1445]

Turnera diffusa

Turnera diffusa (damiana leaf) is considered to be warm and dry.[1446] It is a nervine tonic, antidepressant, anxiolytic, and aphrodisiac,[1447] which is traditionally used to treat sexual dysfunction, and as a tonic for depression and nervous exhaustion in both men and women.[1448,1449]

Turnera diffusa appears to act as an aromatase inhibitor, which helps to improve testosterone levels, while other constituents appear to have an oestrogenic effect.[1450] It is therefore potentially helpful for addressing conditions that are associated with either low testosterone, or low oestrogen levels. In addition, constituents of *Turnera diffusa* bind to progesterone receptors,[1451] which may be beneficial for women with luteal insufficiency and symptoms of premenstrual syndrome.

From an energetic point of view, *Turnera diffusa* appears to nourish the Kidney Yang, and is therefore useful for the treatment of conditions that are associated with Kidney Yang Deficiency, such as fatigue, low libido, premature ejaculation, constipation, and dysuria.[1452] The recommended dose of *Turnera diffusa* is 1.5–3 g per day of dried damiana leaf, or 30–60 ml of a 1:3 tincture.[1453] It is considered to be safe during pregnancy,[1454] and is therefore suitable for use by women who are actively trying to conceive.

Viburnum opulus

Viburnum opulus (cramp bark) is considered to be cool and dry.[1455] It is an antispasmodic herb,[1456,1457,1458] which is traditionally used for cramps and spasms of all kinds.[1459]

However, it is considered to have a particular affinity for the female reproductive organs, and is used interchangeably with *Viburnum prunifolium* for similar purposes.[1460] It has been used both historically and by modern Western herbalists to treat menstrual pain.[1461,1462,1463]

Viburnum opulus may be useful to improve uterine blood flow in cases of spasmodic dysmenorrhoea.[1464] It can also help to reduce pelvic pain in cases of pelvic inflammatory disease, and other painful, spasmodic or inflammatory conditions of the reproductive organs and tissues, such as endometriosis and vaginismus.[1465,1466]

Viburnum opulus is traditionally used for uterine cramps in pregnancy,[1467] and it is widely recommended to prevent miscarriage.[1468,1469,1470] The recommended dose is 1–2 g per day, or 20–45 ml per week of a 1:3 tincture.[1471]

Viburnum prunifolium

Viburnum prunifolium is considered to be cool and dry.[1472] It was historically used by the physiomedicalist and eclectic physicians to treat spasmodic or cramp-like menstrual pains, especially with excessive menstrual flow.[1473] It is still considered to be a uterine antispasmodic, which calms uterine activity in patients with spasmodic dysmenorrhoea,[1474] and is generally considered to be a specific treatment for the relief of menstrual pain.[1475]

Viburnum prunifolium is also a uterine tonic, which improves circulation and nutrition of the reproductive organs, and reduces uterine inflammation.[1476] It tonifies reproductive Qi for treatment of conditions such as PMS and infertility.[1477]

Perhaps as a result of a combination of the above actions, *Viburnum prunifolium* has been widely used to prevent miscarriage.[1478,1479,1480,1481] It is also useful for morning sickness and various other conditions arising in pregnancy.[1482] The recommended dose is 1–2 g per day, or 20–45 ml per week of a 1:3 tincture.[1483]

Vitex agnus-castus

Vitex agnus-castus (chaste berry) is considered to be warm and dry.[1484] It is traditionally used for its beneficial effect on the female hormonal system.[1485] A great deal of modern research has been conducted on the use of *Vitex agnus-castus* for various endocrine problems, including numerous clinical trials.[1486] However, its precise mechanism of action, and its active constituents have not been fully established.[1487]

It is considered by many herbalists to be normalising or amphoteric in its action on the endocrine system. However, clinical experience shows that it is more effective for problems which occur in the premenstrual or luteal phase, indicating that it exerts a particular influence on the corpus luteum and progesterone function;[1488] and has specific indications, rather than having an overall "balancing" effect.

Vitex agnus-castus addresses a wide range of the problems affecting the female reproductive system during the luteal phase, such as premenstrual mood disturbance, fluid retention, and mastalgia due to poor progesterone function, and hyperprolactinaemia,[1489,1490,1491] possibly as a result of modulation of several different types of hormone receptors, such as dopaminergic and opioid receptors.[1492] It has been shown to increase ovulation and conception in infertile women with hyperprolactinaemia and luteal phase dysfunction,[1493] and is widely recommended by herbalists for the treatment of infertility.[1494]

Vitex agnus-castus appears to have dopaminergic properties.[1495] This causes inhibition of prolactin release from the anterior pituitary, which leads to an increase in luteinising hormone (LH), promoting corpus luteum development in the luteal phase, and thereby increasing levels of progesterone.[1496]

Hypothalamic amenorrhoea is associated with low LH.[1497] Therefore, *Vitex agnus-castus* may help to reverse hypothalamic amenorrhoea due to improved LH secretion.[1498] Improved luteal function also leads to an increase in progesterone levels, which is useful for conditions involving oestrogen excess, such as endometriosis and uterine fibroids. *Vitex agnus-castus* also reduces bleeding in menorrhagia (which is often associated with conditions such as uterine fibroids) particularly after several months of use.[1499]

In addition to its effects on the female reproductive system, *Vitex agnus-castus* has also been shown to be effective for acne in both men and women, which may be associated with conditions involving androgen excess. It also increases melatonin secretion and can help with insomnia,[1500] which is frequently associated with reproductive hormone imbalances in conditions such as premenstrual syndrome and ovarian insufficiency.

Vitex agnus-castus is traditionally used to decrease libido in men, and may therefore be useful in some cases of premature ejaculation. It is also useful in cases of erectile dysfunction and infertility in men, where these are due to hyperprolactinaemia.[1501]

Vitex agnus-castus is considered to be safe during pregnancy,[1502] and where a woman is taking it before conception for luteal insufficiency, it is important to continue, in order to ensure effective corpus luteum function in the early stages of pregnancy.

The common practice among herbalists of prescribing *Vitex agnus-castus* as a single dose first thing in the morning has no clinical or pharmacological basis.[1503] It is said to be based on the notion that the pituitary gland is more "active" in the morning. However, in reality, the pituitary gland is active throughout the day and night, secreting various pituitary hormones in a variety of different rhythms. While the amplitude of adrenocorticotrophic hormone (ACTH) secretion peaks in the early morning (leading to increased secretion of cortisol from the adrenal glands), pulsatile secretion of LH occurs approximately once every one to one and a half hours, throughout each twenty-four hour period,[1504] and LH pulses are of greater magnitude during the night.[1505] Therefore administration of *Vitex agnus-castus* as part of an overall prescription is likely to be just as effective as a single dose in the morning.

Very low doses (38–120 mg per day of dried herb or 0.75–2.5 ml per week of a 1:3 tincture) may increase prolactin levels.[1506] This may be useful to increase milk supply in women who are breastfeeding, but can be counterproductive in the treatment of conditions involving hyperprolactinaemia or poor progesterone function.

Low doses of *Vitex agnus-castus* (equivalent to 200–500 mg a day of dried herb or 4–10 ml per week of a 1:3 tincture) are generally sufficient for conditions resulting from latent hyperprolactinaemia or luteal phase dysfunction, such as menstrual cycle irregularities, premenstrual syndrome, mastalgia, perimenopausal symptoms, and infertility related to hyperprolactinaemia. Higher doses (2.5–5 g per day of dried herb, or 17.5–35 ml per week of a 1:1 fluid extract), may be required to reduce prolactin levels in cases of hyperprolactinaemia, or to exert a significant oestrogen or androgen antagonist effect in conditions involving excess oestrogen (such as endometriosis or uterine fibroids), or hyperandrogenism (such as acne or excessive male sex drive).[1507]

Withania somnifera

Withania somnifera (ashwagandha root) is an Ayurvedic herb, which reduces Vata and Kapha, but increases Pitta. It is considered to be a rejuvinative tonic to the reproductive and nervous systems, and is used to treat conditions such as nervous exhaustion and infertility.[1508]

Withania somnifera has been traditionally used to enhance reproductive function. It is considered to have aphrodisiac effects and has been used to promote conception.[1509] It is a nourishing herb, which is useful for treating anaemia,[1510] and for patients with low body weight and athletic exertion.[1511] It may therefore be useful for hypothalamic amenorrhoea, which is associated with insufficient nutrition or overexercise.

Withania somnifera also possesses hypoglycaemic activity that is comparable to oral hypoglycaemic drugs.[1512] Since improved insulin sensitivity is associated with improved ovulatory function and fertility,[1513] this may be one of the mechanisms by which *Withania somnifera* can help to promote conception.

Withania somnifera has nervine and adaptogenic properties and is therefore useful during episodes of prolonged stress. It is a relaxing herb, which can be used to reduce tension, improve sleep patterns,[1514] and help to prevent stress-induced hormonal changes.[1515] *Withania somnifera* has also been shown to improve sexual function and diminished sexual distress in women with dyspareunia and/or vaginismus due to psychogenic causes.[1516]

Adaptogens and adrenal tonics, such as *Withania somnifera*, improve adrenal function,[1517] and may thereby help to increase adrenal production of progesterone and its metabolites. *Withania somnifera* has also been shown to increase levels of DHEA.[1518]

DHEA is essential for oestrogen production in the ovary. It also enhances insulin-like growth factor (IGF-I), which is involved in follicular growth; and improves AMH levels, which reflects an increased number of developing primary follicles. DHEA may also improve ovarian reserve by increasing recruitment of follicles from the dormant primordial follicular pool; and reducing apoptosis (the process by which recruited follicles are destroyed).[1519]

Increasing DHEA levels with *Withania somnifera* may therefore be very beneficial for women with low ovarian reserve or primary ovarian insufficiency, to increase the number of available follicles and improve egg quality. DHEA supplementation has been shown to significantly improve outcomes in women undergoing in vitro fertilisation or intracytoplasmic sperm injection (IVF/ICSI),[1520] and it is possible that *Withania somnifera* may also have a beneficial effect as a result of its ability to improve endogenous DHEA.

Withania somnifera is also traditionally used in Ayurvedic medicine for the treatment of male sexual dysfunction and infertility. It is a relaxing adaptogen, which makes it particularly useful for men suffering from nervous exhaustion, stress, and anxiety.[1521] It is particularly suited to men suffering from Vata disturbance.[1522]

Withania somnifera improves LH and androgen production,[1523] reduces oxidative stress, and improves semen quality,[1524] increasing semen volume, sperm count, and motility.[1525] However, there have been anecdotal reports of *Withania* decreasing sperm motility in some individuals.

Withania somnifera can also reduce autoimmunity,[1526] and increase thyroid function in both men and women with hypothyroidism.[1527] In addition, it improves white blood cell count,[1528] which is a useful adjunct in cases of chronic infection.

The recommended dose of ashwagandha is 3–9 g per day of the dried root,[1529] or 15–45 ml per week of a 1:1 fluid extract.[1530] Ashwagandha is considered to be safe to use during pregnancy,[1531] and was traditionally used during pregnancy to strengthen the uterus and nourish the blood.[1532]

Zingiber officinale

Zingiber officinale (ginger root) is a diffusive circulatory stimulant,[1533] which is traditionally used to stimulate the peripheral circulation, particularly in individuals with cold extremities.[1534] It can also be used to improve pelvic circulation and thereby relieve uterine ischaemia, which may be responsible for dysmenorrhoea.[1535] It is particularly useful for dysmenorrhoea that is better for application of warmth.[1536]

Zingiber officinale has been shown to reduce the production of prostaglandin PGE2,[1537] which helps to reduce inflammation and excessive uterine contractions. It is therefore useful for reducing pelvic pain not only in cases of dysmenorrhoea, but also in other painful, spasmodic, or inflammatory conditions of the reproductive organs and tissues, such as pelvic inflammatory disease, endometriosis, and vaginismus.[1538,1539]

Zingiber officinale has been shown to significantly reduce nausea and vomiting in early pregnancy,[1540,1541] and may be prescribed in combination with *Ballota nigra* and *Matricaria recutita* for this purpose with excellent results. It is considered to be hot and dry, and is useful for treating conditions associated with Kidney Yang Deficiency and Uterus Cold.[1542] It is also used in traditional Chinese medicine as part of formulae to treat Qi Stagnation and remove excess Dampness.[1543]

The recommended dose of *Zingiber officinale* is 250 mg–1 g per day of dried ginger root (or an equivalent quantity of fresh root), or 5–20 ml per week of a 1:3 tincture.

Notes

1024. Mills, S. (1991). *The Essential Book of Herbal Medicine*. London: Pengiun Arkana.

1025. Wood, M. (2004). *The Practice of Traditional Western Herbalism: Basic Doctrine, Energetics and Classification*. Berkeley, CA: North Atlantic.

1026. Rogers, C. (1999). *The Woman's Guide to Herbal Medicine* [online]. Available from http://womans-herbal-guide.com/publications (accessed 27 January 2009).

1027. Cox, E., & Takov, V. (2019). Embryology, ovarian follicle development. *StatPearls* [online]. Available from https://ncbi.nlm.nih.gov/books/NBK532300/ (accessed 3 April 2020).

1028. Erickson, G. (2008). Follicle growth and development. *Global Libary of Women's Medicine* [online]. Available from: https://glowm.com (accessed 3 April 2020).

1029. Rogers, C. (1999). *The Woman's Guide to Herbal Medicine* [online]. Available from http://womans-herbal-guide.com/publications (accessed 27 January 2009).

1030. Daya, S. (2009). Luteal support: Progestogens for pregnancy protection. *Maturitas*, 65(1): S29–S34.

1031. Schindler, A. E. (2004). First trimester endocrinology: consequences for diagnosis and treatment of pregnancy failure. *Gynecological Endocrinology*, 18(1): 51–57.

1032. Wuttke, W., Pitzel, L., Seidlova-Wuttke, D., & Hinney, B. (2001). LH pulses and the corpus luteum: the luteal phase deficiency (LPD). *Vitamins & Hormones*, 63: 131–158.

1033. Glenville, M. (2000). *Natural Solutions to Infertility*. London: Piatkus.

1034. Shinde, P., Patil, P., & Bairaji, V. (2012). Herbs in pregnancy and lactation: a review appraisal. *International Journal of Pharmaceutical Sciences and Research*, 3(9): 3001–3006.

1035. Mills, S., & Bone, K. (2005). *The Essential Guide to Herbal Safety*. London: Churchill Livingstone.

1036. Ernst, E. (2002). Herbal medicinal products during pregnancy: are they safe? *BJOG: An International Journal of Obstetrics and Gynaecology*, 109(227–235).

1037. Holmes, P. (2007). *The Energetics of Western Herbs: A Materia Medica Integrating Western & Chinese Herbal Therapeutics, Volume 2* (4th edn). Santa Rosa, CA: Snow Lotus.

1038. Mills, S. (1991). *The Essential Book of Herbal Medicine*. London: Penguin Arkana.

1039. Heron, S. (1989). Botanical treatment of chronic gynecological conditions: infertility, endometriosis, and symptoms of menopause. In: Tierra, M. (1992). *American Herbalism* (pp. 122–143). Trumansberg, NY: The Crossing Press.

1040. Trickey, R. (2003). *Women, Hormones & the Menstrual Cycle*. Sydney, Australia: Allen & Unwin.

1041. Holmes, P. (2007). *The Energetics of Western Herbs: A Materia Medica Integrating Western & Chinese Herbal Therapeutics, Volume 2* (4th edn). Santa Rosa, CA: Snow Lotus.

1042. Lapraz, J. C. (2008). *Clinical Phytotherapy and Osteoporosis*. London: British Endobiogenic Medicine Society.

1043. Hoffman, D. (2009). Infertility [online]. Available from http://healthy.net/scr/Article.asp?id=1182 (accessed 28 January 2009).

1044. Wood, M. (2004). *The Practice of Traditional Western Herbalism: Basic Doctrine, Energetics and Classification*. Berkeley, CA: North Atlantic.

1045. Weiss, R. (1988). *Herbal Medicine*. Gothenburg, Sweden: Arcanum.

1046. Wood, M. (2004). *The Practice of Traditional Western Herbalism: Basic Doctrine, Energetics and Classification*. Berkeley, CA: North Atlantic.

1047. Hoffman, D. (2003). *Medical Herbalism: The Science and Practice of Herbal Medicine*. Rochester, VT: Healing Arts.

1048. Frawley, D., & Lad, V. (2001). *The Yoga of Herbs: An Ayurvedic Guide to Herbal Medicine*. Twin Lakes, WI: Lotus.

1049. Holmes, P. (2007). *The Energetics of Western Herbs: A Materia Medica Integrating Western & Chinese Herbal Therapeutics, Volume 2* (4th edn). Santa Rosa, CA: Snow Lotus.

1050. Mills, S., & Bone, K. (2005). *The Essential Guide to Herbal Safety*. London: Churchill Livingstone.

1051. Bone, K. (2003). *A Clinical Guide to Blending Liquid Herbs*. London: Churchill Livingstone.

1052. Holmes, P. (2007). *The Energetics of Western Herbs: A Materia Medica Integrating Western & Chinese Herbal Therapeutics, Volume 2* (4th edn). Santa Rosa, CA: Snow Lotus.

1053. Felter, H. W., & Lloyd, J. U. (1898). *King's American Dispensatory* [online]. Available from http://henriettesherbal.com/eclectic/kings/index.html (accessed 5 March 2020).

1054. Fang, Y. Zhao, L. Yan, F., Xia, X., Xu, D., & Cui, X. (2010). Escin improves sperm quality in male patients with varicocele-associated infertility. *Phytomedicine, 17*(3–4): 192–196.

1055. Mills, S. (1991). *The Essential Book of Herbal Medicine*. London: Penguin Arkana.

1056. Mills, S., & Bone, K. (2005). *The Essential Guide to Herbal Safety*. London: Churchill Livingstone.

1057. Mills, S. (1991). *The Essential Book of Herbal Medicine*. London: Penguin Arkana.

1058. Weiss, R., & Fintelmann, V. (2000). *Herbal Medicine* (2nd edn). Stuttgart, Germany: Thieme.

1059. Holmes, P. (2007). *The Energetics of Western Herbs: A Materia Medica Integrating Western & Chinese Herbal Therapeutics, Volume 2* (4th edn). Santa Rosa, CA: Snow Lotus.

1060. Grieve, M. (1931). *A Modern Herbal* [online]. Available from http://botanical.com (accessed 3 March 2020).

1061. Hoffman, D. (1990). *The New Holistic Herbal*. Shaftesbury, UK: Element.

1062. Wood, M. (2004). *The Practice of Traditional Western Herbalism: Basic Doctrine, Energetics and Classification*. Berkeley, CA: North Atlantic.

1063. Lapraz, J. C. (2008). *Clinical Phytotherapy and Osteoporosis*. London: British Endobiogenic Medicine Society.

1064. Wood, M. (1997). *The Book of Herbal Wisdom: Using Plants as Medicines*. Berkeley, CA: North Atlantic.

1065. Shinde, P., Patil, P., & Bairaji, V. (2012). Herbs in pregnancy and lactation: a review appraisal. *International Journal of Pharmaceutical Sciences and Research, 3*(9): 3001–3006.

1066. Pole, S. (2006). *Ayurvedic Medicine: The Principles of Traditional Practice*. London: Churchill Livingstone.

1067. Pole, S. (2006). *Ayurvedic Medicine: The Principles of Traditional Practice*. London: Churchill Livingstone.

1068. Bone, K., & Mills, S. (2013). *Principles and Practice of Phytotherapy: Modern Herbal Medicine*. London: Churchill Livingstone.

1069. Mills, S., & Bone, K. (2005). *The Essential Guide to Herbal Safety*. London: Churchill Livingstone.

1070. Holmes, P. (2007). *The Energetics of Western Herbs: A Materia Medica Integrating Western & Chinese Herbal Therapeutics, Volume 1* (4th edn). Santa Rosa, CA: Snow Lotus.

1071. Grieve, M. (1931). *A Modern Herbal* [online]. Available from: http://botanical.com (accessed 3 March 2020).

1072. Lloyd Brothers Pharmacists Inc. (1913). *A Treatise on Pulsatilla* [online]. Available from http://herbaltherapeutics.net/Pulsatilla.doc.pdf (accessed 6 March 2020).

1073. Hoffman, D. (1990). *The New Holistic Herbal*. Shaftesbury, UK: Element.

1074. Trickey, R. (2003). *Women, Hormones & the Menstrual Cycle*. Sydney, Australia: Allen & Unwin.

1075. Grieve, M. (1931). *A Modern Herbal* [online]. Available from http://botanical.com (accessed 3 March 2020).

1076. Lloyd Brothers Pharmacists Inc. (1913). *A Treatise on Pulsatilla* [online]. Available from http://herbaltherapeutics.net/Pulsatilla.doc.pdf (accessed 6 March 2020).

1077. Bartram, T. (1995). *Encyclopedia of Herbal Medicine*. Christchurch, UK: Grace.

1078. Mills, S., & Bone, K. (2005). *The Essential Guide to Herbal Safety*. London: Churchill Livingstone.

1079. Shinde, P., Patil, P., & Bairaji, V. (2012). Herbs in pregnancy and lactation: a review appraisal. *International Journal of Pharmaceutical Sciences and Research*, 3(9): 3001–3006.

1080. Bone, K. (2003). *A Clinical Guide to Blending Liquid Herbs*. London: Churchill Livingstone.

1081. Holmes, P. (2007). *The Energetics of Western Herbs: A Materia Medica Integrating Western & Chinese Herbal Therapeutics, Volume 2* (4th edn). Santa Rosa, CA: Snow Lotus.

1082. Frawley, D., & Lad, V. (2001). *The Yoga of Herbs: An Ayurvedic Guide to Herbal Medicine*. Twin Lakes, WI: Lotus.

1083. Rogers, C. (1999). *The Woman's Guide to Herbal Medicine* [online]. Available from http://womans-herbal-guide.com/publications (accessed 27 January 2009).

1084. Chevallier, A. (1996). *The Encyclopedia of Medicinal Plants*. Oxford: Blackwell.

1085. Holmes, P. (2007). *The Energetics of Western Herbs: A Materia Medica Integrating Western & Chinese Herbal Therapeutics, Volume 1* (4th edn). Santa Rosa, CA: Snow Lotus.

1086. Mills, S. (1991). *The Essential Book of Herbal Medicine*. London: Penguin Arkana.

1087. Tillotson, A. K. (2001). *The One Earth Herbal Sourcebook*. New York: Kensington.

1088. Trickey, R. (2003). *Women, Hormones & the Menstrual Cycle*. Sydney, Australia: Allen & Unwin.

1089. Yeung, H. C. (1996). *Handbook of Chinese Herbs*. Los Angeles, CA: Institute of Chinese Medicine.

1090. Trickey, R. (2003). *Women, Hormones & the Menstrual Cycle*. Sydney, Australia: Allen & Unwin.

1091. Liu, W., & Gong, C. (2009). Opening the blockage to reproduction: infertility. *Traditional Chinese Medicine Information Page* [online]. Available from http://tcmpage.com/hpinfertility.html (accessed 4 March 2020).

1092. Tillotson, A. K. (2001). *The One Earth Herbal Sourcebook*. New York: Kensington.

1093. Tillotson, A. K. (2001). *The One Earth Herbal Sourcebook*. New York: Kensington.

1094. Liu, W., & Gong, C. (2009). Opening the blockage to reproduction: infertility. *Traditional Chinese Medicine Information Page* [online]. Available from http://tcmpage.com/hpinfertility.html (accessed 4 March 2020).

1095. Mills, S., & Bone, K. (2005). *The Essential Guide to Herbal Safety*. London: Churchill Livingstone.

1096. Pole, S. (2006). *Ayurvedic Medicine: The Principles of Traditional Practice*. London: Churchill Livingstone.

1097. Pole, S. (2006). *Ayurvedic Medicine: The Principles of Traditional Practice*. London: Churchill Livingstone.

1098. Middlebrooks, Z. (2015). An Ayurvedic approach to the treatment of secondary amenorrhoea. *California College of Ayurveda* [online]. Available from https://ayurvedacollege.com/articles/students/Secondary-Amenorrhea (accessed 17 March 2020).

1099. Pole, S. (2006). *Ayurvedic Medicine: The Principles of Traditional Practice*. London: Churchill Livingstone.

1100. Brice-Ytsma, H. & McDermott, A. (2020). *Herbal Medicine in Treating Gynaecological Conditions*. London: Aeon.

1101. Bone, K., & Mills, S. (2013). *Principles and Practice of Phytotherapy: Modern Herbal Medicine*. London: Churchill Livingstone.

1102. Mills, S., & Bone, K. (2005). *The Essential Guide to Herbal Safety*. London: Churchill Livingstone.

1103. Holmes, P. (2007). *The Energetics of Western Herbs: A Materia Medica Integrating Western & Chinese Herbal Therapeutics, Volume 1* (4th edn). Santa Rosa, CA: Snow Lotus.

1104. Mills, S., & Bone, K. (2005). *The Essential Guide to Herbal Safety*. London: Churchill Livingstone.

1105. Hong, C. Y., Ku, J., & Wu, P. (1992). *Astragalus membranaceus* stimulates human sperm motility in vitro. *American Journal of Chinese Medicine*, 20(3–4): 289–294.

1106. Bone, K., & Mills, S. (2013). *Principles and Practice of Phytotherapy: Modern Herbal Medicine*. London: Churchill Livingstone.

1107. Mills, S., & Bone, K. (2005). *The Essential Guide to Herbal Safety*. London: Churchill Livingstone.

1108. Balunas, M. J., Su, B., Brueggemeier, R. W., & Kinghorn, A. D. (2011). Natural products as aromatase inhibitors. *Anti-Cancer Agents in Medicinal Chemistry*, 8(6): 646–682.

1109. Balunas, M. J., Su, B., Brueggemeier, R. W., & Kinghorn, A. D. (2011). Natural products as aromatase inhibitors. *Anti-Cancer Agents in Medicinal Chemistry*, 8(6): 646–682.

1110. Hu, J., Webster, D., Cao, J., & Shao, A. (2018). The safety of green tea and green tea extract consumption in adults – results of a systematic review. *Regulatory Toxicology and Pharmacology*, 95: 412–433.

1111. Lu, J. H., He, J. R., Shen, S. Y., Wei, X.-L., Chen, N.-N., Yuan, M.-Y., Qiu, L., Li, W.-D., Chen, Q-Z., Hu, C.-Y., Xia, H.-M., Bartington, S., Cheng, K. K., Lam, K. B. H., & Qiu, X. (2017). Does tea consumption during early pregnancy have an adverse effect on birth outcomes? *Birth*, 44(3): 281–289.

1112. Bone, K., & Mills, S. (2013). *Principles and Practice of Phytotherapy: Modern Herbal Medicine*. London: Churchill Livingstone.

1113. Brice-Ytsma, H., & McDermott, A. (2020). *Herbal Medicine in Treating Gynaecological Conditions*. London: Aeon.

1114. Felter, H. W., & Lloyd, J. U. (1898). *King's American Dispensatory* [online]. Available from http://henriettesherbal.com/eclectic/kings/index.html (accessed 5 March 2020).

1115. Grieve, M. (1931). *A Modern Herbal* [online]. Available from http://botanical.com (accessed 3 March 2020).

1116. Romm, A. (2016). *Botanical Medicine for Women's Health* (2nd edn). London: Churchill Livingtstone.

1117. Holmes, P. (2007). *The Energetics of Western Herbs: A Materia Medica Integrating Western & Chinese Herbal Therapeutics, Volume 2* (4th edn). Santa Rosa, CA: Snow Lotus.

1118. Mills, S., & Bone, K. (2005). *The Essential Guide to Herbal Safety*. London: Churchill Livingstone.

1119. Dennehy, C. E. (2006). The use of herbs and dietary supplements in gynecology: an evidence-based review. *Journal of Midwifery & Women's Health, 51*: 402–409.

1120. Wuttke, W., Gorkow, C., & Seidlóva-Wuttke, D. (2006). Effects of black cohosh *(Cimicifuga racemosa)* on bone turnover, vaginal mucosa, and various blood parameters in postmenopausal women: a double-blind, placebo-controlled, and conjugated oestrogens-controlled study. *Menopause, 13*(2): 185–196.

1121. Bone, K., & Mills, S. (2013). *Principles and Practice of Phytotherapy: Modern Herbal Medicine*. London: Churchill Livingstone.

1122. Romm, A. (2016). *Botanical Medicine for Women's Health* (2nd edn). London: Churchill Livingstone.

1123. Trickey, R. (2011). *Women, Hormones and the Menstrual Cycle*. Clifton Hill, Victoria, Australia: Melbourne Holistic Health Group.

1124. Dennehy, C. E. (2006). The use of herbs and dietary supplements in gynecology: an evidence-based review. *Journal of Midwifery & Women's Health, 51*: 402–409.

1125. Brice-Ytsma, H., & McDermott, A. (2020). *Herbal Medicine in Treating Gynaecological Conditions*. London: Aeon.

1126. Bone, K. (2003). *A Clinical Guide to Blending Liquid Herbs*. London: Churchill Livingstone.

1127. Mills, S., & Bone, K. (2005). *The Essential Guide to Herbal Safety*. London: Churchill Livingstone.

1128. Trickey, R. (2003). *Women, Hormones & the Menstrual Cycle*. Sydney, Australia: Allen & Unwin.

1129. Felter, H. W., & Lloyd, J. U. (1898) *King's American Dispensatory* [online]. Available from http://henriettesherbal.com/eclectic/kings/index.html (accessed 20 May 2020).

1130. Grieve, M. (1931). *A Modern Herbal* [online]. Available from: http://botanical.com (accessed 20 May 2020).

1131. Davis, P. A., & Yokoyama, W. (2011). Cinnamon intake lowers fasting blood glucose: meta-analysis. *Journal of Medicinal Food, 14*(9): 884–889.

1132. Wang, J. G., Anderson, R. A., Graham, G. M., Chu, M. C., Sauer, M. V., Guarnaccia, M. M., & Lobo, R. A. (2001). The effect of cinnamon extract on insulin resistance parameters in polycystic ovary syndrome: a pilot study. *Nutrition, 17*(4): 315–321.

1133. Chavarro, J. E., Rich-Edwards, J. W., Rosner, B. A., & Willett, W. C. (2009). A prospective study of dietary carbohydrate quantity and quality in relation to risk of ovulatory infertility. *European Journal of Clinical Nutrition, 63*(1): 78–86.

1134. Holmes, P. (2007). *The Energetics of Western Herbs: A Materia Medica Integrating West-ern & Chinese Herbal Therapeutics, Volume 1* (4th edn). Santa Rosa, CA: Snow Lotus.

1135. Liu, W., & Gong, C. (2009). Opening the blockage to reproduction: infertility. *Tra-ditional Chinese Medicine Information Page* [online]. Available from http://tcmpage.com/hpinfertility.html (accessed 4 March 2020).

1136. Frawley, D., & Lad, V. (2001). *The Yoga of Herbs: An Ayurvedic Guide to Herbal Medi-cine*. Twin Lakes, WI: Lotus.

1137. Pole, S. (2006). *Ayurvedic Medicine: The Principles of Traditional Practice*. London: Churchill Livingstone.

1138. De Smet, P. A. G. M., Keller, K., Hänsel, R., & Chandler, R. F. (1992). *Adverse Effects of Herbal Drugs*. Berlin: Springer.

1139. Bone, K. (2003). *A Clinical Guide to Blending Liquid Herbs*. London: Churchill Livingstone.

1140. Holmes, P. (2007). *The Energetics of Western Herbs: A Materia Medica Integrating Western & Chinese Herbal Therapeutics, Volume 2* (4th edn). Santa Rosa, CA: Snow Lotus.

1141. Felter, H. W., & Lloyd, J. U. (1898). *King's American Dispensatory* [online]. Available from http://henriettesherbal.com/eclectic/kings/index.html (accessed 20 May 2020).

1142. Romm, A. (2016). *Botanical Medicine for Women's Health* (2nd edn). London: Churchill Livingstone.

1143. Dennehy, C. E. (2006). The use of herbs and dietary supplements in gynecology: an evidence-based review. *Journal of Midwifery & Women's Health*, 51: 402–409.

1144. Brice-Ytsma, H., & McDermott, A. (2020). *Herbal Medicine in Treating Gynaecological Conditions*. London: Aeon.

1145. Ye, Y. B., Tang, X. Y., Verbruggen, M. A., & Su, Y. X. (2006). Soy isoflavones attenu-ate bone loss in early postmenopausal Chinese women: a single-blind randomized, placebo-controlled trial. *European Journal of Nutrition*, 45: 327–334.

1146. Tabakova, P., Dimitrov, M., & Tashkov, B. (2012). Clinical studies on Tribulus ter-restris protodioscin in women with endocrine infertility or menopausal syndrome. *Herbpharm USA* [online]. Available from http://scicompdf.se/tiggarnot/tabakova-HerbPharmUSA.pdf (accessed 2 March 2020).

1147. Bone, K., & Mills, S. (2013). *Principles and Practice of Phytotherapy: Modern Herbal Medicine*. London: Churchill Livingstone.

1148. Bone, K., & Mills, S. (2013). *Principles and Practice of Phytotherapy: Modern Herbal Medicine*. London: Churchill Livingstone.

1149. Brice-Ytsma, H., & McDermott, A. (2020). *Herbal Medicine in Treating Gynaecological Conditions*. London: Aeon.

1150. Tabakova, P., Dimitrov, M., & Tashkov, B. (2012). Clinical studies on Tribulus ter-restris protodioscin in women with endocrine infertility or menopausal syndrome. *Herbpharm USA* [online]. Available from http://scicompdf.se/tiggarnot/tabakova-HerbPharmUSA.pdf (accessed 2 March 2020).

1151. Brice-Ytsma, H., & McDermott, A. (2020). *Herbal Medicine in Treating Gynaecological Conditions*. London: Aeon.

1152. Brice-Ytsma, H., & McDermott, A. (2020). *Herbal Medicine in Treating Gynaecological Conditions*. London: Aeon.

1153. Trickey, R. (2003). *Women, Hormones & the Menstrual Cycle*. Sydney, Australia: Allen & Unwin.
1154. Romm, A. (2016). *Botanical Medicine for Women's Health* (2nd edn). London: Churchill Livingstone.
1155. Bone, K. (2003). *A Clinical Guide to Blending Liquid Herbs*. London: Churchill Livingstone.
1156. Bone, K., & Mills, S. (2013). *Principles and Practice of Phytotherapy: Modern Herbal Medicine*. London: Churchill Livingstone.
1157. Lebovic, D. I., Mueller, M. D., & Taylor, R. N. (2001). Immunobiology of endometriosis. *Fertility and Sterility*, 75(1): 1–10.
1158. Bone, K., & Mills, S. (2013). *Principles and Practice of Phytotherapy: Modern Herbal Medicine*. London: Churchill Livingstone.
1159. Trickey, R. (2011). *Women, Hormones and the Menstrual Cycle*. Clifton Hill, Victoria, Australia: Melbourne Holistic Health Group.
1160. Bone, K., & Mills, S. (2013). *Principles and Practice of Phytotherapy: Modern Herbal Medicine*. London: Churchill Livingstone.
1161. Bone, K., & Mills, S. (2013). *Principles and Practice of Phytotherapy: Modern Herbal Medicine*. London: Churchill Livingstone.
1162. Holmes, P. (2007). *The Energetics of Western Herbs: A Materia Medica Integrating Western & Chinese Herbal Therapeutics, Volume 2* (4th edn). Santa Rosa, CA: Snow Lotus.
1163. Mills, S., & Bone, K. (2005). *The Essential Guide to Herbal Safety*. London: Churchill Livingstone.
1164. Bone, K. (2003). *A Clinical Guide to Blending Liquid Herbs*. London: Churchill Livingstone.
1165. Panossian, A., & Wagner, H. (2005). Stimulating effect of adaptogens: an overview with particular reference to their efficacy following single dose administration. *Phytotherapy Resources*, 19(10): 819–838.
1166. Chevallier, A. (1996). *The Encyclopedia of Medicinal Plants*. Oxford: Blackwell.
1167. Hoffman, D. (1990). *The New Holistic Herbal*. Shaftesbury, UK: Element.
1168. Holmes, P. (2007). *The Energetics of Western Herbs: A Materia Medica Integrating Western & Chinese Herbal Therapeutics, Volume 1* (4th edn). Santa Rosa, CA: Snow Lotus.
1169. Panossian, A., & Wagner, H. (2005). Stimulating effect of adaptogens: an overview with particular reference to their efficacy following single dose administration. *Phytotherapy Resources*, 19(10): 819–838.
1170. Trickey, R. (2003). *Women, Hormones & the Menstrual Cycle*. Sydney, Australia: Allen & Unwin.
1171. Holmes, P. (2007). *The Energetics of Western Herbs: A Materia Medica Integrating Western & Chinese Herbal Therapeutics, Volume 1* (4th edn). Santa Rosa, CA: Snow Lotus.
1172. Brice-Ytsma, H., & McDermott, A. (2020). *Herbal Medicine in Treating Gynaecological Conditions*. London: Aeon.
1173. Mills, S., & Bone, K. (2005). *The Essential Guide to Herbal Safety*. London: Churchill Livingstone.
1174. Mills, S., & Bone, K. (2005). *The Essential Guide to Herbal Safety*. London: Churchill Livingstone.
1175. Bone, K. (2003). *A Clinical Guide to Blending Liquid Herbs*. London: Churchill Livingstone.

1176. Holmes, P. (2007). *The Energetics of Western Herbs: A Materia Medica Integrating Western & Chinese Herbal Therapeutics, Volume 1* (4th edn). Santa Rosa, CA: Snow Lotus.

1177. Ellingwood, F. (1919). *The American Materia Medica* [online]. Available from http:// henriettesherbal.com/eclectic/ellingwood/index.html (accessed 3 May 2020).

1178. Mills, S., & Bone, K. (2005). *The Essential Guide to Herbal Safety*. London: Churchill Livingstone.

1179. Holmes, P. (2007). *The Energetics of Western Herbs: A Materia Medica Integrating Western & Chinese Herbal Therapeutics, Volume 1* (4th edn). Santa Rosa, CA: Snow Lotus.

1180. Bone, K., & Mills, S. (2013). *Principles and Practice of Phytotherapy: Modern Herbal Medicine*. London: Churchill Livingstone.

1181. Lagrue, G., Behar, A., Kazandjian, M., & Rahbar, K. (1986). Idiopathic cyclic edema. The role of capillary hyperpermeability and its correction by Ginkgo biloba extract. *Presse Médicale, 15*(31): 1550–1553.

1182. Bone, K., & Mills, S. (2013). *Principles and Practice of Phytotherapy: Modern Herbal Medicine*. London: Churchill Livingstone.

1183. Cohen, A., & Bartlik, B. (1998). Ginkgo biloba for antidepressant-induced sexual dysfunction. *Journal of Sex and Marital Therapy, 24*(2): 139–143.

1184. Bone, K. (2003). *A Clinical Guide to Blending Liquid Herbs*. London: Churchill Livingstone.

1185. Dennehy, C. E. (2006). The use of herbs and dietary supplements in gynecology: an evidence-based review. *Journal of Midwifery & Women's Health, 51*: 402–409.

1186. Brice-Ytsma, H., & McDermott, A. (2020). *Herbal Medicine in Treating Gynaecological Conditions*. London: Aeon.

1187. Ye, Y. B., Tang, X. Y., Verbruggen, M. A., & Su, Y. X. (2006). Soy isoflavones attenuate bone loss in early postmenopausal Chinese women: a single-blind randomized, placebo-controlled trial. *European Journal of Nutrition, 45*: 327–334.

1188. Tabakova, P., Dimitrov, M., & Tashkov, B. (2012). Clinical studies on Tribulus terrestris protodioscin in women with endocrine infertility or menopausal syndrome. *Herbpharm USA* [online]. Available from http://scicompdf.se/tiggarnot/tabakova-HerbPharmUSA.pdf (accessed 2 March 2020).

1189. Bone, K., & Mills, S. (2013). *Principles and Practice of Phytotherapy: Modern Herbal Medicine*. London: Churchill Livingstone.

1190. Bone, K., & Mills, S. (2013). *Principles and Practice of Phytotherapy: Modern Herbal Medicine*. London: Churchill Livingstone.

1191. Zhang, X., Shu, X. O., Li, H., Yang, G., Li, Q., Gao, Y.-T., & Zheng, W. (2005). Prospective cohort study of soy food consumption and risk of bone fracture among postmenopausal women. *Archives of Internal Medicine, 165*(16): 1890–1895.

1192. Brice-Ytsma, H., & McDermott, A. (2020). *Herbal Medicine in Treating Gynaecological Conditions*. London: Aeon.

1193. Tabakova, P., Dimitrov, M., & Tashkov, B. (2012). Clinical studies on Tribulus terrestris protodioscin in women with endocrine infertility or menopausal syndrome. *Herbpharm USA* [online]. Available from http://scicompdf.se/tiggarnot/tabakova-HerbPharmUSA.pdf (accessed 2 March 2020).

1194. Dennehy, C. E. (2006). The use of herbs and dietary supplements in gynecology: an evidence-based review. *Journal of Midwifery & Women's Health, 51*: 402–409.

1195. Verheus, M., van Gils, C. H., Keinan-Boker, L., Grace, P. B., Bingham, S. A., & Peeters, P. H. M. (2007). Plasma phytoestrogens and subsequent breast cancer risk. *Journal of Clinical Oncology*, 25(6): 648–655.

1196. Trickey, R. (2003). *Women, Hormones & the Menstrual Cycle*. Sydney, Australia: Allen & Unwin.

1197. Brice-Ytsma, H., & McDermott, A. (2020). *Herbal Medicine in Treating Gynaecological Conditions*. London: Aeon.

1198. Setchell, K. D. R., Brown, N. M., Zimmer-Nechemias, L., Brashear, W. T., Wolfe, B. E., Kirschner, A. S., & Heubi, J. E. (2002). Evidence for the lack of absorption of soy isoflavone glycosides in humans, supporting the crucial role of intestinal metabolism for bioavailability. *American Journal of Clinical Nutrition*, 76(2): 447–453.

1199. Brice-Ytsma, H., & McDermott, A. (2020). *Herbal Medicine in Treating Gynaecological Conditions*. London: Aeon.

1200. Tsangalis, D., Wilcox, G., Shah, N. P., & Stojanovska, L. (2005). Bioavailability of isoflavone phytoestrogens in postmenopausal women consuming soya milk fermented with probiotic bifidobacteria. *British Journal of Nutrition*, 93(6): 867–877.

1201. Pitchford, P. (2002). *Healing with Whole Foods* (3rd edn). Berkeley, CA: North Atlantic.

1202. Trickey, R. (2003). *Women, Hormones & the Menstrual Cycle*. Sydney, Australia: Allen & Unwin.

1203. Felter, H. W., & Lloyd, J. U. (1898). *King's American Dispensatory* [online]. Available from http://henriettesherbal.com/eclectic/kings/index.html (accessed 5 March 2020).

1204. Hoffman, D. (1990). *The New Holistic Herbal*. Shaftesbury, UK: Element.

1205. Frawley, D., & Lad, V. (2001). *The Yoga of Herbs: An Ayurvedic Guide to Herbal Medicine*. Twin Lakes, WI: Lotus.

1206. Mills, S. (1991). *The Essential Book of Herbal Medicine*. London: Penguin Arkana.

1207. Mills, S. (1991). *The Essential Book of Herbal Medicine*. London: Penguin Arkana.

1208. Mills, S. (1991). *The Essential Book of Herbal Medicine*. London: Penguin Arkana.

1209. Grant, P., & Ramasamy, S. (2012). An update on plant derived anti-androgens. *International Journal of Endocrinology and Metabolism*, 10(2): 497–502.

1210. Bone, K. (2003). *A Clinical Guide to Blending Liquid Herbs*. London: Churchill Livingstone.

1211. Blumenthal, M. (1998). *The Complete Commision E Monographs: Therapeutic Guide to Herbal Medicines*. Philadelphia, PA: Lippincott Williams & Wilkins.

1212. Mills, S., & Bone, K. (2005). *The Essential Guide to Herbal Safety*. London: Churchill Livingstone.

1213. Grieve, M. (1931). *A Modern Herbal* [online]. Available from http://botanical.com (accessed 3 March 2020).

1214. Holmes, P. (2007). *The Energetics of Western Herbs: A Materia Medica Integrating Western & Chinese Herbal Therapeutics, Volume 2* (4th edn). Santa Rosa, CA: Snow Lotus.

1215. Trickey, R. (2011). *Women, Hormones and the Menstrual Cycle*. Clifton Hill, Victoria, Australia: Melbourne Holistic Health Group.

1216. Heyerick, A., Vervarcke, S., Depypere, H., Bracke, M., & De Keukeleire, D. (2006). A first prospective, randomized, double-blind, placebo-controlled study on the use of a standardized hop extract to alleviate menopausal discomforts. *Maturitas*, 54(2): 164–175.

1217. Morali, G., Polatti, F., Metelitsa, E. N., Mascarucci, P., Magnani, P., & Marre, G. B. (2006). Open, non-controlled clinical studies to assess the efficacy and safety of a medical device in form of gel topically and intravaginally used in postmenopausal women with genital atrophy. *Arzneimittelforschung, 56*(3): 230–238.

1218. Trickey, R. (2011). *Women, Hormones and the Menstrual Cycle.* Clifton Hill, Victoria, Australia: Melbourne Holistic Health Group.

1219. Füssel, A., Wolf, A., & Brattström, A. (2000). Effect of a fixed valerian-hop extract combination (Ze 91019) on sleep polygraphy in patients with non-organic insomnia: a pilot study. *European Journal of Medical Research, 5*(9): 385–390.

1220. Brice-Ytsma, H., & McDermott, A. (2020). *Herbal Medicine in Treating Gynaecological Conditions.* London: Aeon.

1221. Brice-Ytsma, H., & McDermott, A. (2020). *Herbal Medicine in Treating Gynaecological Conditions.* London: Aeon.

1222. Mills, S., & Bone, K. (2005). *The Essential Guide to Herbal Safety.* London: Churchill Livingstone.

1223. Bone, K., & Mills, S. (2013). *Principles and Practice of Phytotherapy: Modern Herbal Medicine.* London: Churchill Livingstone.

1224. Holmes, P. (2007). *The Energetics of Western Herbs: A Materia Medica Integrating Western & Chinese Herbal Therapeutics, Volume 2* (4th edn). Santa Rosa, CA: Snow Lotus.

1225. Cook, W. (1869). *The Physiomedical Dispensatory* [online]. Available from http://henriettesherbal.com/eclectic/cook/index.html (accessed 5 March 2020).

1226. Felter, H. W., & Lloyd, J. U. (1898). *King's American Dispensatory* [online]. Available from http://henriettesherbal.com/eclectic/kings/index.html (accessed 20 May 2020).

1227. Bone, K. (2003). *A Clinical Guide to Blending Liquid Herbs.* London: Churchill Livingstone.

1228. Bone, K., & Mills, S. (2013). *Principles and Practice of Phytotherapy: Modern Herbal Medicine.* London: Churchill Livingstone.

1229. Felter, H. W., & Lloyd, J. U. (1898). *King's American Dispensatory* [online]. Available from http://henriettesherbal.com/eclectic/kings/index.html (accessed 20 May 2020).

1230. Trickey, R. (2011). *Women, Hormones and the Menstrual Cycle.* Clifton Hill, Victoria, Australia: Melbourne Holistic Health Group.

1231. Holmes, P. (2007). *The Energetics of Western Herbs: A Materia Medica Integrating Western & Chinese Herbal Therapeutics, Volume 2* (4th edn). Santa Rosa, CA: Snow Lotus.

1232. Felter, H. W., & Lloyd, J. U. (1898). *King's American Dispensatory* [online]. Available from http://henriettesherbal.com/eclectic/kings/index.html (accessed 20 May 2020).

1233. Mills, S., & Bone, K. (2005). *The Essential Guide to Herbal Safety.* London: Churchill Livingstone.

1234. Holmes, P. (2007). *The Energetics of Western Herbs: A Materia Medica Integrating Western & Chinese Herbal Therapeutics, Volume 1* (4th edn). Santa Rosa, CA: Snow Lotus.

1235. Mills, S. (1991). *The Essential Book of Herbal Medicine.* London: Penguin Arkana.

1236. Grieve, M. (1931). *A Modern Herbal* [online]. Available from http://botanical.com (accessed 3 March 2020).

1237. Linde, K., Ramirez, G., Mulrow, C. D., Pauls, A., Weidenhammer, W., & Melchart, D. (1996). St John's wort for depression: an overview and meta-analysis of randomised clinical trials. *British Medical Journal*, *313*(7052): 253–258.

1238. Linde, K., Berner, M. M., & Kriston, L. (2008). St John's wort for major depression. *Cochrane Database of Systematic Reviews*, *8*(4): CD000448.

1239. Rahimi, R., Nikfar, S., & Abdollahi, M. (2009). Efficacy and tolerability of Hypericum perforatum in major depressive disorder in comparison with selective serotonin reuptake inhibitors: a meta-analysis. *Progress in Neuro-psychopharmacology & Biological Psychiatry*, *33*(1): 118–127.

1240. Dennehy, C. E. (2006). The use of herbs and dietary supplements in gynecology: an evidence-based review. *Journal of Midwifery & Women's Health*, *51*: 402–409.

1241. Grube, B., Walper, A., & Wheatley, D. (1999). "St. John's wort extract: efficacy for menopausal symptoms of psychological origin." *Advances in Therapy*, *16*(4): 177–186.

1242. Briggs, M., & Briggs, M. (1972). Relationship between monoamine oxidase activity and sex hormone concentration in human blood plasma. *Journal of Reproduction and Fertility*, *29*(3): 447–450.

1243. van Die, M. D., Bone, K. M., Burger, H. G., Reece, J. E., & Teede, H. J. (2009). Effects of a combination of Hypericum perforatum and Vitex agnus-castus on PMS-like symptoms in late-perimenopausal women: findings from a subpopulation analysis. *Journal of Alternative and Complementary Medicine*, *15*(9): 1045–1048.

1244. Mills, S. (1991). *The Essential Book of Herbal Medicine*. London: Penguin Arkana.

1245. Hoffman, D. (1990). *The New Holistic Herbal*. Shaftesbury, UK: Element.

1246. Grieve, M. (1931). *A Modern Herbal* [online]. Available from http://botanical.com (accessed 3 March 2020).

1247. Bone, K., & Mills, S. (2013). *Principles and Practice of Phytotherapy: Modern Herbal Medicine*. London: Churchill Livingstone.

1248. Brice-Ytsma, H., & McDermott, A. (2020). *Herbal Medicine in Treating Gynaecological Conditions*. London: Aeon.

1249. Mills, S., & Bone, K. (2005). *The Essential Guide to Herbal Safety*. London: Churchill Livingstone.

1250. Mills, S., & Bone, K. (2005). *The Essential Guide to Herbal Safety*. London: Churchill Livingstone.

1251. Cook, W. (1869). *The Physiomedical Dispensatory* [online]. Available from http://henriettesherbal.com/eclectic/cook/index.html (accessed 5 March 2020).

1252. Grieve, M. (1931). *A Modern Herbal* [online]. Available from http://botanical.com (accessed 3 March 2020).

1253. Hoffman, D. (1990). *The New Holistic Herbal*. Shaftesbury, UK: Element.

1254. Ellingwood, F. (1919). *The American Materia Medica* [online]. Available from http://henriettesherbal.com/eclectic/ellingwood/index.html (accessed 3 May 2020).

1255. Cook, W. (1869). *The Physiomedical Dispensatory* [online]. Available from http://henriettesherbal.com/eclectic/cook/index.html (accessed 5 March 2020).

1256. Bartram, T. (1995). *Encyclopedia of Herbal Medicine*. Christchurch, UK: Grace.

1257. Weiss, R., & Fintelmann, V. (2000). *Herbal Medicine* (2nd edn). Stuttgart, Germany: Thieme.

1258. Hoffman, D. (1990). *The New Holistic Herbal.* Shaftesbury, UK: Element.

1259. Mills, S., & Bone, K. (2005). *The Essential Guide to Herbal Safety.* London: Churchill Livingstone.

1260. Trickey, R. (2003). *Women, Hormones & the Menstrual Cycle.* Sydney, Australia: Allen & Unwin.

1261. Cook, W. (1869). *The Physiomedical Dispensatory* [online]. Available from http://henriettesherbal.com/eclectic/cook/index.html (accessed 5 March 2020).

1262. Hoffman, D. (1990). *The New Holistic Herbal.* Shaftesbury, UK: Element.

1263. Holmes, P. (2007). *The Energetics of Western Herbs: A Materia Medica Integrating Western & Chinese Herbal Therapeutics, Volume 2* (4th edn). Santa Rosa, CA: Snow Lotus.

1264. Bone, K. (2003). *A Clinical Guide to Blending Liquid Herbs.* London: Churchill Livingstone.

1265. Meissner, H. O., Kapczynski, W., Mscisz, A., & Lutomski, J. (2005). Use of gelatinized maca (Lepidium peruvianum) in early postmenopausal women. *International Journal of Biomedical Science,* 1(1): 33–45.

1266. Meissner, H. O., Reich-Bilinska, H., Mscisz, A., & Kedzia, B. (2006). Therapeutic effects of pre-gelatinized maca (Lepidium peruvianum chacon) used as a non-hormonal alternative to HRT in perimenopausal omen – clinical pilot study. *International Journal of Biomedical Science,* 2(2): 143–159.

1267. Meissner, H. O., Reich-Bilinska, H., Mscisz, A., & Kedzia, B. (2006). Therapeutic effects of pre-gelatinized maca (Lepidium peruvianum chacon) used as a non-hormonal alternative to HRT in perimenopausal women – clinical pilot study. *International Journal of Biomedical Science,* 2(2): 143–159.

1268. Meissner, H. O., Mscisz, A., Reich-Bilinska, H., Kapczynski, W., Mrozikiewicz, P., Bobkiewicz-Kozlowska, T., Kedzia, B., Lowicka, A., & Barchia, I. (2006). Hormone-balancing effect of pre-gelatinized organic maca (Lepidium peruvianum chacon): (III) Clinical responses of early-postmenopausal women to maca in double blind, randomized, lacebo-controlled, crossover configuration, outpatient study. *International Journal of Biomedical Science,* 2(4): 375–394.

1269. Meissner, H. O., Reich-Bilinska, H., Mscisz, A., & Kedzia, B. (2006). Therapeutic effects of pre-gelatinized maca (Lepidium peruvianum chacon) used as a non-hormonal alternative to HRT in perimenopausal women – clinical pilot study. *International Journal of Biomedical Science,* 2(2): 143–159.

1270. Shin, B. C., Lee, M. S., Yang, E. J., Lim, H.-S., & Ernst, E. (2010). Maca (*L. meyenii*) for improving sexual function: a systematic review. *BMC Complementary and Alternative Medicine,* 10: 44.

1271. Lee, M. S., Lee, H. W., You, S., & Ha, K.-T. (2016). The use of maca (Lepidium meyenii) to improve semen quality: a systematic review. *Maturitas,* 92: 64–69.

1272. Gonzales-Arimborgo, C., Yupanqui, I., Montero, E., Alarcón-Yaquetto, D. E., Zevallos-Concha, A., Caballero, L., Gasco, M., Zhao, J., Khan, I. A., & Gonzales, G. F. (2016). Acceptability, safety, and efficacy of oral administration of extracts of black or red maca (Lepidium meyenii) in adult human subjects: a randomized, double-blind, placebo-controlled study. *Pharmaceuticals (Basel),* 9(3): 49.

1273. Dording, C. M., Fisher, L. Papakostas, G., Farabaugh, A., Sonawalla, S., Fava, M., & Mischoulon, D. (2008). A double-blind, randomized, pilot dose-finding study of maca root (L. meyenii) for the management of SSRI-induced sexual dysfunction. *CNS Neuroscience & Therapeutics, 14*(3): 182–191.

1274. Dini, A., Migliuolo, G., Rastrelli, L., Saturnino, P., & Schettino, O. (1994). Chemical composition of Lepidium meyenii. *Food Chemistry, 49*: 347.

1275. Meissner, H. O., Reich-Bilinska, H., Mscisz, A., & Kedzia, B. (2006). Therapeutic effects of pre-gelatinized maca (Lepidium peruvianum chacon) used as a non-hormonal alternative to HRT in perimenopausal women – clinical pilot study. *International Journal of Biomedical Science, 2*(2): 143–159.

1276. Dording, C. M., Fisher, L. Papakostas, G., Farabaugh, A., Sonawalla, S., Fava, M., & Mischoulon, D. (2008). A double-blind, randomized, pilot dose-finding study of maca root (L. meyenii) for the management of SSRI-induced sexual dysfunction. *CNS Neuroscience & Therapeutics, 14*(3): 182–191.

1277. Valerio, L. G., & Gonzales, G. F. (2005). Toxicological aspects of the South American herbs cat's claw (Uncaria tomentosa) and maca (Lepidium meyenii): a critical synopsis. *Toxicological Reviews, 24*(1): 11–35.

1278. Brice-Ytsma, H., & McDermott, A. (2020). *Herbal Medicine in Treating Gynaecological Conditions*. London: Aeon.

1279. Lephart, E. D. (2015). Modulation of aromatase by phytoestrogens. *Enzyme Research* [online]. Available from https://hindawi.com/journals/er/2015/594656/ (accessed 2 March 2020).

1280. Pino, A. M., Valladares, L. E., Palma, M. A., Mancilla, A. M., Yáñez, M., & Albala, C. (2000). Dietary isoflavones affect sex hormone-binding globulin levels in postmenopausal women. *Journal of Clinical Endocrinology & Metabolism, 85*(8): 2797–2800.

1281. Brooks, J. D., Ward, W. E., Lewis, J. E., Hilditch, J., Nickell, L., Wong, E., & Thompson, L. U. (2004). Supplementation with flaxseed alters estrogen metabolism in postmenopausal women to a greater extent than does supplementation with an equal amount of soy. *American Journal of Clinical Nutrition, 79*(2): 318–325.

1282. Brice-Ytsma, H., & McDermott, A. (2020). *Herbal Medicine in Treating Gynaecological Conditions*. London: Aeon.

1283. Brice-Ytsma, H., & McDermott, A. (2020). *Herbal Medicine in Treating Gynaecological Conditions*. London: Aeon.

1284. Weiss, R. (1988). *Herbal Medicine*. Gothenburg, Sweden: Arcanum.

1285. Holmes, P. (2007). *The Energetics of Western Herbs: A Materia Medica Integrating Western & Chinese Herbal Therapeutics, Volume 2* (4th edn). Santa Rosa, CA: Snow Lotus.

1286. Felter, H. W., & Lloyd, J. U. (1898). *King's American Dispensatory* [online]. Available from http://henriettesherbal.com/eclectic/kings/index.html (accessed 5 March 2020).

1287. Chevallier, A. (1996). *The Encyclopedia of Medicinal Plants*. Oxford: Blackwell.

1288. Hoffman, D. (1990). *The New Holistic Herbal*. Shaftesbury, UK: Element.

1289. Amsterdam, J. D., Li, Y., Soeller, I., Rockwell, K., Mao, J. J., & Shults, J. (2009). A randomized, double-blind, placebo-controlled trial of oral Matricaria recutita (chamomile) extract therapy for generalized anxiety disorder. *Journal of Clinical Psychopharmacology, 29*(4): 378–382.

1290. Mills, S. (1991). *The Essential Book of Herbal Medicine*. London: Penguin Arkana.

1291. Mills, S., & Bone, K. (2005). *The Essential Guide to Herbal Safety*. London: Churchill Livingstone.

1292. Cook, W. (1869). *The Physiomedical Dispensatory* [online]. Available from http://henriettesherbal.com/eclectic/cook/index.html (accessed 5 March 2020).

1293. Felter, H. W., & Lloyd, J. U. (1898). *King's American Dispensatory* [online]. Available from http://henriettesherbal.com/eclectic/kings/index.html (accessed 5 March 2020).

1294. Mills, S. (1991). *The Essential Book of Herbal Medicine*. London: Penguin Arkana.

1295. Akbarzadeh, M., Dehghani, M., Moshfeghy, Z., Emamghoreishi, M., Tavakoli, P., & Zare, N. (2015). Effect of *Melissa officinalis* capsule on the intensity of premenstrual syndrome symptoms in high school girl students. *Nursing and Midwifery Studies*, 4(2): e27001.

1296. Kennedy, D. O., Little, W., & Scholey, A. B. (2004). Attenuation of laboratory-induced stress in humans after acute administration of Melissa officinalis (lemon balm). *Psychosomatic Medicine*, 66(4): 607–613.

1297. Holmes, P. (2007). *The Energetics of Western Herbs: A Materia Medica Integrating Western & Chinese Herbal Therapeutics, Volume 2* (4th edn). Santa Rosa, CA: Snow Lotus.

1298. Yarnell, E. (2006). Botanical medicine for thyroid regulation. *Alternative and Complementary Therapies*, 12(3): 107–112.

1299. Mills, S., & Bone, K. (2005). *The Essential Guide to Herbal Safety*. London: Churchill Livingstone.

1300. Holmes, P. (2007). *The Energetics of Western Herbs: A Materia Medica Integrating Western & Chinese Herbal Therapeutics, Volume 2* (4th edn). Santa Rosa, CA: Snow Lotus.

1301. Mills, S., & Bone, K. (2005). *The Essential Guide to Herbal Safety*. London: Churchill Livingstone.

1302. Grieve, M. (1931). *A Modern Herbal* [online]. Available from http://botanical.com (accessed 3 March 2020).

1303. Cook, W. (1869). *The Physiomedical Dispensatory* [online]. Available from http://henriettesherbal.com/eclectic/cook/index.html (accessed 5 March 2020).

1304. Holmes, P. (2007). *The Energetics of Western Herbs: A Materia Medica Integrating Western & Chinese Herbal Therapeutics, Volume 1* (4th edn). Santa Rosa, CA: Snow Lotus.

1305. Felter, H. W., & Lloyd, J. U. (1898). *King's American Dispensatory* [online]. Available from http://henriettesherbal.com/eclectic/kings/index.html (accessed 5 March 2020).

1306. D'Cruz, S. C., Vaithinathan, S., Jubendradass, R., & Mathur, P. P. (2010). Effects of plant products on the testes. *Asian Journal of Andrology*, 12(4): 468–479.

1307. Grant, G. (2010). Spearmint herbal tea has significant anti-androgen effects in polycystic ovarian syndrome. A randomized controlled trial. *Phytotherapy Research*, 24(2): 186–188.

1308. Romm, A. (2020). 5 safe herbs for a more comfortable pregnancy and birth [online]. Available from https://avivaromm.com/5-safe-herbs-for-a-more-comfortable-pregnancy-and-better-birth/ (accessed 5 June 2020).

1309. Pole, S. (2006). *Ayurvedic Medicine: The Principles of Traditional Practice*. London: Churchill Livingstone.

1310. Frawley, D., & Lad, V. (2001). *The Yoga of Herbs: An Ayurvedic Guide to Herbal Medicine*. Twin Lakes, WI: Lotus.

1311. Pole, S. (2006). *Ayurvedic Medicine: The Principles of Traditional Practice*. London: Churchill Livingstone.

1312. Pole, S. (2006). *Ayurvedic Medicine: The Principles of Traditional Practice*. London: Churchill Livingstone.

1313. Cook, W. (1869). *The Physiomedical Dispensatory* [online]. Available from http://henriettesherbal.com/eclectic/cook/index.html (accessed 5 March 2020).

1314. Felter, H. W., & Lloyd, J. U. (1898). *King's American Dispensatory* [online]. Available from http://henriettesherbal.com/eclectic/kings/index.html (accessed 5 March 2020).

1315. Grieve, M. (1931). *A Modern Herbal* [online]. Available from http://botanical.com (accessed 3 March 2020).

1316. Trickey, R. (2003). *Women, Hormones & the Menstrual Cycle*. Sydney, Australia: Allen & Unwin.

1317. Holmes, P. (2007). *The Energetics of Western Herbs: A Materia Medica Integrating Western & Chinese Herbal Therapeutics, Volume 2* (4th edn). Santa Rosa, CA: Snow Lotus.

1318. Trickey, R. (2003). *Women, Hormones & the Menstrual Cycle*. Sydney, Australia: Allen & Unwin.

1319. Trickey, R. (2011). *Women, Hormones and the Menstrual Cycle*. Clifton Hill, Victoria, Australia: Melbourne Holistic Health Group.

1320. Grant, P., & Ramasamy, S. (2012). An update on plant derived anti-androgens. *International Journal of Endocrinology and Metabolism*, 10(2): 497–502.

1321. Holmes, P. (2007). *The Energetics of Western Herbs: A Materia Medica Integrating Western & Chinese Herbal Therapeutics, Volume 2* (4th edn). Santa Rosa, CA: Snow Lotus.

1322. Liu, W., & Gong, C. (2009). Opening the blockage to reproduction: infertility. *Traditional Chinese Medicine Information Page* [online]. Available from http://tcmpage.com/hpinfertility.html (accessed 4 March 2020).

1323. Tillotson, A. K. (2009). Female infertility. [Online] Available from http://oneearthherbs.squarespace.com/diseases/female-infertility.html (accessed 28 January 2009).

1324. Holmes, P. (2007). *The Energetics of Western Herbs: A Materia Medica Integrating Western & Chinese Herbal Therapeutics, Volume 1* (4th edn). Santa Rosa, CA: Snow Lotus.

1325. Liu, W., & Gong, C. (2009). Opening the blockage to reproduction: infertility. *Traditional Chinese Medicine Information Page* [online]. Available from http://tcmpage.com/hpinfertility.html (accessed 4 March 2020).

1326. Bone, K. (2003). *A Clinical Guide to Blending Liquid Herbs*. London: Churchill Livingstone.

1327. Holmes, P. (2007). *The Energetics of Western Herbs: A Materia Medica Integrating Western & Chinese Herbal Therapeutics, Volume 2* (4th edn). Santa Rosa, CA: Snow Lotus.

1328. Bone, K., & Mills, S. (2013). *Principles and Practice of Phytotherapy: Modern Herbal Medicine*. London: Churchill Livingstone.

1329. Bone, K. (2003). *A Clinical Guide to Blending Liquid Herbs*. London: Churchill Livingstone.

1330. Mills, S., & Bone, K. (2005). *The Essential Guide to Herbal Safety*. London: Churchill Livingstone.

1331. Hosoi, M., Belcaro, G., Saggino, A., Luzzi, R., Dugall, M., & Feragalli, B. (2018). Pycnogenol® supplementation in minimal cognitive dysfunction. *Journal of Neurosurgical Sciences, 62*(3): 279–284.

1332. Arcangeli, P. (2000). Pycnogenol® in chronic venous insufficiency. *Fitoterapia, 71*(3): 236–244.

1333. Luzzi, R., Belcaro, G., Hosoi, M., Feragalli, B., Cornelli, U., Dugall, M., & Ledda, A. (2017). Normalization of cardiovascular risk factors in pre-menopausal women with Pycnogenol. *Minerva Ginecologica, 69*(1): 29–34.

1334. Kohama, T., Suzuki, N., Ohno, S., & Inoue, M. (2004). Analgesic efficacy of French maritime pine bark extract in dysmenorrhea: an open clinical trial. *Journal of Reproductive Medicine, 49*(10): 828–832.

1335. Kohama, T., Herai, K., & Inoue, M. (2007). Effect of French maritime pine bark extract on endometriosis as compared with leuprorelin acetate. *Journal of Reproductive Medicine, 52*(8): 703–708.

1336. Luzzi, R., Belcaro, G., Hosoi, M., Feragalli, B., Cornelli, U., Dugall, M., & Ledda, A. (2017). Normalization of cardiovascular risk factors in pre-menopausal women with Pycnogenol. *Minerva Ginecologica, 69*(1): 29–34.

1337. Bottari, A., Belcaro, G., Ledda, A., Luzzi, R., Cesarone, M. R., & Dugall, M. (2013). Lady Prelox® improves sexual function in generally healthy women of reproductive age. *Minerva Ginecologica, 65*(4): 435–444.

1338. Belcaro, G., Cornelli, U., Luzzi, R., Cesarone, M. R., Dugall, M., Feragalli, B., Errichi, S., Ippolito, E., Grossi, M. G., Hosoi, M., Cornelli, M., & Gizzi, G. (2013). Pycnogenol supplementation improves health risk factors in subjects with metabolic syndrome. *Phytotherapy Research, 27*(10): 1572–1578.

1339. Stanislavov, R., Niklova, V., & Rohdewald, P. (2008). Improvement of erectile function with Prelox: a randomized, double-blind, placebo-controlled, crossover trial. *International Journal of Impotence Research, 20*(2): 173–178.

1340. Stanislavov, R., Nikolova, V., & Rohdewald, P. (2009). Improvement of seminal parameters with Prelox: a randomized, double-blind, placebo-controlled, crossover trial. *Phytotherapy Research, 23*(3): 297–302.

1341. American Botanical Council Proprietary Botanical Ingredient Scientific and Clinical Monograph for Pycnogenol® (French maritime pine bark extract) [online]. Available from http://abc.herbalgram.org/ (accessed 7 June 2020).

1342. Holmes, P. (2007). *The Energetics of Western Herbs: A Materia Medica Integrating Western & Chinese Herbal Therapeutics, Volume 2* (4th edn). Santa Rosa, CA: Snow Lotus.

1343. Liu, W., & Gong, C. (2009). Opening the blockage to reproduction: infertility. *Traditional Chinese Medicine Information Page* [online]. Available from http://tcmpage.com/hpinfertility.html (accessed 4 March 2020).

1344. Maciocia, G. (2004). *Diagnosis in Chinese Medicine: A Comprehensive Guide*. London: Churchill Livingstone.

1345. Yu, Q. (2018). Traditional Chinese medicine: perspectives on and treatment of menopausal symptoms. *Climacteric, 21*(2): 93–95.

1346. Maciocia, G. (2012). On blood deficiency. *European Journal of Oriental Medicine, 7*(1): 6–12.

1347. Bone, K. (2003). *A Clinical Guide to Blending Liquid Herbs.* London: Churchill Livingstone.

1348. Mills, S., & Bone, K. (2005). *The Essential Guide to Herbal Safety.* London: Churchill Livingstone.

1349. Cook, W. (1869). *The Physiomedical Dispensatory* [online]. Available from http://henriettesherbal.com/eclectic/cook/index.html (accessed 5 March 2020).

1350. Holmes, P. (2007). *The Energetics of Western Herbs: A Materia Medica Integrating Western & Chinese Herbal Therapeutics, Volume 1* (4th edn). Santa Rosa, CA: Snow Lotus.

1351. BHMA (1991). *British Herbal Pharmacopoeia.* Bournemouth, UK: British Herbal Medicine Association.

1352. Bozin, B., Mimica-Dukic, N., Samojlik, I., & Jovin, E. (2007). Antimicrobial and antioxidant properties of rosemary and sage (*Rosmarinus officinalis* L. and *Salvia officinalis* L., Lamiaceae) essential oils. *Journal of Agricultural and Food Chemistry, 55*(19): 7879–7885.

1353. Cook, W. (1869). *The Physiomedical Dispensatory* [online]. Available from http://henriettesherbal.com/eclectic/cook/index.html (accessed 5 March 2020).

1354. Mills, S. (1991). *The Essential Book of Herbal Medicine.* London: Penguin Arkana.

1355. Bone, K. (2003). *A Clinical Guide to Blending Liquid Herbs.* London: Churchill Livingstone.

1356. Bone, K., & Mills, S. (2013). *Principles and Practice of Phytotherapy: Modern Herbal Medicine.* London: Churchill Livingstone.

1357. Holmes, P. (2007). *The Energetics of Western Herbs: A Materia Medica Integrating Western & Chinese Herbal Therapeutics, Volume 2* (4th edn). Santa Rosa, CA: Snow Lotus.

1358. Frawley, D., & Lad, V. (2001). *The Yoga of Herbs: An Ayurvedic Guide to Herbal Medicine.* Twin Lakes, WI: Lotus.

1359. Wood, M. (2004). *The Practice of Traditional Western Herbalism: Basic Doctrine, Energetics and Classification.* Berkeley, CA: North Atlantic.

1360. Holmes, P. (2007). *The Energetics of Western Herbs: A Materia Medica Integrating Western & Chinese Herbal Therapeutics, Volume 2* (4th edn). Santa Rosa, CA: Snow Lotus.

1361. Bone, K. (2003). *A Clinical Guide to Blending Liquid Herbs.* London: Churchill Livingstone.

1362. Holmes, P. (2007). *The Energetics of Western Herbs: A Materia Medica Integrating Western & Chinese Herbal Therapeutics, Volume 2* (4th edn). Santa Rosa, CA: Snow Lotus.

1363. Trickey, R. (2003). *Women, Hormones & the Menstrual Cycle.* Sydney, Australia: Allen & Unwin.

1364. Rogers, C. (1999). *The Woman's Guide to Herbal Medicine* [online]. Available from http://womans-herbal-guide.com/publications (accessed 27 January 2009).

1365. Hoffman, D. (1990). *The New Holistic Herbal.* Shaftesbury, UK: Element.

1366. Mills, S. (1991). *The Essential Book of Herbal Medicine.* London: Penguin Arkana.

1367. Tillotson, A. K. (2001). *The One Earth Herbal Sourcebook.* New York: Kensington.

1368. Bartram, T. (1995). *Encyclopedia of Herbal Medicine.* Christchurch, UK: Grace.

1369. Bone, K. (2003). *A Clinical Guide to Blending Liquid Herbs.* London: Churchill Livingstone.

1370. Mills, S., & Bone, K. (2005). *The Essential Guide to Herbal Safety.* London: Churchill Livingstone.

1371. Engels, G. (2010). Sage. *HerbalGram, 89*: 1–4.

1372. Kavvadias, D., Monschein, V. S., Sand, P., Riederer, P., & Schreier, P. (2003). Constituents of sage (*Salvia officinalis*) with in vitro affinity to human brain benzodiazepine receptor. *Planta Medica, 69*(2): 113–117.

1373. Heffner, L. J., & Schust, D. J. (2014). *The Reproductive System at a Glance*. Oxford: John Wiley & Sons.

1374. Rahte, S., Evans, R., Eugster, P. J., Marcourt, L., Wolfender, J.-L., Kortenkamp, A., & Tasdemir, D. (2013). Salvia officinalis for hot flushes: towards determination of mechanism of activity and active principles. *Planta Medica, 79*(9): 753–760.

1375. Moss, L., Rouse, M., Wesnes, K. A., & Moss, M. (2010). Differential effects of the aromas of Salvia species on memory and mood. *Human Psychopharmacology, 25*(5): 388–396.

1376. Bone, K. (2003). *A Clinical Guide to Blending Liquid Herbs*. London: Churchill Livingstone.

1377. Mills, S., & Bone, K. (2005). *The Essential Guide to Herbal Safety*. London: Churchill Livingstone.

1378. Trickey, R. (2011). *Women, Hormones and the Menstrual Cycle*. Clifton Hill, Victoria, Australia: Melbourne Holistic Health Group.

1379. Bone, K., & Mills, S. (2013). *Principles and Practice of Phytotherapy: Modern Herbal Medicine*. London: Churchill Livingstone.

1380. Holmes, P. (2007). *The Energetics of Western Herbs: A Materia Medica Integrating Western & Chinese Herbal Therapeutics, Volume 1* (4th edn). Santa Rosa, CA: Snow Lotus.

1381. Holmes, P. (2007). *The Energetics of Western Herbs: A Materia Medica Integrating Western & Chinese Herbal Therapeutics, Volume 1* (4th edn). Santa Rosa, CA: Snow Lotus.

1382. Liu, W., & Gong, C. (2009). Opening the blockage to reproduction: infertility. *Traditional Chinese Medicine Information Page* [online]. Available from http://tcmpage.com/hpinfertility.html (accessed 4 March 2020).

1383. Trickey, R. (2011). *Women, Hormones and the Menstrual Cycle*. Clifton Hill, Victoria, Australia: Melbourne Holistic Health Group.

1384. Bone, K., & Mills, S. (2013). *Principles and Practice of Phytotherapy: Modern Herbal Medicine*. London: Churchill Livingstone.

1385. Brice-Ytsma, H., & McDermott, A. (2020). *Herbal Medicine in Treating Gynaecological Conditions*. London: Aeon.

1386. Bone, K. (2003). *A Clinical Guide to Blending Liquid Herbs*. London: Churchill Livingstone.

1387. Grieve, M. (1931). *A Modern Herbal* [online]. Available from http://botanical.com (accessed 3 March 2020).

1388. Holmes, P. (2007). *The Energetics of Western Herbs: A Materia Medica Integrating Western & Chinese Herbal Therapeutics, Volume 1* (4th edn). Santa Rosa, CA: Snow Lotus.

1389. Dueck, C. A., Matt, K. S., Manore, M. M., & Skinner, J. S. (1996). Treatment of athletic amenorrhoea with a diet and training intervention program. *International Journal of Sports Nutrition, 6*(1): 24–40.

1390. Ellingwood, F. (1919) *The American Materia Medica* [online]. Available from http://henriettesherbal.com/eclectic/ellingwood/index.html (accessed 3 May 2020).

1391. Trickey, R. (2011). *Women, Hormones and the Menstrual Cycle*. Clifton Hill, Victoria, Australia: Melbourne Holistic Health Group.

1392. Holmes, P. (2007). *The Energetics of Western Herbs: A Materia Medica Integrating Western & Chinese Herbal Therapeutics, Volume 1* (4th edn). Santa Rosa, CA: Snow Lotus.

1393. Bone, K. (2003). *A Clinical Guide to Blending Liquid Herbs*. London: Churchill Livingstone.

1394. Mills, S., & Bone, K. (2005). *The Essential Guide to Herbal Safety*. London: Churchill Livingstone.

1395. Ellingwood, F. (1919). *The American Materia Medica* [online]. Available from http://henriettesherbal.com/eclectic/ellingwood/index.html (accessed 3 May 2020).

1396. Grieve, M. (1931). *A Modern Herbal* [online]. Available from http://botanical.com (accessed 3 March 2020).

1397. Felter, H. W., & Lloyd, J. U. (1898). *King's American Dispensatory* [online]. Available from http://henriettesherbal.com/eclectic/kings/index.html (accessed 5 March 2020).

1398. Ellingwood, F. (1919). *The American Materia Medica* [online]. Available from http://henriettesherbal.com/eclectic/ellingwood/index.html (accessed 3 March 2020).

1399. Grieve, M. (1931). *A Modern Herbal* [online]. Available from http://botanical.com (accessed 3 March 2020).

1400. Romm, A. (2016). *Botanical Medicine for Women's Health* (2nd edn). London: Churchill Livingstone.

1401. Ellingwood, F. (1919). *The American Materia Medica* [online]. Available from http://henriettesherbal.com/eclectic/ellingwood/index.html (accessed 3 March 2020).

1402. Bone, K., & Mills, S. (2013). *Principles and Practice of Phytotherapy: Modern Herbal Medicine*. London: Churchill Livingstone.

1403. Bone, K., & Mills, S. (2013). *Principles and Practice of Phytotherapy: Modern Herbal Medicine*. London: Churchill Livingstone.

1404. Trickey, R. (2011). *Women, Hormones and the Menstrual Cycle*. Clifton Hill, Victoria, Australia: Melbourne Holistic Health Group.

1405. Institute for Quality and Efficiency in Health Care (2014). Benign enlarged prostate: medication and herbal products. *PubMed Health* [online]. Available from ncbi.nlm.nih.gov (accessed 27 July 2015).

1406. Trickey, R. (2011). *Women, Hormones and the Menstrual Cycle*. Clifton Hill, Victoria, Australia: Melbourne Holistic Health Group.

1407. Bone, K. (2003). *A Clinical Guide to Blending Liquid Herbs*. London: Churchill Livingstone.

1408. Mills, S., & Bone, K. (2005). *The Essential Guide to Herbal Safety*. London: Churchill Livingstone.

1409. Holmes, P. (2007). *The Energetics of Western Herbs: A Materia Medica Integrating Western & Chinese Herbal Therapeutics, Volume 2* (4th edn). Santa Rosa, CA: Snow Lotus.

1410. Cook, W. (1869). *The Physiomedical Dispensatory* [online]. Available from http://henriettesherbal.com/eclectic/cook/index.html (accessed 5 March 2020).

1411. Grieve, M. (1931). *A Modern Herbal* [online]. Available from http://botanical.com (accessed 3 March 2020).

1412. Felter, H. W., & Lloyd, J. U. (1898). *King's American Dispensatory* [online]. Available from http://henriettesherbal.com/eclectic/kings/index.html (accessed 5 March 2020).

1413. Holmes, P. (2007). *The Energetics of Western Herbs: A Materia Medica Integrating Western & Chinese Herbal Therapeutics, Volume 2* (4th edn). Santa Rosa, CA: Snow Lotus.

1414. Bone, K. (2003). *A Clinical Guide to Blending Liquid Herbs*. London: Churchill Livingstone.

1415. Hoffman, D. (1990). *The New Holistic Herbal*. Shaftesbury, UK: Element.

1416. Mills, S. (1991). *The Essential Book of Herbal Medicine*. London: Penguin Arkana.

1417. Schütz, K., Carle, R., & Schieber, A. (2006). Taraxacum – a review on its phytochemical and pharmacological profile. *Journal of Ethnopharmacology, 107*(3): 313–323.

1418. Glenville, M. (2000). *Natural Solutions to Infertility*. London: Piatkus.

1419. Hudson, T. (2008). *Women's Encyclopedia of Natural Medicine*. New York: McGraw Hill.

1420. Balunas, M. J., Su, B., Brueggemeier, R. W., & Kinghorn, A. D. (2011). Natural products as aromatase inhibitors. *Anti-Cancer Agents in Medicinal Chemistry, 8*(6): 646–682.

1421. Bone, K. (2003). *A Clinical Guide to Blending Liquid Herbs*. London: Churchill Livingstone.

1422. Mills, S., & Bone, K. (2005). *The Essential Guide to Herbal Safety*. London: Churchill Livingstone.

1423. Brice-Ytsma, H., & McDermott, A. (2020). *Herbal Medicine in Treating Gynaecological Conditions*. London: Aeon.

1424. Tabakova, P., Dimitrov, M., & Tashkov, B. (2012). Clinical studies on Tribulus terrestris protodioscin in women with endocrine infertility or menopausal syndrome. *Herbpharm USA* [online]. Available from http://scicompdf.se/tiggarnot/tabakova-HerbPharmUSA.pdf (accessed 2 March 2020).

1425. Pole, S. (2006). *Ayurvedic Medicine: The Principles of Traditional Practice*. London: Churchill Livingstone.

1426. Thirunavukkarasu, M., Sellandi, M., Thakar, A. B., & Baghel, M. S. (2012). Clinical study of *Tribulus Terrestris* Linn. in oligozoospermia: a double blind study. *Ayu, 33*(3): 356–364.

1427. Pole, S. (2006). *Ayurvedic Medicine: The Principles of Traditional Practice*. London: Churchill Livingstone.

1428. Mills, S., & Bone, K. (2005). *The Essential Guide to Herbal Safety*. London: Churchill Livingstone.

1429. Pole, S. (2006). *Ayurvedic Medicine: The Principles of Traditional Practice*. London: Churchill Livingstone.

1430. Gogte, V. V. M. (2000). *Ayurvedic Pharmacology & Therapeutic Uses of Medicinal Plants – Dravyagunavignyan*. New Delhi: Chaukhamba.

1431. Pole, S. (2006). *Ayurvedic Medicine: The Principles of Traditional Practice*. London: Churchill Livingstone.

1432. Bensky, D., Gamble, A., & Kaptchuk, T. J. (1993). *Chinese Herbal Medicine: Material Medica*. Seattle, WA: Eastland.

1433. Pole, S. (2006). *Ayurvedic Medicine: The Principles of Traditional Practice*. London: Churchill Livingstone.

1434. Brice-Ytsma, H., & McDermott, A. (2020). *Herbal Medicine in Treating Gynaecological Conditions*. London: Aeon.

1435. Tabakova, P., Dimitrov, M., & Tashkov, B. (2012). Clinical studies on Tribulus terrestris protodioscin in women with endocrine infertility or menopausal syndrome. *Herbpharm USA* [online]. Available from http://scicompdf.se/tiggarnot/tabakova-HerbPharmUSA.pdf (accessed 2 March 2020).

1436. Pole, S. (2006). *Ayurvedic Medicine: The Principles of Traditional Practice.* London: Churchill Livingstone.

1437. Mills, S., & Bone, K. (2005). *The Essential Guide to Herbal Safety.* London: Churchill Livingstone.

1438. Felter, H. W., & Lloyd, J. U. (1898). *King's American Dispensatory* [online]. Available from http://henriettesherbal.com/eclectic/kings/index.html (accessed 5 March 2020).

1439. Grieve, M. (1931). *A Modern Herbal* [online]. Available from http://botanical.com (accessed 3 March 2020).

1440. Ellingwood, F. (1919). *The American Materia Medica* [online]. Available from http://henriettesherbal.com/eclectic/ellingwood/index.html (accessed 3 March 2020).

1441. Trickey, R. (2011). *Women, Hormones and the Menstrual Cycle.* Clifton Hill, Victoria, Australia: Melbourne Holistic Health Group.

1442. Dennehy, C. E. (2006). The use of herbs and dietary supplements in gynecology: an evidence-based review. *Journal of Midwifery & Women's Health, 51:* 402–409.

1443. Brice-Ytsma, H., & McDermott, A. (2020). *Herbal Medicine in Treating Gynaecological Conditions.* London: Aeon.

1444. Shinde, P., Patil, P., & Bairaji, V. (2012).Herbs in pregnancy and lactation: a review appraisal. *International Journal of Pharmaceutical Sciences and Research, 3(9):* 3001–3006.

1445. Trickey, R. (2011). *Women, Hormones and the Menstrual Cycle.* Clifton Hill, Victoria, Australia: Melbourne Holistic Health Group.

1446. Holmes, P. (2007). *The Energetics of Western Herbs: A Materia Medica Integrating Western & Chinese Herbal Therapeutics, Volume 1* (4th edn). Santa Rosa, CA: Snow Lotus.

1447. Brice-Ytsma, H., & McDermott, A. (2020). *Herbal Medicine in Treating Gynaecological Conditions.* London: Aeon.

1448. Chevallier, A. (1996). *The Encyclopedia of Medicinal Plants.* New York: DK.

1449. Bown, D. (1995). *Encyclopaedia of Herbs and Their Uses.* New York: DK.

1450. Zhao, J., Dasmahapatra, A., Khan, S., & Khan, I. A. (2008). Anti-aromatase activity of the constituents from damiana (Turnera diffusa). *Journal of Ethnopharmacology, 120(3):* 387–393.

1451. Zava, D. T., Dollbaum, C. M., & Blen, M. (1998). Estrogen and progestin bioactivity of foods, herbs, and spices. *Proceedings of the Society for Experimental Biology and Medicine, 217(3):* 369–378.

1452. Holmes, P. (2007). *The Energetics of Western Herbs: A Materia Medica Integrating Western & Chinese Herbal Therapeutics, Volume 1* (4th edn). Santa Rosa, CA: Snow Lotus.

1453. Bone, K. (2003). *A Clinical Guide to Blending Liquid Herbs.* London: Churchill Livingstone.

1454. Mills, S., & Bone, K. (2005). *The Essential Guide to Herbal Safety.* London: Churchill Livingstone.

1455. Holmes, P. (2007). *The Energetics of Western Herbs: A Materia Medica Integrating Western & Chinese Herbal Therapeutics, Volume 2* (4th edn). Santa Rosa, CA: Snow Lotus.

1456. Cook, W. (1869). *The Physiomedical Dispensatory* [online]. Available from http://henriettesherbal.com/eclectic/cook/index.html (accessed 5 March 2020).
1457. Hoffman, D. (2009). Infertility [online]. Available from http://healthy.net/scr/Article.asp?id=1182 (accessed 28 January 2009).
1458. Mills, S. (1991). *The Essential Book of Herbal Medicine*. London: Penguin Arkana.
1459. Grieve, M. (1931). *A Modern Herbal* [online]. Available from http://botanical.com (accessed 3 March 2020).
1460. Felter, H. W., & Lloyd, J. U. (1898). *King's American Dispensatory* [online]. Available from http://henriettesherbal.com/eclectic/kings/index.html (accessed 5 March 2020).
1461. Cook, W. (1869). *The Physiomedical Dispensatory* [online]. Available from http://henriettesherbal.com/eclectic/cook/index.html (accessed 5 March 2020).
1462. Hoffman, D. (2009). Infertility [online]. Available from http://healthy.net/scr/Article.asp?id=1182 (accessed 28 January 2009).
1463. Mills, S. (1991). *The Essential Book of Herbal Medicine*. London: Penguin Arkana.
1464. Trickey, R. (2003). *Women, Hormones & the Menstrual Cycle*. Sydney, Australia: Allen & Unwin.
1465. Bone, K., & Mills, S. (2013). *Principles and Practice of Phytotherapy: Modern Herbal Medicine*. London: Churchill Livingstone.
1466. Romm, A. (2016). *Botanical Medicine for Women's Health* (2nd edn). London: Churchill Livingstone.
1467. Cook, W. (1869). *The Physiomedical Dispensatory* [online]. Available from http://henriettesherbal.com/eclectic/cook/index.html (accessed 5 March 2020).
1468. Ellingwood, F. (1919). *The American Materia Medica* [online]. Available from http://henriettesherbal.com/eclectic/ellingwood/index.html (accessed 3 May 2020).
1469. Tillotson, A. K. (2009). Female infertility [online]. Available from http://oneearthherbs.squarespace.com/diseases/female-infertility.html (accessed 28 January 2009).
1470. Trickey, R. (2003). *Women, Hormones & the Menstrual Cycle*. Sydney, Australia: Allen & Unwin.
1471. Bone, K. (2003). *A Clinical Guide to Blending Liquid Herbs*. London: Churchill Livingstone.
1472. Holmes, P. (2007). *The Energetics of Western Herbs: A Materia Medica Integrating Western & Chinese Herbal Therapeutics, Volume 2* (4th edn). Santa Rosa, CA: Snow Lotus.
1473. Felter, H. W., & Lloyd, J. U. (1898). *King's American Dispensatory* [online]. Available from http://henriettesherbal.com/eclectic/kings/index.html (accessed 5 March 2020).
1474. Trickey, R. (2003). *Women, Hormones & the Menstrual Cycle*. Sydney, Australia: Allen & Unwin.
1475. Chevallier, A. (1996). *The Encyclopedia of Medicinal Plants*. Oxford: Blackwell.
1476. Felter, H. W., & Lloyd, J. U. (1898). *King's American Dispensatory* [online]. Available from http://henriettesherbal.com/eclectic/kings/index.html (accessed 5 March 2020).
1477. Holmes, P. (2007). *The Energetics of Western Herbs: A Materia Medica Integrating Western & Chinese Herbal Therapeutics, Volume 2* (4th edn). Santa Rosa, CA: Snow Lotus.

1478. Cook, W. (1869). *The Physiomedical Dispensatory* [online]. Available from http://henriettesherbal.com/eclectic/cook/index.html (accessed 5 March 2020).

1479. Felter, H. W., & Lloyd, J. U. (1898). *King's American Dispensatory* [online]. Available from http://henriettesherbal.com/eclectic/kings/index.html (accessed 5 March 2020).

1480. Mills, S. (1991). *The Essential Book of Herbal Medicine*. London: Penguin Arkana.

1481. Trickey, R. (2003). *Women, Hormones & the Menstrual Cycle*. Sydney, Australia: Allen & Unwin.

1482. Ellingwood, F. (1919). *The American Materia Medica* [online]. Available from http://henriettesherbal.com/eclectic/ellingwood/index.html (accessed 3 May 2020).

1483. Bone, K. (2003). *A Clinical Guide to Blending Liquid Herbs*. London: Churchill Livingstone.

1484. Holmes, P. (2007). *The Energetics of Western Herbs: A Materia Medica Integrating Western & Chinese Herbal Therapeutics, Volume 1* (4th edn). Santa Rosa, CA: Snow Lotus.

1485. Chevallier, A. (1996). *The Encyclopedia of Medicinal Plants*. Oxford: Blackwell.

1486. Blumenthal, M. (1998). *The Complete Commision E Monographs:Therapeutic Guide to Herbal Medicines*. Philadelphia, PA: Lippincott Williams & Wilkins.

1487. Newall, C. A., Anderson, L. A., & Phillipson, J. D. (1996). *Herbal Medicines: a Guide for Health-care Professionals*. London: Pharmaceutical Press.

1488. Mills, S. (1991). *The Essential Book of Herbal Medicine*. London: Penguin Arkana.

1489. Berger, D., Schaffner, W., Schrader, E., Meier, B., & Brattstron, A. (2000). Efficacy of Vitex agnus castus L. extract Ze 440 in patients with pre-menstrual syndrome (PMS). *Archives of Gynecology and Obstetrics, 264*(3): 150–153.

1490. Gardiner, P. (2000). Chasteberry (*Vitex agnus castus*). *The Longwood Herbal Taskforce* [online]. Available from http://longwoodherbal.org/vitex/vitex.pdf (accessed 28 February 2012).

1491. Schellenberg, R. (2001). Treatment for the premenstrual syndrome with agnus castus fruit extract: prospective, randomised, placebo controlled study. *British Medical Journal, 322*(7279): 134–137.

1492. Webster, D. E., Dentali, S. J., Farnsworth, N. R., & Wang, Z. J. (2008). Chaste tree fruit and premenstrual syndrome (Chapter 12). In: D. Mischoulon & J. F. Rosenbaum (Eds.), *Natural Medications for Psychiatric Disorders: Considering the Alternatives*. Riverwoods, IL: Wolters Kluwer Health.

1493. Webster, D. E., Dentali, S. J., Farnsworth, N. R., & Wang, Z. J. (2008). Chaste tree fruit and premenstrual syndrome (Chapter 12). In: D. Mischoulon & J. F. Rosenbaum (Eds.), *Natural Medications for Psychiatric Disorders: Considering the Alternatives*. Riverwoods, IL: Wolters Kluwer Health.

1494. Christie, S., & Walker, A. F. (1997). Vitex agnus castus L.: (1) A review of its traditional and modern therapeutic use; (2) current use from a survey of practitioners. *European Journal of Herbal Medicine, 3*(3): 29–45.

1495. Gardiner, P. (2000). Chasteberry (*Vitex agnus castus*). *The Longwood Herbal Taskforce* [online]. Available from http://longwoodherbal.org/vitex/vitex.pdf (accessed 28 February 2012).

1496. Milowicz, A., & Jedrzejuk, D. (2006). Premenstrual syndrome: From etiology to treatment. *Maturitas, 55*(1): s47–s54.

1497. Dueck, C. A., Matt, K. S., Manore, M. M., & Skinner, J. S. (1996). Treatment of athletic amenorrhoea with a diet and training intervention program. *International Journal of Sports Nutrition, 6*(1): 24–40.

1498. Milowicz, A., & Jedrzejuk, D. (2006). Premenstrual syndrome: From etiology to treatment. *Maturitas, 55*(1): s47–s54.

1499. Zamani, M., Mansour Ghanaei, M. M., Farimany, M., & Nasr Elahi, S. H. (2007). Efficacy of mefenamic acid and vitex in reduction of menstrual blood loss and Hb changes in patients with a complain of menorrhagia. *Iranian Journal of Obstetrics, Gynecology and Infertility, 10*(1): 79–86.

1500. Brice-Ytsma, H., & McDermott, A. (2020). *Herbal Medicine in Treating Gynaecological Conditions.* London: Aeon.

1501. Bone, K., & Mills, S. (2013). *Principles and Practice of Phytotherapy (Second Edition).* London: Churchill Livingstone.

1502. Mills, S., & Bone, K. (2005). *The Essential Guide to Herbal Safety.* London: Churchill Livingstone.

1503. Bone, K., & Mills, S. (2013). *Principles and Practice of Phytotherapy (Second Edition).* London: Churchill Livingstone.

1504. Reame, N., Sauder, S. E., Kelch, R. P., & Marshall, J. C. (1984). Pulsatile gonadotropin secretion during the human menstrual cycle: evidence for altered frequency of gonadotropin-releasing hormone secretion. *Journal of Clinical Endocrinology and Metabolism, 59*(2): 328–337.

1505. Rossmanith, W. G., & Lauritzen, C. (2009). The luteinizing hormone pulsatile secretion: diurnal excursions in normally cycling and postmenopausal women. *Gynecological Endocrinology, 5*(4): 249–265.

1506. Bone, K., & Mills, S. (2013). *Principles and Practice of Phytotherapy* (2nd edn). London: Churchill Livingstone.

1507. Bone, K., & Mills, S. (2013). *Principles and Practice of Phytotherapy* (2nd edn). London: Churchill Livingstone.

1508. Frawley, D., & Lad, V. (2001). *The Yoga of Herbs: An Ayurvedic Guide to Herbal Medicine.* Twin Lakes, WI: Lotus.

1509. Pole, S. (2006). *Ayurvedic Medicine: The Principles of Traditional Practice.* London: Churchill Livingstone.

1510. Pole, S. (2006). *Ayurvedic Medicine: The Principles of Traditional Practice.* London: Churchill Livingstone.

1511. Pole, S. (2006). *Ayurvedic Medicine: The Principles of Traditional Practice.* London: Churchill Livingstone.

1512. Andallu, B., & Radhika, B. (2000). Hypoglycemic, diuretic and hypocholesterolemic effect of winter cherry (Withania somnifera, Dunal) root. *Indian Journal of Experimental Biology, 38*(6): 607–609.

1513. Chavarro, J. E., Rich-Edwards, J. W., Rosner, B. A., & Willett, W. C. (2009). A prospective study of dietary carbohydrate quantity and quality in relation to risk of ovulatory infertility. *European Journal of Clinical Nutrition, 63*(1): 78–86.

1514. Trickey, R. (2003). *Women, Hormones & the Menstrual Cycle.* Sydney, Australia: Allen & Unwin.

1515. Trickey, R. (2003). *Women, Hormones & the Menstrual Cycle.* Sydney, Australia: Allen & Unwin.

1516. Dongre, S., Langade, D., & Bhattacharyya, S. (2015). Efficacy and safety of ashwagandha (Withania somnifera) root extract in improving sexual function in women: a pilot study. *BioMed Research International*, 284154.

1517. Tillotson, A. K. (2009). Female infertility [online]. Available from http://oneearthherbs.squarespace.com/diseases/female-infertility.html (accessed 28 February 2009).

1518. Lopresti, A. L., Smith, S. J., Malvi, H., & Kodgule, R. (2019). An investigation into the stress-relieving and pharmacological actions of an ashwagandha (*Withania somnifera*) extract. A randomized, double-blind, placebo-controlled study. *Medicine (Baltimore)*, 98(37): e17186.

1519. Naredi, N., Sandeep, K., Jamwal, V. D. S., Nagraj, N., & Raj, S. (2015). Dehydroepiandrosterone: a panacea for the ageing ovary? *Medical Journal Armed Forces India*, 71(3): 274–277.

1520. Xu, L., Hu., C., Liu, Q., & Li, Y. (2019). The effect of dehydroepiandrosterone (DHEA) supplementation on IVF or ICSI: a meta-analysis of randomized controlled trials. *Geburtshilfe und Frauenheilkunde*, 79(7): 705–712.

1521. Ambiye, V. R., Langade, D., Dongre, S., Aptikar, P., Kulkarni, M., & Dongre, A. (2013). Clinical evaluation of the spermatogenic activity of the root extract of ashwagandha (*Withania somnifera*) in oligospermic males: a pilot study. *Evidence-Based Complementary and Alternative Medicine* [online]. Available from http://ncbi.nlm.nih.gov/pmc/articles/PMC3863556/#!po=3.84615 (accessed 15 July 2015).

1522. Ambiye, V. R., Langade, D., Dongre, S., Aptikar, P., Kulkarni, M., & Dongre, A. (2013). Clinical evaluation of the spermatogenic activity of the root extract of ashwagandha (*Withania somnifera*) in oligospermic males: a pilot study. *Evidence-Based Complementary and Alternative Medicine* [online]. Available from http://ncbi.nlm.nih.gov/pmc/articles/PMC3863556/#!po=3.84615 (accessed 15 July 2015).

1523. Ambiye, V. R., Langade, D., Dongre, S., Aptikar, P., Kulkarni, M., & Dongre, A. (2013). Clinical evaluation of the spermatogenic activity of the root extract of ashwagandha (*Withania somnifera*) in oligospermic males: a pilot study. *Evidence-Based Complementary and Alternative Medicine* [online]. Available from http://ncbi.nlm.nih.gov/pmc/articles/PMC3863556/#!po=3.84615 (accessed 15 July 2015).

1524. Ahmad, M. K., Mahdi, A. A., Shukla, K. K., Islam, N., Rajender, S., Madhukar, D., Shankhwar, S. N., & Ahmad, S. (2010). Withania somnifera improves semen quality by regulating reproductive hormone levels and oxidative stress in seminal plasma of infertile males. *Fertility and Sterility*, 94(3): 989–996.

1525. Ambiye, V. R., Langade, D., Dongre, S., Aptikar, P., Kulkarni, M., & Dongre, A. (2013). Clinical evaluation of the spermatogenic activity of the root extract of ashwagandha (*Withania somnifera*) in oligospermic males: a pilot study. *Evidence-Based Complementary and Alternative Medicine* [online]. Available from http://ncbi.nlm.nih.gov/pmc/articles/PMC3863556/#!po=3.84615 (accessed 15 July 2015).

1526. Pole, S. (2006). *Ayurvedic Medicine: The Principles of Traditional Practice*. London: Churchill Livingstone.

1527. Romm, A. (2016). *Botanical Medicine for Women's Health* (2nd edn). London: Churchill Livingstone.

1528. Tillotson, A. K. (2001). *The One Earth Herbal Sourcebook*. New York: Kensington.

1529. Pole, S. (2006). *Ayurvedic Medicine: The Principles of Traditional Practice*. London: Churchill Livingstone.

1530. Bone, K. (2003). *A Clinical Guide to Blending Liquid Herbs*. London: Churchill Livingstone.

1531. Mills, S., & Bone, K. (2005). *The Essential Guide to Herbal Safety*. London: Churchill Livingstone.

1532. Pole, S. (2006). *Ayurvedic Medicine: The Principles of Traditional Practice*. London: Churchill Livingstone.

1533. Mills, S. (1991). *The Essential Book of Herbal Medicine*. London: Penguin Arkana.

1534. Felter, H. W., & Lloyd, J. U. (1898). *King's American Dispensatory* [online]. Available from http://henriettesherbal.com/eclectic/kings/index.html (accessed 5 March 2020).

1535. Beers, M. H., & Berkow, R. (1999). *The Merck Manual of Diagnosis and Therapy*. Kenilworth, NJ: Merck.

1536. Trickey, R. (2003). *Women, Hormones & the Menstrual Cycle*. Sydney, Australia: Allen & Unwin.

1537. Gonlachanvit, S., Chen, Y. H., Hasler, W. L., Sun, W. M., & Owyang, C. (2003). Ginger reduces hyperglycemia-evoked gastric dysrhythmias in healthy humans: possible role of endogenous prostaglandins. *Journal of Pharmacology and Experimental Therapeutics, 307*(3): 1098–1103.

1538. Bone, K., & Mills, S. (2013). *Principles and Practice of Phytotherapy: Modern Herbal Medicine*. London: Churchill Livingstone.

1539. Romm, A. (2016). *Botanical Medicine for Women's Health* (2nd edn). London: Churchill Livingstone.

1540. Ensiyeh, J., & Sakineh, M. A. C. (2009). Comparing ginger and vitamin B6 for the treatment of nausea and vomiting in pregnancy: a randomised controlled trial. *Midwifery, 25*(6): 649–653.

1541. Keating, A., & Chez, R. A. (2002). Ginger syrup as an antiemetic in early pregnancy. *Alternative Therapies in Health and Medicine, 8*(5): 89–91.

1542. Holmes, P. (2007). *The Energetics of Western Herbs: A Materia Medica Integrating Western & Chinese Herbal Therapeutics, Volume 1* (4th edn). Santa Rosa, CA: Snow Lotus.

1543. Liu, W., & Gong, C. (2009). Opening the blockage to reproduction: infertility. *Traditional Chinese Medicine Information Page* [online]. Available from http://tcmpage.com/hpinfertility.html (accessed 4 July 2011).

INDEX

311